Anti-Tumor Necrosis Factor Therapy in Inflammatory Bowel Disease

Frontiers of Gastrointestinal Research

Vol. 34

Series Editor

Choitsu Sakamoto Tokyo

Anti-Tumor Necrosis Factor Therapy in Inflammatory Bowel Disease

Volume Editors

Gerhard Rogler Zurich
Hans Herfarth Chapel Hill, N.C.
Toshifumi Hibi Tokyo
Ole Haagen Nielsen Copenhagen

26 figures, 17 in color, and 15 tables, 2015

KARGER

Basel · Freiburg · Paris · London · New York · Chennai · New Delhi · Bangkok · Beijing · Shanghai · Tokyo · Kuala Lumpur · Singapore · Sydney

Frontiers of Gastrointestinal Research

Gerhard Rogler
Klinik für Gastroenterologie und Hepatologie
Universitäts Spital Zürich
CH–8091 Zurich (Switzerland)

Hans Herfarth
Division of Gastroenterology and Hepatology
UNC School of Medicine
Chapel Hill, NC 27599-7080 (USA)

Toshifumi Hibi
Center for Advanced IBD Research and Treatment
Kitasato Institute Hospital
Tokyo, Minato-ku 108-8642 (Japan)

Ole Haagen Nielsen
Dept. of Gastroenterology, Medical Section
Herlev Hospital
University of Copenhagen (Denmark)

Library of Congress Cataloging-in-Publication Data

Anti-tumor necrosis factor therapy in inflammatory bowel disease / volume editors, Gerhard Rogler, Toshifumi Hibi, Hans Herfarth, Ole Haagen Nielsen.
p. ; cm. -- (Frontiers of gastrointestinal research, ISSN 0302-0665 ; vol. 34)
Includes bibliographical references and indexes.
ISBN 978-3-318-05473-6 (hard cover : alk. paper) -- ISBN 978-3-318-05474-3 (electronic version)
I. Rogler, G. (Gerhard), editor. II. Hibi, Toshifumi, 1947- , editor. III. Herfarth, H., editor. IV. Nielsen, Ole Haagen, editor. V. Series: Frontiers of gastrointestinal research ; v. 34. 0302-0665
[DNLM: 1. Inflammatory Bowel Diseases--therapy. 2. Tumor Necrosis Factors. W1 FR946E v.34 2015 / WI 420]
RC862.I53
616.3'44--dc23

2015017502

Bibliographic Indices. This publication is listed in bibliographic services, including Current Contents® and Index Medicus.

www.karger.com
Printed in Germany on acid-free and non-aging paper (ISO 9706) by Kraft Druck GmbH, Ettlingen
ISSN 0302–0665
e-ISSN 1622–3754
ISBN 978–3–318–05473–6
e-ISBN 978–3–318–05474–3

KARGER 125 YEARS

Contents

Preface

The introduction of anti TNF antibodies into the treatment of patients with inflammatory bowel disease about fifteen years ago has dramatically changed the field of IBD therapy. This treatment option has significantly improved the quality of life for patients with severe Crohn's disease and ulcerative colitis. Extensive research has been performed analyzing the mode of action of anti TNF antibodies in vitro and in vivo, positioning this therapeutic approach in current treatment strategies and analyzing the side effects of anti-TNF strategies and various other aspects, such as monitoring of therapy. With the introduction of anti-TNF antibody biosimilars the field has become more complex and new questions have been raised.

Surprisingly so far there have been no attempt to provide a comprehensive overview on all aspects of TNF action, mechanisms of anti TNF therapy, treatment strategies, side effects, monitoring, biosimilars and many other aspects that are important with respect to anti TNF therapy. This monograph for the first time makes the effort to cover all those important aspects and answer questions that are associated with them. It is the first text book written by experts in the field that tries to bridge basic research on TNF action and on properties of the different antibodies to frequent questions regarding treatment strategies, stop options, etc. The authors have included newest results; the single chapters are focused and to the point; and the information given is helpful and precise.

We hope that this wide-ranging overview on anti-TNF therapy in inflammatory bowel disease will help clinicians and guide them to the optimal treatment decision. At the end we hope to improve the quality of life of patients with inflammatory bowel disease with the information provided in this monograph.

Gerhard Rogler, Zurich, Switzerland
Hans Herfarth, Chapel Hill, N.C., USA
Toshifumi Hibi, Tokyo, Japan
Ole Haagen Nielsen, Copenhagen, Denmark

Rogler G, Herfarth H, Hibi T, Nielsen OH (eds): Anti-Tumor Necrosis Factor Therapy in Inflammatory Bowel Disease.
Front Gastrointest Res. Basel, Karger, 2015, vol 34, pp 1–8 (DOI: 10.1159/000381380)

The Effect of TNF-α on the Regulation of Epithelial Function in Inflammatory Bowel Disease

Kiichiro Tsuchiya

Department of Advanced Therapeutics for Gastrointestinal Diseases, Graduate School of Tokyo Medical and Dental University, Tokyo, Japan

Abstract

TNF-α is a crucial cytokine in inflammatory bowel disease (IBD) because anti-TNF-α therapy very effectively mitigates the disease. Inhibiting TNF-α induces not only the suppression of inflammation but also mucosal healing, suggesting that TNF-α may be involved in the mucosal damage observed in IBD. Although it has not been completely elucidated how TNF-α damages intestinal epithelial cells (IECs), recent reports have shown various effects of TNF-α on IECs that may be involved in the pathogenesis of IBD. In this section, we review the various functions of TNF-α in IECs, such as barrier function, cell survival, differentiation, and carcinogenesis, in IBD.

Introduction

The gut epithelium undergoes continual renewal throughout adult life to maintain the proper architecture and function of intestinal crypts [1]. The epithelial layer is a highly dynamic tissue with high epithelial cell turnover, which is effectuated by cell shedding at the villus tip, the constant proliferation of stem cells, and the transient amplification of cells along the crypt-villus axis. This process involves highly coordinated regulation of the induction of cellular differentiation, and the cessation of proliferation is affected by various intracellular signaling pathways such as Notch, Wnt, and bone morphogenetic protein [2, 3]. Recent studies have shown that dysregulation of the differentiation system for prompt intestinal epithelial cell (IEC) formation induces the pathology of inflammatory bowel disease (IBD) [4, 5] because a central function of IECs is to control the mucosal barrier, which is essential for maintaining the luminal environment [6]. In particular, aberrant Notch signaling induced by inflammation in patients with ulcerative colitis (UC) leads to the lack of IEC differentiation, resulting in goblet cell depletion [4]. Goblet cells play a role in the mucosal barrier by secreting glycoprotein-rich mucus into the intestinal lumen, suggesting that inflammation may damage the mucosal barrier [7]. In addition, Paneth cells at the base of crypts in the small intestine secrete antimicrobial agents that prevent the gut microbiota from invading the body [8, 9]. The number of Paneth cells is also reduced in ileal lesions of patients with Crohn's disease (CD) [10]. Moreover, the recognition of bacteria by Paneth cells is weakened because of the genetic mutation of NOD2 or autophagy-related genes [11], indicating that the barrier function is impaired by both inflammation and genetic factors. Taken together, inflammation of the intestine in IBD patients may directly cause the dysfunction of IECs, although the precise mechanism remains unknown. TNF-α is an important proinflammatory cytokine that plays a central role in intestinal inflammation [12] because elevated serum levels of TNF-α in IBD patients have previously been reported [13]. Moreover, single nucleotide polymorphisms identified in genome-wide association studies indicated genes such as RELA, NFKB1, TNFSF15 [14], and TNFAIP3/A20 [15] as potential risk alleles; these results link alterations in TNF-α signaling to IBD. Antibodies targeting TNF-α have been the most successful approach in the clinical management of IBD, highlighting the importance and the clinical relevance of TNF-α function to not only intestinal inflammation but also mucosal healing [16–18]. In this section, we review TNF-α as a controller of multiple cellular processes, such as inflammatory mediator production, cell proliferation, cell survival, carcinogenesis, and different cell death modalities, that are intricately linked to the epithelial response to injury.

TNF-α Signaling Pathways in Intestinal Epithelial Cells

TNF-α is produced by immune cells and stromal cells invading the inflamed mucosa and by the intestinal epithelium stimulated via Toll-like receptors. The transmembrane protein pro-TNF-α is cleaved by a disintegrin and metallopeptidase domain 17 [19], releasing a biologically active trimeric form [20]. Both receptors for TNF-α, TNFRSF1A (TNF-R1) and TNFRSF1B (TNF-R2), are expressed in IECs and transmit the intracellular signaling of TNF-α [21–23]. The cytoplasmic domains of TNF-R1 and TNF-R2 are known to be associated with TNF receptor-associated factor 2, which induces the activation of IKK. Activated IKK subsequently induces the phosphorylation of IκB, resulting in the activation of NF-κB, which consists of p50 and RelA/p65, because of the dissociation of the IκB/NF-κB complex. TNF-R1 signaling leads to a variety of intracellular events, eventually activating two major transcription factors, NF-κB and c-Jun. Ligand-activated TNF-R1 is recognized by the adaptor protein TNF receptor-associated death domain (TRADD), which recruits additional adaptor proteins such as receptor-interacting serine/threonine kinase 1 (RIPK1) [24] and TNF receptor-associated factor 2 [25] to form a membrane-bound complex. Furthermore, TRADD interacts with the adaptor protein Fas-associated death domain (FADD) via death domains, leading to the recruitment of caspase-8 to a cytoplasmic complex. Caspase-8 plays a central role in the regulation of cell death pathways such as apoptosis and necroptosis [26]. However, TNFR2, which is not coupled with the FADD/TRADD complex, does not induce proapoptotic signaling upon interaction with TNF-α. TNF-R2 has been shown to mediate the upregulation of myosin light chain kinase (MLCK), which increases paracellular permeability via the regulation of tight junctions (TJs) [27–29].

The Regulation of Intestinal Epithelial Cell Differentiation by TNF-α

IECs consist of five types of cells: goblet cells, entero-endocrine cells, Paneth cells, Tuft cells, and enterocytes [30]. These secretory cells play a role in the mucosal barrier by secreting a variety of peptides depending on the cell type [31]. The dysregulation of IEC has been reported in IBD; for instance, aberrant Notch signaling may induce the proliferation of IECs to maintain the mucosa, although the differentiation of IECs is suppressed, as shown by goblet cell depletion [32, 33]. In a dextran sulfate sodium (DSS) colitis model, treatment with a Notch signaling inhibitor, which induces goblet cell differentiation, worsens the mucosal damage and consequently suppresses cell proliferation [4], suggesting that Notch signaling may not serve as a target for mucosal healing in UC. Another report indicated that caudal type homeobox 2 (CDX2) expression is reduced in the mucosa in UC [34], indicating that the dysregulation of the molecular mechanisms underlying intestinal differentiation may be critical for the pathogenesis of UC. CDX2 is an intestine-specific transcription factor that is essential for the regulation of genes related to epithelial functions. CDX2 is a crucial regulator of intestinal epithelial function, including the control of the balance between IEC differentiation and proliferation [35]. We have previously reported that CDX2 directly induces Atonal homolog 1 (Atoh1) expression by binding to the 3′ region of the Atoh1 gene but that HES1 directly suppresses Atoh1 expression by binding to the 5′ promoter region of the Atoh1 gene [33]. Moreover, we have shown that CDX2 can induce Atoh1 expression despite HES1 expression via Notch signaling activation, suggesting that CDX2 may promote both the proliferation and the differentiation of IECs. Therefore, the reduced CDX2 expression level in the mucosa in IBD indicates that the dysregulation of the molecular mechanism underlying intestinal differentiation may be critical for the pathogenesis of IBD. A previous report has shown that TNF-α suppresses the expression of CDX2 in a colonic cell line [36], suggesting that the overexpression of TNF-α in IECs may induce goblet cell depletion in IBD. In a mouse model, intestine-specific TNF-α overexpression induced Crohn's-like ileitis [20, 37], supporting the concept that the local TNF-α microenvironment in IECs is the determining factor for the development of an inflammatory phenotype.

TNF-α in Tight Junction Modulation

TJs between adjacent IECs regulate the semi-permeable barrier in the intestine [38]. The selectivity of TJs controls the trafficking of luminal antigens through the mucosa and facilitates the interaction between the bacterial flora and the mucosal immune system [38]. TNF-α regulates intestinal permeability by mediating TJ remodeling following the activation of MLCK. The phosphorylation of the regulatory light-chain of myosin II by MLCK induces actomyosin ring contraction. The redistribution of peri-junctional actin, ZO-1, claudin, and occludin from the TJ complex subsequently causes an increase in paracellular flux [39, 40]. Mice expressing constitutively active MLCK display increased barrier permeability and inflammatory cytokine production. Moreover, patients with CD have increased intestinal expression and activity of MLCK [41], implicating a TNF-mediated pathway in the reduced barrier function that is a feature of IBD. Therefore, factors that control TNF-induced changes in IEC TJs may play critical roles in barrier function and in the prevention of IBD. Kolodziej et al. demonstrated that TNFAIP3, also known as A20, plays a direct role in IEC function by controlling the TNF-induced increases in the permeability of TJs between IECs [42]. TNFAIP3 regulates NF-kB activation via TNF-α, resulting in increased sensitivity of IECs to apoptosis, which further demonstrates the importance of TNFAIP3 in IECs.

Apoptosis and Necroptosis of Intestinal Epithelial Cells by TNF-α

Cell death mechanisms have been associated with the development of IBD in humans and mice because high levels of apoptosis have been observed in IECs of patients with IBD. For many years, the death of IECs has been known to be a consequence of TNF-α-mediated stimulation. TNF-α induces extrinsic caspase-dependent apoptosis, which is brought about by cell signaling via TNF-R1, inducing the cleavage and activation of caspase-3 due to the homodimerization of caspase-8, thereby promoting the canonical extrinsic apoptosis pathway [43].

In addition, necroptosis, a relatively novel programmed necrosis-like pathway associated with caspase-independent cell death via the TNF-α receptor, appears to be linked to the pathogenesis of CD and is seen in animal models of intestinal inflammation [44]. A central molecule in necroptosis is receptor-interacting serine/threonine kinase 3 (RIPK3), which phosphorylates mixed lineage kinase domain-like protein and forms a complex called the necroptosome following its interaction with deubiquitylated RIPK1. Two independent groups recently assessed the role of programmed necrosis in IBD. Becker et al. demonstrated that mice carrying a conditional deletion of caspase-8 in IECs developed terminal ileitis and were highly susceptible to DSS colitis due to the impairment of Paneth cells and the induction of necroptosis by TNF-α in association with increased RIPK3 expression [45]. Moreover, RIPK3 is highly expressed and necroptosis is increased in Paneth cells in the terminal ileum of CD patients, indicating dysregulated antimicrobial immune cell functions in the intestinal epithelium. In addition, Welz et al. showed the necroptotic loss of Paneth cells in FADD-deficient mice with intestinal inflammation [46], suggesting a potential role of necroptosis in the pathogenesis of IBD. Moreover, Dannappel et al. demonstrated that both RIPK1-dependent and RIPK1-independent pathways drive RIPK3-mediated necroptosis [24]. RIPK1 has the capacity to either inhibit or induce apoptosis and necroptosis, suggesting that RIPK1 may be a novel target for IBD as a key regulator of immunity and homeostasis of the mucosal barrier.

The Carcinogenesis of Colitis-Associated Colon Cancer by TNF-α

The inflammation of the entire colon for more than 10 years after the onset of UC raises the risk of colitis-associated cancer (CAC) in patients with UC [47]. The risk of colorectal cancer is 20- to 30-fold higher in UC patients than in the control population [48].

Understanding the pathogenesis of colon carcinogenesis in UC at the molecular and cellular levels is crucial. Oral administration of DSS solution to rodents is widely employed to simulate human UC because it can cause acute inflammation and ulceration in the entire colon similar to that observed in UC patients. Moreover, prior administration of azoxymethane (AOM), which induces tumors in the distal colon of rodents, can accelerate and increase the incidence of DSS-induced colon carcinogenesis to a very high rate after three successive rounds of DSS ingestion [49]. The inactivation of IKKβ in either myeloid cells or IECs using conditional deficient mice can reduce the incidence and the development of colon carcinogenesis induced by the combined treatment of AOM and DSS [49]. Moreover, in IECs, IKKβ contributes to tumor initiation and promotion by suppressing apoptosis; however, IKKβ is not required for inflammation per se. Taken together, the induction of NF-κB by inflammatory stimuli may play a crucial role in colon carcinogenesis. However, the molecules that enhance the peak of NF-κB signaling during the course of colon carcinogenesis remains to be identified. NF-κB activation is required for the expression of many proinflammatory molecules, including cytokines and adhesion molecules. Among these cytokines, TNF-α can further augment NF-κB activation in various cell types after binding to either TNF receptor p55 (TNF-Rp55) or TNF-Rp75. Popivanova et al. demonstrated the roles of the TNF-α/TNF-Rp55 axis in colon carcinogenesis induced by AOM and DSS using TNF-Rp55$^{-/-}$ mice and the specific human TNF-α antagonist etanercept [50]. They showed the crucial involvement of TNF-α in the initiation of CAC. Moreover, blocking TNF-α reversed carcinoma progression, even after colon carcinoma was established. In addition, we have demonstrated that blocking TNF-α in vivo inhibited its signaling via TNF-R2, which was significantly upregulated during colitis, resulting in the reduction of

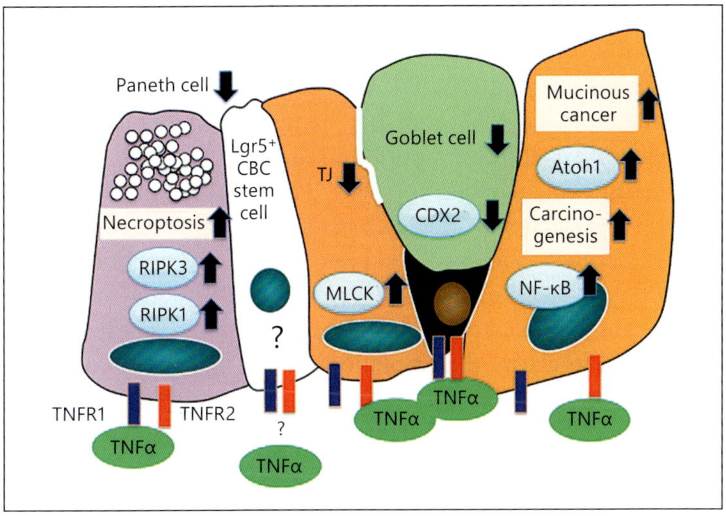

Fig. 1. Schematic representation of the multiple functions of TNF-α in intestinal epithelial cells.

the development and progression of CAC. It has been suggested that drugs targeting TNF-α may be useful for the treatment of CAC.

The clinical features of CAC are markedly different from those of sporadic colon cancer. CAC has been considered to be more malignant than sporadic cancer because of its chemoresistance and poor prognosis [51]. Moreover, the pathological findings of CAC are often classified as undifferentiated mucinous-type carcinoma [52–54], and the molecular mechanisms underlying CAC, such as the acquisition of a mucinous form, invasion, metastasis, and chemoresistance, should be characterized and clarified.

Muc2 mRNA is upregulated in response to TNF-α via a MAPK-dependent pathway in the colon cancer cell line HT29 [55, 56]. Another study demonstrated that TNF-α stimulation induced a goblet-cell-like phenotype in a human adenocarcinoma cell line [57], suggesting a role of TNF-α in IEC differentiation toward the mucinous lineage. In addition, the mucinous phenotype of IECs has been reported to be regulated by Atoh1 [58], which is a basic helix-loop-helix type transcription factor and which is among the genes that are essential for the differentiation toward secretory lineages. Subsequently, we demonstrated that the Atoh1 protein is actively degraded by the GSK3-mediated ubiquitin-proteasomal pathway, resulting in a nonmucinous phenotype in sporadic cancer [59]. In contrast, another group has reported that the Atoh1 protein is expressed in mucinous cancer cells [60], suggesting that Atoh1 may also regulate the mucinous phenotype of colon cancer. We now have evidence that the stabilization of the Atoh1 protein by TNF-α in colon cancer cells induces not only the mucinous phenotype but also cancer stemness, resulting in the acquisition of malignant potential such as tumor formation and chemoresistance (unpublished data). These results suggest that TNF-α may cause not only the carcinogenesis but also the malignant potential of CAC.

Conclusion and Future Directions

We reviewed the multiple functions and diverse effects of TNF-α on IECs in view of the pathogenesis of IBD. TNF-α induces multiple intracellular signaling cascades that determine crucial aspects of cell fate, such as survival, death, and proliferation, via its selective binding to TNF-α receptors (fig. 1). The most important factor involved in the fate of IECs is the regulation of NF-κB signaling via TNF-α. The response of IECs to TNF-α may be altered by various conditions, such as the expression and distribution of TNF receptors, the ubiquitination state of signaling components, crosstalk with Toll-like receptors and the specific cell type. In particular, necroptosis of Paneth cells induced by TNF-α may influence stem cell maintenance because Paneth cells support neighboring stem cells by supplying Wnt3A. In the future, the effect of TNF-α on intestinal stem cells should be assessed to clarify the regulation of IEC fate and its association with IBD.

However, it is suggested that the fate of IECs may be modulated by the signaling state of TNF-α. Therefore, we should carefully estimate the intestinal situation to assess outcomes related to the responses of IECs to TNF-α stimulation. The recent establishment of in vitro culture systems for IECs, such as a mini-gut [61, 62], may be helpful to assess the effect of TNF-α on IECs alone because these systems enable the exclusion of the effects of TNF-α on the other immune regulatory cells such as T cells, B cells, and macrophages. Using this in vitro culture system, it was recently reported that the ligation of NOD2 to muramyl dipeptide mediates stem cell survival against oxidative stress [63]. It would be desirable to reveal the intestinal stem cell behaviors influenced by TNF-α using this system.

Furthermore, attention should be given to the possibility that TNF-α influences the level of CAC malignancy. Because CAC prevention and therapy remains to be established, the precise mechanisms of cell signaling via TNF-α in CAC should be urgently assessed to enable the discovery of novel therapeutic targets.

References

1 Booth C, Brady G, Potten CS: Crowd control in the crypt. Nat Med 2002;8:1360–1361.

2 Haramis AP, Begthel H, van den Born M, van Es J, Jonkheer S, Offerhaus GJ, Clevers H: De novo crypt formation and juvenile polyposis on BMP inhibition in mouse intestine. Science 2004;303:1684–1686.

3 Nakamura T, Tsuchiya K, Watanabe M: Crosstalk between Wnt and Notch signaling in intestinal epithelial cell fate decision. J Gastroenterol 2007;42:705–710.

4 Okamoto R, Tsuchiya K, Nemoto Y, Akiyama J, Nakamura T, Kanai T, Watanabe M: Requirement of Notch activation during regeneration of the intestinal epithelia. Am J Physiol Gastrointest Liver Physiol 2009;296:G23–G35.

5 Dahan S, Roda G, Pinn D, Roth-Walter F, Kamalu O, Martin A, Mayer L: Epithelial: lamina propria lymphocyte interactions promote epithelial cell differentiation. Gastroenterology 2008;134:192–203.

6 Dignass AU: Mechanisms and modulation of intestinal epithelial repair. Inflamm Bowel Dis 2001;7:68–77.

7 Simoneau A, Herring-Gillam FE, Vachon PH, Perreault N, Basora N, Bouatrouss Y, Pageot LP, Zhou J, Beaulieu JF: Identification, distribution, and tissular origin of the alpha5(IV) and alpha6(IV) collagen chains in the developing human intestine. Dev Dyn 1998;212:437–447.

8 Wehkamp J, Chu H, Shen B, Feathers RW, Kays RJ, Lee SK, Bevins CL: Paneth cell antimicrobial peptides: topographical distribution and quantification in human gastrointestinal tissues FEBS Lett 2006;580:5344–5350.

9 Chu H, Pazgier M, Jung G, Nuccio SP, Castillo PA, de Jong MF, Winter MG, Winter SE, Wehkamp J, Shen B, Salzman NH, Underwood MA, Tsolis RM, Young GM, Lu W, Lehrer RI, Bäumler AJ, Bevins CL: Human α-defensin 6 promotes mucosal innate immunity through self-assembled peptide nanonets. Science 2012;337:477–481.

10 Jager S, Stange EF, Wehkamp J: Inflammatory bowel disease: an impaired barrier disease. Langenbecks Arch Surg 2013;398:1–12.

11 Fritz T, Niederreiter L, Adolph T, Blumberg RS, Kaser A: Crohn's disease: NOD2, autophagy and ER stress converge. Gut 2011;60:1580–1588.

12 Panja A, Goldberg S, Eckmann L, Krishen P, Mayer L: The regulation and functional consequence of proinflammatory cytokine binding on human intestinal epithelial cells. J Immunol 1998;161:3675–3684.

13 Reinecker HC, Steffen M, Witthoeft T, Pflueger I, Schreiber S, MacDermott RP, Raedler A: Enhanced secretion of tumour necrosis factor-alpha, IL-6, and IL-1 beta by isolated lamina propria mononuclear cells from patients with ulcerative colitis and Crohn's disease. Clin Exp Immunol 1993;94:174–181.

14 Hirano A, Yamazaki K, Umeno J, Ashikawa K, Aoki M, Matsumoto T, Nakamura S, Ninomiya T, Matsui T, Hirai F, Kawaguchi T, Takazoe M, Tanaka H, Motoya S, Kiyohara Y, Kitazono T, Nakamura Y, Kamatani N, Kubo M: Association study of 71 European Crohn's disease susceptibility loci in a Japanese population. Inflamm Bowel Dis 2013;19:526–533.

15 Jostins L, Ripke S, Weersma RK, Duerr RH, McGovern DP, Hui KY, Lee JC, Schumm LP, Sharma Y, Anderson CA, Essers J, Mitrovic M, Ning K, Cleynen I, Theatre E, Spain SL, Raychaudhuri S, Goyette P, Wei Z, Abraham C, Achkar JP, Ahmad T, Amininejad L, Ananthakrishnan AN, Andersen V, Andrews JM, Baidoo L, Balschun T, Bampton PA, Bitton A, Boucher G, Brand S, Büning C, Cohain A, Cichon S, D'Amato M, De Jong D, Devaney KL, Dubinsky M, Edwards C, Ellinghaus D, Ferguson LR, Franchimont D, Fransen K, Gearry R, Georges M, Gieger C, Glas J, Haritunians T, Hart A, Hawkey C, Hedl M, Hu X, Karlsen TH, Kupcinskas L, Kugathasan S, Latiano A, Laukens D, Lawrance IC, Lees CW, Louis E, Mahy G, Mansfield J, Morgan AR, Mowat C, Newman W, Palmieri O, Ponsioen CY, Potocnik U, Prescott NJ, Regueiro M, Rotter JI, Russell RK, Sanderson JD, Sans M, Satsangi J, Schreiber S, Simms LA, Sventoraityte J, Targan SR, Taylor KD, Tremelling M, Verspaget HW, De Vos M, Wijmenga C, Wilson DC, Winkelmann J, Xavier RJ, Zeissig S, Zhang B, Zhang CK, Zhao H, Silverberg MS, Annese V, Hakonarson H, Brant SR, Radford-Smith G, Mathew CG, Rioux JD, Schadt EE, Daly MJ, Franke A, Parkes M, Vermeire S, Barrett JC, Cho JH: Host-microbe interactions have shaped the genetic architecture of inflammatory bowel disease. Nature 2012;491:119–124.

16 Marini M, Bamias G, Rivera-Nieves J, Moskaluk CA, Hoang SB, Ross WG, Pizarro TT, Cominelli F: TNF-alpha neutralization ameliorates the severity of murine Crohn's-like ileitis by abrogation of intestinal epithelial cell apoptosis. Proc Natl Acad Sci U S A 2003;100: 8366–8371.

17 Fischer A, Gluth M, Pape UF, Wiedenmann B, Theuring F, Baumgart DC: Adalimumab prevents barrier dysfunction and antagonizes distinct effects of TNF-alpha on tight junction proteins and signaling pathways in intestinal epithelial cells. Am J Physiol Gastrointest Liver Physiol 2013;304:G970–G979.

18 Neurath MF: New targets for mucosal healing and therapy in inflammatory bowel diseases. Mucosal Immunol 2014; 7:6–19.

19 Lisi S, D'Amore M, Sisto M: ADAM17 at the interface between inflammation and autoimmunity. Immunol Lett 2014;162: 159–169.

20 Roulis M, Armaka M, Manoloukos M, Apostolaki M, Kollias G: Intestinal epithelial cells as producers but not targets of chronic TNF suffice to cause murine Crohn-like pathology. Proc Natl Acad Sci U S A 2011;108:5396–5401.

21 Onizawa M, Nagaishi T, Kanai T, Nagano K, Oshima S, Nemoto Y, Yoshioka A, Totsuka T, Okamoto R, Nakamura T, Sakamoto N, Tsuchiya K, Aoki K, Ohya K, Yagita H, Watanabe M: Signaling pathway via TNF-alpha/NF-kappaB in intestinal epithelial cells may be directly involved in colitis-associated carcinogenesis. Am J Physiol Gastrointest Liver Physiol 2009;296:G850–G859.

22 Li J, Yin Q, Wu H: Structural basis of signal transduction in the TNF receptor superfamily. Adv Immunol 2013;119: 135–153.

23 Workman LM, Habelhah H: TNFR1 signaling kinetics: spatiotemporal control of three phases of IKK activation by posttranslational modification. Cell Signal 2013;25:1654–1664.

24 Dannappel M, Vlantis K, Kumari S, Polykratis A, Kim C, Wachsmuth L, Eftychi C, Lin J, Corona T, Hermance N, Zelic M, Kirsch P, Basic M, Bleich A, Kelliher M, Pasparakis M: RIPK1 maintains epithelial homeostasis by inhibiting apoptosis and necroptosis. Nature 2014;513:90–94.

25 Awane M, Andres PG, Li DJ, Reinecker HC: NF-kappa B-inducing kinase is a common mediator of IL-17-, TNF-alpha-, and IL-1 beta-induced chemokine promoter activation in intestinal epithelial cells. J Immunol 1999;162:5337–5344.

26 Gunther C, Martini E, Wittkopf N, Amann K, Weigmann B, Neumann H, Waldner MJ, Hedrick SM, Tenzer S, Neurath MF, Becker C: Caspase-8 regulates TNF-alpha-induced epithelial necroptosis and terminal ileitis. Nature 2011;477:335–339.

27 Ye D, Ma I, Ma TY: Molecular mechanism of tumor necrosis factor-alpha modulation of intestinal epithelial tight junction barrier. Am J Physiol Gastrointest Liver Physiol 2006;290:G496–G504.

28 Wang F, Graham WV, Wang Y, Witkowski ED, Schwarz BT, Turner JR: Interferon-gamma and tumor necrosis factor-alpha synergize to induce intestinal epithelial barrier dysfunction by up-regulating myosin light chain kinase expression. Am J Pathol 2005;166:409–419.

29 Boivin MA, Ye D, Kennedy JC, Al-Sadi R, Shepela C, Ma TY: Mechanism of glucocorticoid regulation of the intestinal tight junction barrier. Am J Physiol Gastrointest Liver Physiol 2007;292:G590–G598.

30 Cheng H, Leblond C: Origin, differentiation and renewal of the four main epithelial cell types in the mouse small intestine. V. Unitarian theory of the origin of the four epithelial cell types. Am J Anat 1974;141:537–561.

31 Potten CS, Booth C, Pritchard DM: The intestinal epithelial stem cell: the mucosal governor. Int J Exp Pathol 1997;78: 219–243.

32 Fre S, Huyghe M, Mourikis P, Robine S, Louvard D, Artavanis-Tsakonas S: Notch signals control the fate of immature progenitor cells in the intestine. Nature 2005;435:964–968.

33 Zheng X, Tsuchiya K, Okamoto R, Iwasaki M, Kano Y, Sakamoto N, Nakamura T, Watanabe M: Suppression of hath1 gene expression directly regulated by hes1 via notch signaling is associated with goblet cell depletion in ulcerative colitis. Inflamm Bowel Dis 2011;17: 2251–2260.

34 Coskun M: The role of CDX2 in inflammatory bowel disease. Dan Med J 2014; 61:B4820.

35 Verzi MP, Shin H, He HH, Sulahian R, Meyer CA, Montgomery RK, Fleet JC, Brown M, Liu XS, Shivdasani RA: Differentiation-specific histone modifications reveal dynamic chromatin interactions and partners for the intestinal transcription factor CDX2. Dev Cell 2010;19:713–726.

36 Coskun M, Olsen AK, Holm TL, Kvist PH, Nielsen OH, Riis LB, Olsen J, Troelsen JT: TNF-α-induced down-regulation of CDX2 suppresses MEP1A expression in colitis. Biochim Biophys Acta 2012;1822:843–851.

37 Bamias G, Dahman MI, Arseneau KO, Guanzon M, Gruska D, Pizarro TT, Cominelli F: Intestinal-specific TNFalpha overexpression induces Crohn's-like ileitis in mice. PLoS One 2013;8:e72594.

38 Su L, Shen L, Clayburgh DR, Nalle SC, Sullivan EA, Meddings JB, Abraham C, Turner JR: Targeted epithelial tight junction dysfunction causes immune activation and contributes to development of experimental colitis. Gastroenterology 2009;136:551–563.

39 Liu H, Li M, Wang P, Wang F: Blockade of hypoxia-inducible factor-1alpha by YC-1 attenuates interferon-gamma and tumor necrosis factor-alpha-induced intestinal epithelial barrier dysfunction. Cytokine 2011;56:581–588.
40 Bruewer M, Luegering A, Kucharzik T, Parkos CA, Madara JL, Hopkins AM, Nusrat A: Proinflammatory cytokines disrupt epithelial barrier function by apoptosis-independent mechanisms. J Immunol 2003;171:6164–6172.
41 Gilbert S, Zhang R, Denson L, Moriggl R, Steinbrecher K, Shroyer N, Lin J, Han X: Enterocyte STAT5 promotes mucosal wound healing via suppression of myosin light chain kinase-mediated loss of barrier function and inflammation. EMBO Mol Med 2012;4:109–124.
42 Kolodziej LE, Lodolce JP, Chang JE, Schneider JR, Grimm WA, Bartulis SJ, Zhu X, Messer JS, Murphy SF, Reddy N, Turner JR, Boone DL: TNFAIP3 maintains intestinal barrier function and supports epithelial cell tight junctions. PLoS One 2011;6:e26352.
43 Inagaki-Ohara K, Yada S, Takamura N, Reaves M, Yu X, Liu E, Rooney I, Nicholas S, Castro A, Ware CF, Green DR, Lin T: p53-dependent radiation-induced crypt intestinal epithelial cells apoptosis is mediated in part through TNF-TNFR1 system. Oncogene 2001;20:812–818.
44 Nunes T, Bernardazzi C, de Souza HS: Cell death and inflammatory bowel diseases: apoptosis, necrosis, and autophagy in the intestinal epithelium. Biomed Res Int 2014;2014:218493.
45 Becker C, Watson AJ, Neurath MF: Complex roles of caspases in the pathogenesis of inflammatory bowel disease. Gastroenterology 2013;144:283–293.
46 Welz PS, Wullaert A, Vlantis K, Kondylis V, Fernandez-Majada V, Ermolaeva M, Kirsch P, Sterner-Kock A, van Loo G, Pasparakis M: FADD prevents RIP3-mediated epithelial cell necrosis and chronic intestinal inflammation. Nature 2011;477:330–334.
47 Wong N, Harrison D: Colorectal neoplasia in ulcerative colitis-recent advances. Histopathology 2001;39:221–234.
48 Eaden JA, Abrams KR, Mayberry JF: The risk of colorectal cancer in ulcerative colitis: a meta-analysis. Gut 2001;48:526–535.
49 Greten F, Eckmann L, Greten T, Park J, Li Z, Egan L, Kagnoff M, Karin M: IKKbeta links inflammation and tumorigenesis in a mouse model of colitis-associated cancer. Cell 2004;118:285–296.
50 Popivanova BK, Kitamura K, Wu Y, Kondo T, Kagaya T, Kaneko S, Oshima M, Fujii C, Mukaida N: Blocking TNF-alpha in mice reduces colorectal carcinogenesis associated with chronic colitis. J Clin Invest 2008;118:560–570.
51 Ullman TA, Itzkowitz SH: Intestinal inflammation and cancer. Gastroenterology 2011;140:1807–1816.
52 Qizilbash AH: Pathologic studies in colorectal cancer. A guide to the surgical pathology examination of colorectal specimens and review of features of prognostic significance. Pathol Annu 1982;17:1–46.
53 Kano Y, Tsuchiya K, Zheng X, Horita N, Fukushima K, Hibiya S, Yamauchi Y, Nishimura T, Hinohara K, Gotoh N, Suzuki S, Okamoto R, Nakamura T, Watanabe M: The acquisition of malignant potential in colon cancer is regulated by the stabilization of Atonal homolog 1 protein. Biochem Biophys Res Commun 2013;432:175–181.
54 Laureti S, Ugolini F, D'Errico A, Rago S, Poggioli G: Adenocarcinoma below ileoanal anastomosis for ulcerative colitis: report of a case and review of the literature. Dis Colon Rectum 2002;45:418–421.
55 Dharmani P, Leung P, Chadee K: Tumor necrosis factor-alpha and Muc2 mucin play major roles in disease onset and progression in dextran sodium sulphate-induced colitis. PLoS One 2011;6:e25058.
56 McElroy SJ, Prince LS, Weitkamp JH, Reese J, Slaughter JC, Polk DB: Tumor necrosis factor receptor 1-dependent depletion of mucus in immature small intestine: a potential role in neonatal necrotizing enterocolitis. Am J Physiol Gastrointest Liver Physiol 2011;301:G656–G666.
57 Zhu YQ, Tan XD: TFF3 modulates NF-{kappa}B and a novel negative regulatory molecule of NF-{kappa}B in intestinal epithelial cells via a mechanism distinct from TNF-{alpha}. Am J Physiol Cell Physiol 2005;289:C1085–C1093.
58 Yang Q, Bermingham N, Finegold M, Zoghbi H: Requirement of Math1 for secretory cell lineage commitment in the mouse intestine. Science 2001;294:2155–2158.
59 Tsuchiya K, Nakamura T, Okamoto R, Kanai T, Watanabe M: Reciprocal targeting of Hath1 and beta-catenin by Wnt glycogen synthase kinase 3beta in human colon cancer. Gastroenterology 2007;132:208–220.
60 Park ET, Oh HK, Gum JR, Crawley SC, Kakar S, Engel J, Leow CC, Gao WQ, Kim YS: HATH1 expression in mucinous cancers of the colorectum and related lesions. Clinical Cancer Research 2006;12:5403–5410.
61 Sato T, Vries RG, Snippert HJ, van de Wetering M, Barker N, Stange DE, van Es JH, Abo A, Kujala P, Peters PJ, Clevers H: Single Lgr5 stem cells build crypt-villus structures in vitro without a mesenchymal niche. Nature 2009;459:262–265.
62 Yui S, Nakamura T, Sato T, Nemoto Y, Mizutani T, Zheng X, Ichinose S, Nagaishi T, Okamoto R, Tsuchiya K, Clevers H, Watanabe M: Functional engraftment of colon epithelium expanded in vitro from a single adult $Lgr5^+$ stem cell. Nat Med 2012;18:618–623.
63 Nigro G, Rossi R, Commere PH, Jay P, Sansonetti PJ: The cytosolic bacterial peptidoglycan sensor Nod2 affords stem cell protection and links microbes to gut epithelial regeneration. Cell Host Microbe 2014;15:792–798.

Kiichiro Tsuchiya, MD, PhD, Associate Professor
Department of Advanced Therapeutics for Gastrointestinal Diseases
Department of Gastroenterology and Hepatology, Tokyo Medical and Dental University (TMDU)
1-5-45 Yushima, Bunkyo-ku
Tokyo 113-8510 (Japan)
E-Mail kii.gast@tmd.ac.jp

Rogler G, Herfarth H, Hibi T, Nielsen OH (eds): Anti-Tumor Necrosis Factor Therapy in Inflammatory Bowel Disease.
Front Gastrointest Res. Basel, Karger, 2015, vol 34, pp 9–26 (DOI: 10.1159/000381381)

Physiological Role of TNF in Mucosal Immunology: Regulation of Macrophage/Dendritic Cell Function

Aymeric Rivollier[a] • J. Marsal[b] • William W. Agace[a, c]

[a]Section of Immunology and Vaccinology, National Veterinary Institute, Technical University of Denmark, Frederiksberg, Denmark; [b]Department of Gastroenterology, Skåne University Hospital, Lund, and [c]Immunology Section, Lund University, Lund, Sweden

Abstract

Intestinal mononuclear phagocytes, comprising macrophages (Mϕs) and dendritic cells (DCs), play important roles in the generation and the regulation of immune responses to intestinal antigens, and alterations in the development and/or the function of these cells are thought to contribute to the pathogenesis of inflammatory bowel disease. In this review, we discuss the role of tumor necrosis factor-α (TNF) in regulating multiple aspects of intestinal Mϕ and DC physiology, including their differentiation, migration, maturation, survival and effector functions. In inflammatory bowel disease, TNF signaling has been implicated in reprogramming monocyte differentiation from the anti-inflammatory Mϕ lineage towards the pro-inflammatory mononuclear phagocyte lineage. These cells become a major source of TNF and, thus, may contribute to the chronic inflammatory process. Finally, we highlight some of the important gaps in our current knowledge regarding the role of TNF in Mϕ and DC physiology and suggest important directions for future research in this field.

Introduction

The maintenance of gastrointestinal (GI) tract homeostasis is critically dependent on the capacity of its immune system to remain tolerant to harmless dietary and commensal microorganism-derived antigens while maintaining the ability to generate protective immune responses towards harmful intestinal pathogens [1]. Intestinal mononuclear phagocytes (MPs), including macrophages (Mϕs) and dendritic cells (DCs), are believed to play a key role in this process and to play pro-inflammatory roles in the setting of chronic intestinal inflammation. A deeper understanding of the factors that control the development and the function of MP subsets in the steady state and how their roles are modified in the inflammatory setting will provide important insights into the biology of these cells. Such information may in turn result in new strategies for the treatment of inflammatory bowel disease (IBD).

Tumor necrosis factor-α (TNF) acts as a key modulator of immune and stromal cell biology by regulating genes responsible for inflammation, proliferation, differentiation and apoptosis [2]. It is synthesized as a monomeric protein that is inserted into the cell membrane as a homotrimer (mTNF), which is cleaved by the matrix metalloprotease TNF-converting enzyme (TACE) into a soluble trimeric form (sTNF). Both sTNF and mTNF are biologically active and can bind to and signal through two different transmembrane TNF receptors (TNF-Rs): TNF-R1 (also known as p55) and TNF-R2 (also known as p75). These receptors have distinct expression patterns and affinities for mTNF and sTNF [3]. While TNF-R1 is constitutively expressed on most cell types and preferentially binds to sTNF, TNF-R2 expression is highly regulated. TNF-R2 is typically expressed in hematopoietic and endothelial cells and binds to mTNF with higher affinity than sTNF [3, 4]. Both TNF-R1 and TNF-R2 can be cleaved from the cell surface by TACE in response to inflammatory signals. The resulting cleaved extracellular domains of TNF-R1 and TNF-R2 (soluble TNF-R (sTNF-R)1 and sTNF-R2) retain the ability to bind to and neutralize sTNF and, thus, function as endogenous TNF inhibitors [3–5]. An additional level of complexity of TNF biology is that mTNF can itself function as a receptor. The binding of mTNF to TNF-Rs or anti-TNF agents induces reverse signaling into the cell through this membrane-anchored ligand [3, 6, 7].

Here, we review the state-of-the-art literature on the role of TNF signaling in the regulation of intestinal Mϕ and DC biology and discuss how the currently used anti-TNF therapies might be affecting these cells in IBD patients to modulate disease progression. Unfortunately, the vast majority of studies assessing the impact of TNF on MP biology have not taken into account the phenotypic, functional and ontogenic heterogeneity of intestinal MPs (see below). Studies that do so are urgently required for a more complete understanding of the impact of TNF and anti-TNF therapies on MP-mediated intestinal immune homeostasis and inflammation.

Defining Mononuclear Phagocyte Subsets in the Intestinal Mucosa

The intestinal MP population contains several subsets of Mϕs and DCs [8–10], whose identification requires simultaneous examination of several surface biomarkers [9, 10]. Recent ontogeny studies support such heterogeneity in the MP compartment and distinguish classical DC (cDC) subsets (arising from blood-circulating committed DC precursors) from intestinal Mϕs, which are the progeny of monocytes [11–14] (fig. 1). Intestinal cDCs are located within gut-associated lymphoid tissue (lymphoid structures associated with the intestinal mucosa, including Peyer's patches and isolated lymphoid follicles) and diffusely throughout the intestinal lamina propria (LP). cDCs act as sentinels and sensors to monitor the luminal content of the intestine by sampling bacteria and food antigens, and these cells constitutively migrate to intestinal draining lymph nodes (for example, the mesenteric lymph nodes (MLNs) or the caudal lymph nodes), where they present antigens to naïve T cells and initiate adaptive immune responses [9, 15]. cDCs display poor phagocytic abilities, develop in response to the cytokine Fms-related tyrosine kinase 3 ligand and express the DC-specific transcription factor Zbtb46 [16]. cDCs are characterized by high expression of CD11c and major histocompatibility complex class II (MHC-II) and a lack of the high-affinity immunoglobulin G receptor FcγR1, which marks cells of the monocyte/Mϕ lineage in the steady state [17]. Importantly, the intestinal cDC compartment is itself heterogeneous: several surface markers appear to define at least three functionally specialized cDC subsets requiring distinct transcription factors for their development in mice and their counterparts in humans (fig. 1).

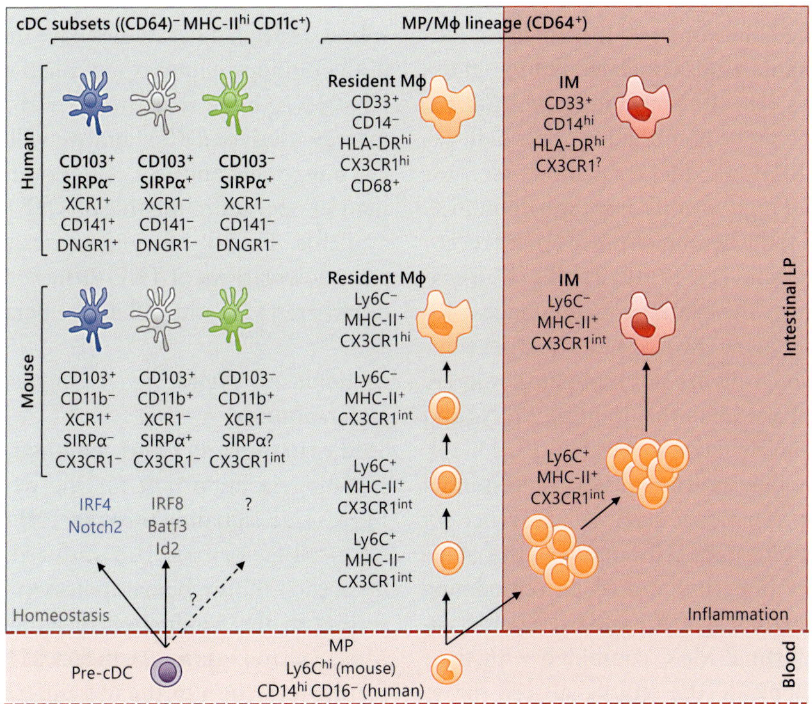

Fig. 1. Comparative overview of the phenotype of classical dendritic cell (DC; cDC) and monocyte-derived mononuclear phagocyte (MP) subsets in mice and humans. Intestinal lamina propria (LP) cDC subsets arise from blood-circulating committed DC precursors (pre-cDCs), in contrast to circulating monocytes, which generate tissue-resident macrophages (Mϕ). cDCs are characterized by high expression of CD11c and major histocompatibility complex class II (MHC-II) and the lack of expression of the high-affinity immunoglobulin G receptor FcγR1 (CD64), which marks cells of the Mϕ/monocyte lineage. In the homeostatic LP, several cDC subsets with different functions can be identified in mice and humans by their differential expression of the αE and αM integrins (CD103 and CD11b, respectively), signal regulatory protein-α, the chemokine receptor XCR1, CD141 and DNGR1. The indicated transcription factors IRF4, Notch2, IRF8, Batf3 and Id2 have been implicated in regulating the development of each subset. There are marked differences in the ratio of CD103^{+}CD11b^{+} to CD103^{+}CD11b^{-} DCs along the length of the mouse intestine. CD103^{+}CD11b^{+} DCs represent the majority of DCs in the small intestine but are rarely present in the colon [117]. Whether these differential localizations contribute to regional immune specializations remains to be more clearly assessed. In the small intestine, the numbers of CD103^{+}CD11b^{+} DCs in different segments of the intestine correlate with the presence of T helper 17 cells, and our group has reported a role of these DCs in intestinal T helper 17 cell homeostasis [117]. In contrast, blood-circulating monocytes generate tissue-resident Mϕs via a series of fractalkine receptor (CX3CR1)$^{intermediate\ (int)}$ cells. Resident Mϕs can be identified by their high expression of CD64, MHC-II and CX3CR1, as well as the hemoglobin scavenger receptor and macrosialin (CD68), in both mice and humans. Additional useful markers of these cells include the myeloid marker CD33 and the co-receptor for lipopolysaccharide CD14 in humans and the Mer tyrosine kinase receptor and the mannose receptor CD206 in mice. When homeostasis is perturbed by inflammation, monocytes and their CX3CR1^{int} derivatives accumulate in large numbers in the LP at the expenses of tissue-resident Mϕs and generate inflammatory monocytes, which are Ly6C^{-}MHC-II^{+}CX3CR1^{int} in mice and CD33^{+}CD14^{hi}HLA-DR^{hi} in humans. Whether the differentiation and functions of the pre-cDC-derived cDC subsets are also perturbed during inflammation remains to be established.

Intestinal Mϕs are found throughout the GI tract and represent the majority (>80%) of MPs in the noninflamed intestinal LP [13], but these cells are rarely present in gut-associated lymphoid tissue and MLNs [18]. In both mice and humans, intestinal Mϕs can be identified by their high expression of MHC-II, the fractalkine receptor (CX3CR1), the high-affinity immunoglobulin G receptor FcγR1, the hemoglobin scavenger receptor, and macrosialin [11, 17, 19–21] (fig. 1). Intestinal Mϕs require the cytokine macrophage colony-stimulating factor (M-CSF) for their development [22]. These cells are not thought to migrate from the intestinal LP to the draining MLNs and are poor at priming naïve T cells [11, 13, 23–25]. In the steady-state intestine, Mϕs play essential housekeeping functions such as clearance of apoptotic and senescent cells, maintenance of intestinal barrier integrity, and tissue remodeling [26–31]. The high phagocytic and bactericidal capacities of intestinal Mϕs, combined with their positioning beneath the epithelial cell layer, makes them an ideal candidate to eliminate bacteria that breach the epithelial layer [11, 13, 32].

Recent reports have demonstrated that the mucosal Mϕ compartment requires continuous replenishment by blood monocytes that are Ly6C^{hi} in mice and CD14^{hi}CD16^{-} in humans [11, 33]. Under steady-state conditions, these monocytes enter the intestinal mucosa and develop into mature MHC-II^{hi}CX3CR1^{hi} Mϕs within a few days through a series of intermediate cell phenotypes, and an analogous monocyte differentiation process has been suggested to occur in the human intestine [11].

Impact of TNF Signaling on Intestinal Mononuclear Phagocytes

Most studies assessing the role of TNF in intestinal MP development and function have been performed prior to our appreciation of the complexity of this compartment. Given the distinct ontogeny and functionality of intestinal MP subsets (see above), it seems highly likely that the outcome of TNF signaling is distinct for each MP subset. Indeed, most studies have focused on cells of the monocyte lineage (so called monocyte-derived DCs, bone marrow-derived Mϕs or bone marrow-derived DCs), and we will therefore focus our review on these cells, pointing out information relevant to the role of TNF in cDCs when available. Finally, the different signaling pathways downstream of TNF-Rs have been reviewed elsewhere [3, 4] and will not be detailed here.

Mononuclear Phagocyte Development/ Differentiation

Studies in the early 1990s demonstrated that TNF signaling is important for the development of Mϕs. sTNF signaling through TNF-R1 augments stem cell factor- and IL-7-induced myelopoiesis from early mouse hematopoietic progenitors, resulting in the production of almost exclusively Mϕs in vitro [34] (fig. 2). In fact, sTNF is required for the induction of the Mϕ differentiation program. In its absence, precursors fail to enter a differentiation program and instead maintain a proliferative program [35]. Similarly, autocrine TNF signaling strongly potentiates IL-3- and granulocyte M-CSF-dependent early myelopoiesis in vitro and facilitates the development of monocytic cells from human CD34^{+} hematopoietic progenitors while inhibiting granulopoiesis [36]. Cooperation between granulocyte M-CSF and TNF is also crucial for the generation of murine bone marrow-derived DCs as well as human blood CD34^{+} progenitor-derived DCs in vitro [37, 38] (fig. 2). However, further studies are required to assess the respective contributions of sTNF, mTNF, TNF-R1 and TNF-R2 in the generation of intestinal Mϕ and cDC subsets in vivo.

During IBD, increased infiltration of blood monocytes is observed in the intestine. This infiltration is notably driven by TNF signaling in endothelial cells, which induces an upregulation of adhesion molecules (endothelial-leukocyte adhesion molecule-1, vascular cell adhesion

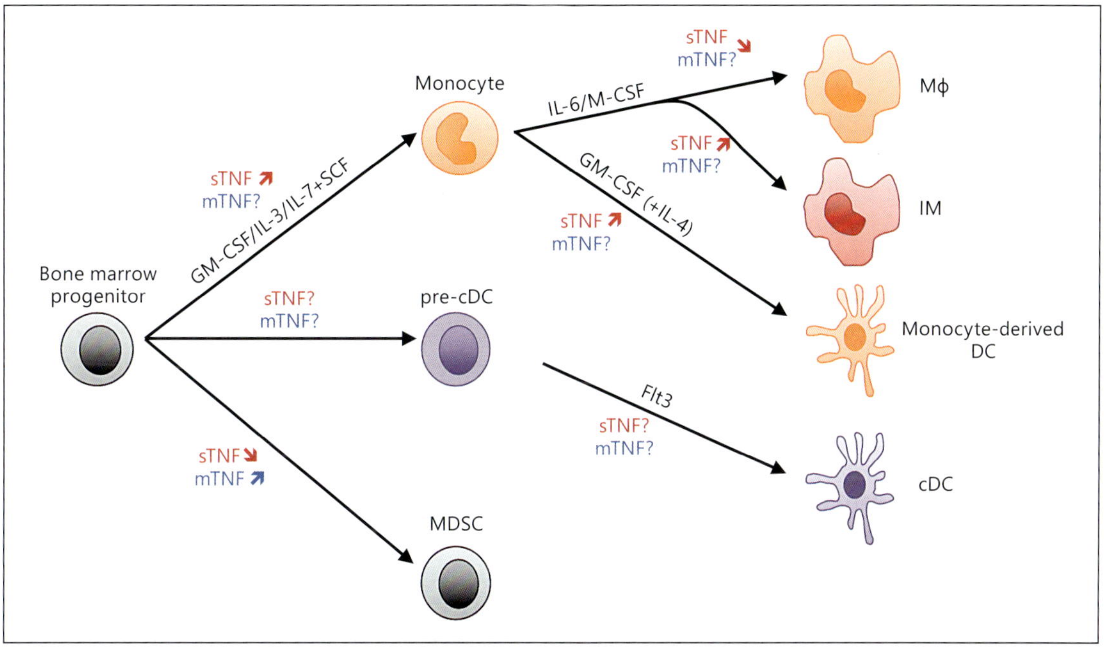

Fig. 2. Proposed roles of TNF signaling in the development of intestinal MP subsets. The figure depicts the role of TNF signaling in the development of MP subsets. Such information should be interpreted with caution, as it is based on studies using in vitro bone marrow derived-, blood CD34$^+$ progenitor derived- or monocyte-derived DCs and Mϕs. A major issue is that the in vivo counterparts of monocyte-derived DCs generated in the presence of granulocyte macrophage colony-stimulating factor ± IL-4 have not been clearly identified in the intestine. These cells are zbtb46$^+$ and, therefore, could be considered as cDCs; however, they are CD64$^+$ and monocyte-derived. Therefore, their classification in the current monocyte/Mϕ/cDC nomenclature is difficult. In addition, the role of TNF signaling in the development of Flt3-dependent cDCs, which are thought to represent the equivalent of steady-state intestinal and lymph node-resident cDCs, has not been investigated. Soluble TNF: sTNF; membrane-bound TNF: mTNF. ↗ indicates a potentiating role; ↘ indicates an inhibitory role; ? indicates not yet investigated. GM-CSF: granulocyte macrophage colony-stimulating factor; IL-3, -7, -6, and -4: interleukin-3, -7, -6, and -4, respectively; SCF: stem cell factor; Flt3: Fms-related tyrosine kinase 3 ligand; pre-cDC: cDC precursor; MDSC: myeloid-derived suppressor cell; IM: inflammatory monocyte.

molecule-1, and intercellular adhesion molecule-1) that are critical for the classical adhesion cascade and for the extravasation of blood monocytes expressing the ligands for these molecules (P-selectin glycoprotein ligand-1, leukocyte function-associated molecule 1, very late antigen-4 and Mac-1/CD11b) [39]. The recruited monocytes do not generate mature anti-inflammatory tissue-resident Mϕs any longer but rather arrest or divert their differentiation process to a more pro-inflammatory subset of MPs [11, 13, 40] (see below). We will hereafter refer to this pro-inflammatory MP subset as inflammatory monocytes (IMs). Interestingly, TNF may represent one of the local microenvironmental factors that switches the differentiation of monocytes from anti-inflammatory Mϕs to pro-inflammatory IMs. Indeed, Chomarat et al. reported that upon contact with resting IL-6-secreting stromal cells such as fibroblasts, human monocytes upregulate their expression of the M-CSF receptor (M-CSFR), allowing them to consume M-CSF in an autocrine fashion and to differentiate into Mϕs [41]. The addition of sTNF blocked this Mϕ differentiation process by decreasing the expression of the M-CSFR and inducing its internalization. Instead, in the presence of sTNF, monocytes differentiated into cells termed DCs by the authors, and these cells shared similarities with the IMs observed in the inflamed mucosa of IBD patients (fig. 2). These cells displayed pro-inflammatory properties and notably stimulated the proliferation of T cells [41]. The relevance of this in vitro data remains to be established in the intestine in vivo, but it represents a potentially interesting mechanism to explain the switch in the monocyte differentiation program in the inflamed intestine.

The balance between sTNF and mTNF may also be critical to the control of the differentiation program of intestinal monocytes. Myeloid-derived suppressor cells (MDSCs), a heterogeneous population of immature myeloid precursors that accumulate in patients and animal models of chronic inflammation or cancer, negatively regulate immune responses [42]. Active MDSCs suppress T cell and DC activation via arginase-1-, nitric oxide-, reactive oxygen species-, cysteine deprivation-, IL-10- or regulatory T cell-dependent mechanisms. In chronic inflammatory disorders, MDSCs seem to appear at relatively late stages of the inflammatory process in response to pro-inflammatory factors, and their appearance may represent a regulatory mechanism developed by the organism to terminate adaptive immune responses [42, 43]. The relationship of MDSC with the other myeloid cell types that accumulate in the inflamed intestine has not been fully elucidated, but some MDSCs might represent monocytes that were prevented from differentiating into Mϕs or IMs. mTNF was recently reported to trigger the accumulation and activation of MDSCs via the TNF-R2 and p38 MAPK pathways, enhancing their suppressive activities [44] (fig. 2). In contrast, sTNF inhibited these processes by signaling via TNF-R1. This study revealed a novel immunosuppressive effect of mTNF and suggested that a balance between sTNF through TNF-R1 and mTNF through TNF-R2 controls the development of monocytes into IMs or MDSCs, respectively. Further characterization of MDSCs and their control by mTNF and sTNF are needed, and given their powerful immune-regulatory properties, MDSCs could also be a target of therapeutic interest in IBD.

Beyond direct TNF signaling in MP biology, signaling induced by the binding of anti-TNF antibodies to monocytes was also reported to control the differentiation of these cells into immunoregulatory Mϕs in healthy donor peripheral blood mononuclear cell cultures. These Mϕs produced high amounts of IL-10, expressed the regulatory Mϕ marker CD206 (a mannose receptor) and were capable of inhibiting the proliferation of activated T cells [45]. Their differentiation required the binding of anti-TNF antibodies to mTNF expressed on T cells and to Fcγ receptors expressed on monocytes. Therefore, only anti-TNF agents containing an Fc portion (infliximab and adalimumab, which are two monoclonal antibodies), but not etanercept (a fusion protein of TNF-R2 and the Fc region of human IgG1) or certolizumab (a Fab' fragment from a humanized IgG1 conjugated to polyethylene glycol), can induce the generation of immunoregulatory Mϕs in vitro. The in vivo relevance of this finding was demonstrated in IBD patients before and after treatment with infliximab [45]. A significant induction of regulatory macrosialin^{+} CD206^{+} Mϕs was observed in patients with mucosal healing after treatment with infliximab, and this induction was absent from patients without mucosal healing. Further, these Mϕs suppressed T cell proliferation and induced wound healing in vitro, suggesting a key role of infliximab-induced Mϕs in mucosal healing.

Classical Dendritic Cell Maturation and Migration

cDCs can exist in different states of maturation/activation. Intestinal cDCs that migrate to MLNs in the steady state [46] have an immature or semi-mature phenotype, express high levels of MHC-II and the chemokine receptor CCR7 but low

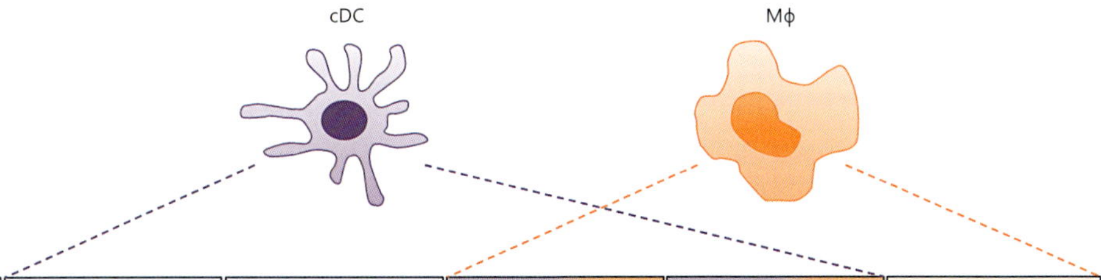

TNF signalling pathway involved	Migration	Maturation	Apoptosis (cDC)	Apoptosis (Mϕ)	Cytokine production (cDC)	Cytokine production (Mϕ)	Autophagy
sTNF/TNF-R1	+	+*in vitro* TNF-independent *in vivo?*	–?	–?	0	0	+
mTNF/TNF-R2	N.D.	N.D.	–?	–?	N.D.	N.D.	N.D.
mTNF-mediated reverse signalling	N.D.	N.D.	–?	–?	–anti-TNF mAb, + mTNF cleavage, + when prior to TNF-R1, –when after TNF-R1	–anti-TNF mAb, + when prior to TNF-R1, –when after TNF-R1	N.D.

Fig. 3. Proposed roles of TNF signaling in intestinal MP biology. The figure depicts the role of TNF signaling in the regulation of MP biology based on evidence obtained using bone marrow derived- or monocyte-derived DCs and Mϕs in vitro or using monocytes in vivo after anti-TNF therapy. Further studies are required to determine the impact of TNF signaling on the regulation of intestinal MP subset functionality in vivo. + indicates a positive contribution of the TNF pathway to the given mechanism; – indicates a negative contribution of the TNF pathway to the given mechanism; 0 indicates no impact of the TNF pathway on the given mechanism; N.D. indicates not yet determined; ? indicates contributions that need to be confirmed. The high frequency of 'N.D.' and '?' in this figure underscores the urgent need for further research efforts addressing the multiple contributions of TNF signaling to intestinal MP biology.

levels of T cell co-stimulatory molecules (CD80, CD86 or CD40), and can induce tolerogenic or hyporesponsive T cells in vivo [47, 48]. In the setting of inflammation or upon exposure to bacteria or pathogen-associated molecular patterns (PAMPs), immature cDCs undergo profound phenotypic changes and acquire a mature phenotype: downregulation of antigen uptake receptors and increased expression of MHC-II, co-stimulatory molecules, and cytokines for optimal T cell activation in MLNs [49]. The cDC maturation process also includes enhanced expression of the chemokine receptor CCR7, which is required for their migration from the intestine to draining MLNs [49].

While multiple studies have illustrated a potent role of TNF as a human and murine DC maturation factor in vitro, the role of TNF in regulating cDC maturation in vivo is less clear. In vitro exogenous sTNF added to human monocyte-derived or mouse bone marrow-derived DC cultures, as well as endogenous TNF produced in these cultures in response to added lipopolysaccharide (LPS), induces DC maturation in a TNF-R1-dependent (but not TNF-R2-dependent) manner [50–54] (fig. 3). sTNF is required for the optimal upregulation of MHC-II and co-stimulatory molecules on DCs. This allows them to efficiently stimulate the proliferation and differentiation of naïve $CD4^+$ T cells into IFNγ-producing T helper 1 (Th1) cells [52, 53, 55, 56] and to efficiently prime virus-specific $CD8^+$ T cells [57]. The sTNF-induced maturation of human monocyte-derived DCs in vitro relies on the activation of the MAPKs extracellular signal-related kinase 2, c-Jun N-terminal kinase and p38 and of the classical NF-κB pathway. Conversely, IL-10 receptor (IL-10R) signaling represses the sTNF-induced maturation program by blocking the activation of these pathways [58, 59]. In vivo, the release of cDCs from the intestine after the administration of LPS or R848 (a toll-like receptor (TLR)7/8 ligand) and their migration to the MLN are TNF-dependent. However, interestingly, the maturation of cDCs in this model seems to be TNF-independent [46, 48]. The full maturation of cDCs was in fact shown to be driven by type I IFN, which is produced by plasmacytoid DCs in MLNs in the case of R848 administration [60]. Hence, it has been suggested that cDC migration and full functional maturation may be two independently regulated events [61], the former of which is TNF-dependent while the latter of which is TNF-independent in vivo. In agreement with this statement, both $TNF^{-/-}$ and $TNF\text{-}R1^{-/-}$ mice in the steady state have normal numbers of mature splenic cDCs, suggesting that TNF is indeed dispensable for the maturation of cDCs in vivo [54, 57]. Additional work is required to determine whether the ability of TNF to drive intestinal LP-cDC migration to draining intestinal lymph nodes in vivo is a direct effect of TNF signaling in these cells or is an indirect effect of TNF signaling via an alternative cell type. In addition, it will be important to dissect the respective contributions of sTNF, mTNF, and their receptors to determine whether these processes are regulated in the same manner in all the migratory cDC subsets. Of note, the amount of TNF-R shedding should also be evaluated in future studies, as TNF-R2 shedding was reported to negatively regulate lung DC activation, controlling their IL-12 production and their migration to lung-draining lymph nodes by limiting the amount of available bioactive sTNF and mTNF during *Mycobacterium tuberculosis* infection [62].

The inhibition of the TNF-induced migration and/or maturation of intestinal cDC subsets may represent a mechanism that contributes to some of the beneficial effects of TNF blockade observed in IBD patients. In this regard, etanercept treatment in psoriasis patients was shown to reduce DC maturation and activation, leading to a reduction in T cell activation [63].

Control of Autophagy in Macrophages

Autophagy is an evolutionarily conserved process whereby cells eliminate their own organelles or cytoplasm by targeting them to lysosomes. During this process, organelles or cytoplasmic material, including protein aggregates and bacteria, are sequestered into double membrane-coated autophagosomes that subsequently fuse with endosomes and lysosomes to form autolysosomes, where lysosomal degradation occurs [64]. Autophagy is a central component of the Mϕ machinery to eradicate intracellular bacterial infections and to degrade bacteria after ingestion. The importance of this microbicidal pathway in the pathogenesis of IBD was highlighted by the discovery that synonymous single nucleotide polymorphisms in the autophagocytic genes ATG16L1 and IRGM are associated with enhanced risk for IBD and by recent functional analyses suggesting that Crohn's disease-associated mutations in autophagy-related genes may impair the ability of Mϕs to eradicate intracellular bacteria [64]. A number of studies using mouse peritoneal Mϕs or human monocyte-derived Mϕs reported that TNF signaling in these cells is required for the phagolysosomal compartment to acidify during infection with the intracellular parasite *Toxoplasma gondii* (reviewed in [65]). Moreover, IFNγ-induced phagosome maturation and autophagy are seemingly dependent upon autocrine TNF secretion by these Mϕs [65]. It will be important to assess whether TNF signaling is required for the autophagic process and for the control of commensal bacterial dissemination by intestinal Mϕs under homeostatic conditions and during IBD and to dissect the respective contributions of sTNF and mTNF to these processes (fig. 3).

Control of Cytokine Production in Monocyte-Derived Macrophages and Dendritic Cells

As described earlier, the binding of TNF-Rs or anti-TNF reagents to mTNF can induce reverse signaling [3]. Reverse signaling is mediated by phosphorylation of the cytoplasmic tail of mTNF, intracellular calcium elevation and activation of the p38 and Erk MAPK pathways [7].

In vitro, mouse cells of the monocyte lineage such as monocytic cell lines, as well as pulmonary, synovial or peritoneal Mϕs and monocytes, were found to be resistant to stimulation with LPS, zymosan or other PAMPs following pre-incubation in anti-TNF antibodies, indicating that reverse signaling through mTNF might serve as a 'silencing signal' in monocyte-derived cells to shut down their subsequent capacity to produce pro-inflammatory cytokines [7] (fig. 3). Reverse signaling through mTNF might also serve as a 'silencing signal' in human monocytes, as the TNF antagonists adalimumab and infliximab, which strongly bind to both mTNF and sTNF, suppress LPS-induced TNF, IL-1b and IL 10 or IL-12 production in these cells, while etanercept, which preferentially binds to sTNF, does not [66, 67]. Both LPS signaling and TNF antagonist-induced reverse signaling via the cytoplasmic tail of mTNF activate the Erk pathway. The silencing signal has been proposed to result from a shortened Erk signal duration induced by reverse signaling, from the inhibition of the nuclear translocation of Erk induced by reverse signaling, or from the fact that reverse signaling and LPS activate two different isoforms of Erk (Erk1 and Erk2) [7]. Besides reverse signaling induced by the binding of anti-TNF antibodies to mTNF, a second reverse signaling pathway was recently described to be functional during LPS-induced maturation of human monocyte-derived DCs. Here, LPS was found to trigger the cleavage of mTNF, releasing sTNF from mature DCs, while the remaining membrane-anchored cytoplasmic tail of mTNF was shown to be cleaved by signal peptide peptidase-like proteases (SPPL2a and SPPL2b), releasing a TNF intracellular domain that translocated to the nucleus and triggered the production of IL-12 [68]. Thus, reverse signaling pathways initiated downstream of mTNF appear to vary depending on the factors present in the human monocyte-derived DC microenvironment; while reverse signaling initiated by anti-TNF antibodies (and potentially TNF-R2) seems to negatively regulate the production of pro-inflammatory cytokines, reverse signaling initiated by the LPS-induced cleavage of mTNF to release sTNF triggers the production of pro-inflammatory cytokines such as IL-12. It remains to be determined whether the cleavage of the cytoplasmic tail of mTNF is required for anti-TNF antibody-induced reverse signaling and signal silencing in monocyte-derived cells. Another unsolved question that could explain some of the observed differences between the different anti-TNF agents is whether the crosslinking of multiple mTNF molecules is required to initiate reverse signaling.

Whether such reverse signaling has pro- or anti-inflammatory effects also appears to be dependent on the cytokine context in which the signaling occurs. Thus, experiments using the human monocytic line U937 suggest that reverse signaling occurring prior to sTNF stimulation enhances the production of inflammatory cytokines induced by sTNF in these cells but that reverse signaling occurring after sTNF stimulation inhibits the sTNF-induced production of inflammatory cytokines [69].

While the in vivo relevance of mTNF-mediated reverse signaling in intestinal MP subsets remains to be demonstrated, such signaling could represent an important mechanism by which sTNF-Rs and TNF-R expressing cells, such as T cells, control the differential production of pro-inflammatory cytokines by cDCs versus monocyte-derived Mϕs or IMs. At least two TNF antagonists showing clinical efficacy in IBD (infliximab and adalimumab) are capable of triggering this pathway and may thereby modulate inflammatory cytokine production by MPs [3, 5–7]. mTNF-mediated reverse signaling as a silencing signal could also be particularly relevant to intestinal Mϕs under homeostatic conditions since these Mϕs, in contrast to their counterparts in other tissues, do not produce pro-inflammatory cytokines upon exposure to bacteria or PAMPs but rather release the immunoregulatory cytokine IL-10 [11, 13, 32, 70–72]. This 'inflammatory anergic' state of intestinal Mϕs is controlled by soluble factors (particularly TGF-β and IL-10) [11, 13, 32, 70–72], notably produced by intestinal stromal cells, but could also involve $Foxp3^+$ regulatory cells (Tregs), which express high levels of TNF-R2 [73, 74] and which could trigger reverse signaling in Mϕs.

Protection of Monocytes/Macrophages/Dendritic Cells from Apoptosis

Apoptosis, a form of programmed cell death, is a natural physiological process that is essential for normal development and for the maintenance of cell homeostasis. In contrast to necrosis, which is a form of traumatic cell death, apoptosis allows the 'silent' elimination of unwanted cells by producing cell fragments (called apoptotic bodies), which are engulfed by phagocytes and are quickly removed before they cause damage. Defective apoptotic processes have been implicated in an extensive variety of diseases [75]. In IBD, the resistance of mucosal T cells to several pro-apoptotic signals, causing their accumulation in the intestinal mucosa, has been proposed as a pathogenic mechanism [5]. TNF signaling has, in multiple in vitro studies, been shown to have anti-apoptotic effects on myeloid cells. For example, LPS, via sTNF/TNF-R1-mediated autocrine signaling, can protect murine bone marrow-derived Mϕs from apoptosis induced by the withdrawal of M-CSF. This mechanism is MyD88-, PI3K-, Erk-, and NF-kB-dependent and is facilitated by the induction of a general cytoprotective program similar to that mediated by M-CSF [76] (fig. 3). The sTNF-induced maturation of mouse bone marrow-derived DCs increases their resistance to apoptosis (induced by prostate cancer cells) by stabilizing their expression of the anti-apoptotic protein Bcl-2 [77]. Similarly, sTNF promotes the survival of mature Langerhans cells migrating from human epidermis explant cultures [78].

Consistent with an anti-apoptotic role of TNF, the anti-TNF agents infliximab and adalimumab induce the apoptosis of circulating blood monocytes from healthy donors and patients with active IBD by upregulating the expression of Bax and Bak, two pro-apoptotic members of the Bcl-2 family, and the release of cytochrome C from the mitochondria into the cytosol [79]. Cytochrome C then activates the pro-apoptotic caspase cascade, including the effector caspase-3, which induces DNA fragmentation. However, studies regarding the mechanisms by which these agents induce apoptosis have generated confusing results. Only the infliximab and adalimumab antibodies, which bind to both mTNF and sTNF, induce the apoptosis of monocytes from healthy donors and from Crohn's disease patients; however, the fusion protein etanercept, which mainly blocks sTNF signaling rather than mTNF, does not [67]. This suggests that the pro-apoptotic activity of infliximab and adalimumab are directly mediated by their ability to induce mTNF-mediated reverse signaling in monocytes or to block mTNF-TNF-R2 intercellular interactions and that sTNF does not play any crucial anti-apoptotic role. However, the latter conclusion is hard to reconcile with the documented anti-apoptotic role of sTNF in myeloid cells mentioned earlier. Infliximab is also able to induce apoptosis in vivo: blood monocyte apoptosis has been shown to occur as early as 4 hours after treatment of active Crohn's disease patients with infliximab, and monocytopenia is commonly observed in IBD patients after treatment with infliximab [79].

Collectively, these results suggest that the induction of monocyte apoptosis could represent an important mechanism by which clinically efficient anti-TNF antibodies dampen the inflammatory process in IBD patients. Further supporting this concept, etanercept, which does not induce monocyte apoptosis as efficiently as infliximab and adalimumab in vitro, is not clinically effective in IBD patients [67]. Whether the apoptosis-inducing capacities of infliximab and adalimumab rely on their capacity to induce mTNF-mediated reverse signaling or to inhibit TNF-R2-mTNF interactions in monocytes and Mϕs, as was shown for T cells [80], remains to be more carefully addressed. Two additional mechanisms by which infliximab binds to mTNF may contribute to monocytopenia include the induction of cell lysis via antibody-dependent cell cytotoxicity and complement-dependent cytotoxicity [5]. Besides the anti-TNF agents used during IBD therapy, the increased amounts of sTNF-Rs released after cleavage by TACE observed in IBD [3, 81] could induce monocyte apoptosis in vivo since sTNF-R1 induces apoptosis in vitro in primary human monocytes through reverse signaling via mTNF [81]. Finally, given the inconsistent results generated from in vitro experiments using sTNF or etanercept, the role of sTNF as an anti-apoptotic agent acting on MPs in vivo requires further investigation.

In conclusion, the apoptotic process may be controlled by at least three TNF signaling pathways: mTNF-mediated reverse signaling, TNF-R2 signaling after mTNF binding or TNF-R1 signaling after sTNF binding. The individual contribution of each one of these pathways in vivo must be carefully addressed in not only circulating blood monocytes but also intestinal LP cDC, Mϕ and IM subsets.

TNF Production by Mononuclear Phagocytes and Its Impact on the Intestinal Microenvironment

Monocyte-Derived Mononuclear Phagocytes Are a Major Source of TNF and a Driving Force of the Inflammatory Process during Inflammatory Bowel Disease

Experimental animal models and patient studies have revealed that major changes occur in the balance of intestinal Mϕ/cDC quantity and function during IBD [1, 82]. In both the human and the mouse inflamed intestine, modifications in local microenvironment factors increase the recruitment of monocytes and alter their normal differentiation process. Indeed, during intestinal inflammation, newly recruited monocytes appear to display a reduced capacity to generate anti-inflammatory mature tissue-resident Mϕs, and these cells arrest and/or divert their differentiation to a pro-inflammatory subset of MPs, which massively expands in the intestine and eventually outnumbers the other cDC and Mϕ subsets [11, 13, 40]. This pro-inflammatory subset, characterized as $Ly6C^{+}MHC\text{-}II^{hi}CX3CR1^{intermediate}$ in mice [11] and $HLA\text{-}DR^{hi}CD33^{+}CD14^{hi}$ in humans [83], is believed to play a central pro-inflammatory role by producing large amounts of TNF and other inflammatory mediators, such as IL-1, IL-6, IL-23, reactive oxygen species and nitric oxide [11, 13, 14, 17, 80, 84–88] (fig. 1). Whether such cells are capable of priming naïve T cells and thus contributing to the initiation of adaptive immune responses is still a matter of debate [8, 13, 23, 40], and this subset has been alternatively called monocyte-derived DCs, IMs or TNF- and iNOS-producing DCs. We refer to this cell subset as IMs in this chapter. Remarkably, resident Mϕs appear to remain inflammatory anergic in the inflamed intestine [11, 13, 17, 40, 88].

The mechanisms by which TNF initiates and amplifies inflammation in IBD patients or mouse models of IBD are still poorly understood. TNF, a 'master regulator' of pro-inflammatory cytokine production, orchestrates inflammatory processes by switching on a TNF-dependent cytokine cascade in an autocrine and paracrine manner [89] (fig. 4). In the intestine, TNF notably promotes the recruitment of neutrophils, induces accelerated loss of enterocytes by apoptosis and increases the proliferation of these cells, leading to enhanced permeability, defective absorptive functions and leakier tight junctions of the epithelium. As a result, TNF not only increases the influx of

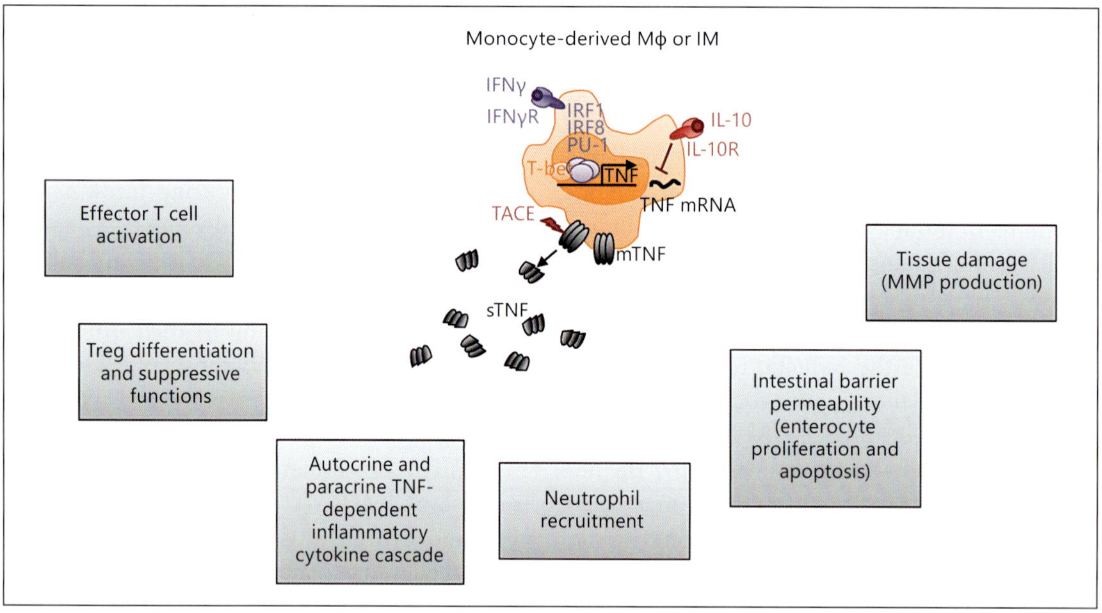

Fig. 4. Control of TNF production by intestinal monocyte-derived MP subsets and the impact of TNF on the intestinal environment. IL-10 signaling via the IL-10 receptor negatively regulates the production of TNF by destabilizing TNF mRNA and repressing its translation. T-bet directly binds to the TNF promoter and inhibits TNF expression. In contrast, IFNγ signaling induces the expression of the transcription factors interferon regulatory factor (IRF)1 and IRF8, which, together with PU.1, bind to the TNF promoter and drive TNF expression. mTNF and sTNF produced by DCs and Mϕs signal in an autocrine and paracrine manner in immune cells and epithelial cells to promote the inflammatory response and the tissue destruction observed during IBD. The potential production of sTNF and mTNF by cDCs and their contribution to IBD pathogenesis remain to be assessed. IFNγ: interferon-gamma; IFNγ-R: interferon-gamma receptor; IRF: interferon regulatory factor; T-bet: T-box expressed in T cells; IL-10: interleukin-10; IL-10R: interleukin-10 receptor; TACE: TNF-converting enzyme; IM: inflammatory monocyte; Treg: foxp3^{+} regulatory T cell; MMP: matrix metalloprotease.

luminal antigens and crypt hyperplasia but also activates endogenous matrix metalloproteases, which results in mucosal damage, ulceration and subsequent fibrosis [90].

Multiple studies have suggested that IM-derived TNF is an important contributor to intestinal inflammation [11, 13, 14, 40, 91, 92]. For example, dextran sulfate sodium-induced colitis is reduced in mice in which monocytes are deficient in TNF production [14] or in mice that have decreased numbers of monocytes in the blood [40, 86]. Further, in the T cell transfer colitis model, the presence of mTNF in recipient mice is sufficient for the development intestinal inflammation in the complete absence of sTNF, while sTNF and mTNF expression by donor T cells is dispensable [90]. Despite these findings, the relative contribution of IM-derived mTNF and sTNF to the inflammatory process has yet to be determined since numerous cells, including epithelial cells, mast cells, neutrophils, eosinophils and T cells, can produce TNF in the intestine.

Finally, multiple studies have pointed out a direct role of mTNF expressed on intestinal MPs in the control of Treg differentiation and suppressive functions [73, 74, 93–96] and in the modulation of effector T cell activation, their sensitivity to Treg suppression [4, 97], and their survival [80] via TNF-R2 in both humans and mice. As these topics are discussed in subsequent chapters of this book, they will not be covered further here. The role of TNF signaling in MPs for the control of intracellular or extracellular bacterial infections will also not be covered here due to space restrictions (for recent reviews of this topic, please see [4, 65, 98]).

Factors Controlling TNF Production by Monocyte-Derived Mononuclear Phagocytes

Although the induction of TNF production is critical for a rapid response to tissue trauma or infection, the prolonged or dysregulated production of TNF, as occurs in IBD, has serious adverse consequences. During IBD, microbial products constantly stimulate the production of TNF by IMs by triggering pattern recognition receptors, including TLRs and nucleotide-binding oligomerization domain-2 [40, 99]. TNF protein production is controlled at the levels of transcription, pre-mRNA processing, mRNA stability, translation and retention at the plasma membrane [3]. Several critical factors have been identified that modulate TNF expression in MPs (fig. 4).

The immunosuppressive cytokine IL-10 has emerged as one of the most important factors regulating intestinal MP-mediated TNF production and ensuring Mϕ quiescence in the face of environmental stimuli. Indeed, mice deficient in IL-10 or with a specific deletion of the IL-10R signaling molecule STAT3 in myeloid cells develop spontaneous colitis [100, 101]. Colonic MPs from these mice display exaggerated pro-inflammatory responses to bacterial products [13, 102–104]. IL-10R deficiency is also associated with an early onset form of severe IBD in humans [105, 106], and Zigmund et al. recently demonstrated that while IL-10 production by intestinal Mϕs is dispensable for the maintenance of intestinal homeostasis, IL-10R receptor expression and signaling in monocytes is critical for their conditioning and their differentiation into intestinal Mϕs. In the absence of IL-10R, monocytes recruited to the intestine differentiated into TNF-producing IMs, leading to the development of spontaneous and severe colitis [107, 108]. The molecular mechanism responsible for the IL-10-mediated inhibition of TNF production has not been addressed directly in the intestine, but a similar mechanism has been described for peritoneal Mϕs, in which IL-10 represses the translation of TNF mRNA through the modulation of the p38 serine/threonine kinase MAPK-activated protein kinase 2 pathway [109]. Like the expression of many other cytokines, TNF expression can be regulated at the post-transcriptional level. AU-rich elements (AREs) residing in the 3′-untranslated region of TNF mRNA are important in controlling its stability and translational activation. The loss of these AREs increases TNF mRNA stability and results in TNF overexpression [110]. While LPS signaling through TLR4 and CD14 induces the phosphorylation of p38 and MAPK-activated protein kinase 2 and stabilizes TNF mRNA for further translation in an ARE-dependent manner, IL-10R signaling inhibits p38 activation, most likely via SOCS-3, and therefore destabilizes TNF mRNA and represses its translation [109].

IFNγ may also represent a key regulator of the production of TNF by myeloid cells in the intestine. TNF was one of the earliest genes described to be activated by IFNγ in mouse peritoneal and bone marrow-derived Mϕs [111, 112]. Using the monocyte/Mϕ cell line RAW 264.7, Vila-del Sol et al. demonstrated that TNF expression induced by IFNγ is regulated at the transcriptional level. This transcriptional regulation by IFNγ is the result of the coordinated recruitment of the transcription factors IFN regulatory factor (IRF)1, IRF8, and, possibly, PU.1 to the TNF promoter in a similar way as has been described for other inflammatory cytokines and chemokines induced by IFNγ, such as IL-12, IL-1β, and RANTES [113]. This mechanism could be relevant to IBD, in which monocytes are recruited to a LP environment enriched in IFNγ produced locally by T and NK cells and differentiate into TNF-producing IMs. Corroborating this idea, in a T cell transfer colitis model, while TNF production by T cells

Box 1. Some outstanding questions about the role of TNF signaling in intestinal MP biology	
1.	What are the expression profiles of mTNF, sTNF, TNF-R1 and TNF-R2 in intestinal MP subsets and their precursors under homeostatic conditions?
2.	How are these expression profiles modulated during intestinal inflammation?
3.	What are the selective contributions of TNF-R1- and TNF-R2-mediated signaling and mTNF-mediated reverse signaling to intestinal monocyte-derived Mϕ and IM development, survival and function?
4.	What are the selective contributions of TNF-R1- and TNF-R2-mediated signaling and mTNF-mediated reverse signaling to intestinal cDC subset development, survival and function?
5.	What is the contribution of the TNF-R shedding process to the control of intestinal MPs during IBD?

themselves is not required for the development of intestinal inflammation, these cells appear to be important for amplifying the production of TNF by IMs [90, 114]. The signals delivered by T cells to amplify TNF production remain to be identified but tentatively include IFNγ.

More recently, the T-box family transcription factor T-bet has surprisingly emerged as a critical regulator of TNF production by colonic MPs. In the absence of adaptive immunity, the loss of T-bet in conventionally raised T-bet$^{-/-}$ × Rag2$^{-/-}$ mice results in a spontaneous and highly penetrant colitis that shares histologic features with ulcerative colitis in humans. Ulcerative colitis in T-bet$^{-/-}$ × Rag2$^{-/-}$ mice is associated with altered colonic barrier function and dysfunctional IMs, which produce high amounts of TNF [115, 116]. In fact, T-bet binds to the mouse TNF promoter at two T-box consensus sites and directly regulates TNF expression in MPs [115]. Interestingly, both the T-bet-deficient genetic background and the modified microbiota composition engendered by T-bet deficiency are required for disease initiation.

Conclusion and Future Directions

TNF shapes the immune system of the GI tract by regulating DC and Mϕ physiology at multiple levels, such as their differentiation, migration, maturation, survival and effector functions. In addition, recent research suggests that during IBD, TNF may be involved in the reprogramming of monocyte differentiation from a Mϕ lineage towards an IM lineage. These IMs become a major source of TNF and thus drive the chronic inflammatory process.

Many of the insights regarding the role of TNF in MP biology have been generated with cell lines or with DCs or Mϕs generated in vitro from blood or bone marrow precursors. It will thus now be important to validate these findings in vivo in animal models of IBD and in IBD patients. Box 1 recapitulates some of the key questions that need to be addressed in order to gain a further understanding of the contribution of the multiple TNF signaling pathways in distinct MP subsets during IBD. TNF signaling is a complex process involving both mTNF and sTNF that can signal via at least three different pathways: TNF-R1, TNF-R2 and mTNF-mediated reverse signaling. To our knowledge, no data are currently available regarding the expression profiles of TNF-R1, TNF-R2 or mTNF by intestinal Mϕ and cDC subsets. Future studies aiming at addressing the role of TNF in intestinal MP biology should thus first concentrate on defining the actual expression profile of TNF-R1, TNF-R2, and mTNF on different subsets of interest in the intestine under homeostatic conditions and during the development of intestinal inflammation. Most anti-TNF agents are potentially able to interfere with the TNF-R1, TNF-R2 and mTNF-mediated reverse signaling pathways, and the studies investigating the role of TNF in MP biology to date have failed to fully dissect the respective contribution of each individual pathway. Further studies using mice expressing mTNF or mice with a deletion of TNF-Rs in specific subsets of cDCs or in monocyte-derived MPs will greatly help to identify the contribution of each of the TNF signaling pathways to the modulation of intestinal MP subset biology in the steady state and during IBD. With the identification of the various cDC, Mϕ and IM subsets in the mouse and the human intestine, such studies may help in the design of more selective treatments for IBD patients.

References

1 Xavier RJ, Podolsky DK: Unravelling the pathogenesis of inflammatory bowel disease. Nature 2007;448:427–434.

2 Leppkes M, Roulis M, Neurath MF, et al: Pleiotropic functions of TNF-alpha in the regulation of the intestinal epithelial response to inflammation. Int Immunol 2014;26:509–515.

3 Tracey D, Klareskog L, Sasso EH, et al: Tumor necrosis factor antagonist mechanisms of action: a comprehensive review. Pharmacol Ther 2008;117:244–279.

4 Kruglov AA, Kuchmiy A, Grivennikov SI, et al: Physiological functions of tumor necrosis factor and the consequences of its pathologic overexpression or blockade: mouse models. Cytokine Growth Factor Rev 2008;19:231–244.

5 Lugering A, Lebiedz P, Koch S, et al: Apoptosis as a therapeutic tool in IBD? Ann N Y Acad Sci 2006;1072:62–77.

6 Eissner G, Kirchner S, Lindner H, et al: Reverse signaling through transmembrane TNF confers resistance to lipopolysaccharide in human monocytes and macrophages. J Immunol 2000;164:6193–6198.

7 Eissner G, Kolch W, Scheurich P: Ligands working as receptors: reverse signaling by members of the TNF superfamily enhance the plasticity of the immune system. Cytokine Growth Factor Rev 2004;15:353–366.

8 Bain CC, Mowat AM: Macrophages in intestinal homeostasis and inflammation. Immunol Rev 2014;260:102–117.

9 Bekiaris V, Persson EK, Agace WW: Intestinal dendritic cells in the regulation of mucosal immunity. Immunol Rev 2014;260:86–101.

10 Persson EK, Scott CL, Mowat AM, et al: Dendritic cell subsets in the intestinal lamina propria: Ontogeny and function. Eur J Immunol 2013;43:3098–3107.

11 Bain CC, Scott CL, Uronen-Hansson H, et al: Resident and pro-inflammatory macrophages in the colon represent alternative context-dependent fates of the same Ly6C(hi) monocyte precursors. Mucosal Immunol 2012;6:498–510.

12 Bogunovic M, Ginhoux F, Helft J, et al: Origin of the lamina propria dendritic cell network. Immunity 2009;31:513–525.

13 Rivollier A, He J, Kole A, et al: Inflammation switches the differentiation program of Ly6Chi monocytes from antiinflammatory macrophages to inflammatory dendritic cells in the colon. J Exp Med 2012;209:139–155.

14 Varol C, Vallon-Eberhard A, Elinav E, et al: Intestinal lamina propria dendritic cell subsets have different origin and functions. Immunity 2009;31:502–512.

15 Persson EK, Jaensson E, Agace WW: The diverse ontogeny and function of murine small intestinal dendritic cell/macrophage subsets. Immunobiology 2010;215:692–697.

16 Satpathy AT, Kc W, Albring JC, et al: Zbtb46 expression distinguishes classical dendritic cells and their committed progenitors from other immune lineages. J Exp Med 2012;209:1135–1152.

17 Tamoutounour S, Henri S, Lelouard H, et al: CD64 distinguishes macrophages from dendritic cells in the gut and reveals the Th1-inducing role of mesenteric lymph node macrophages during colitis. Eur J Immunol 2012;42:3150–3166.

18 Hume DA, Perry VH, Gordon S: The mononuclear phagocyte system of the mouse defined by immunohistochemical localisation of antigen F4/80: macrophages associated with epithelia. Anat Rec 1984;210:503–512.

19 Gautier EL, Shay T, Miller J, et al: Gene-expression profiles and transcriptional regulatory pathways that underlie the identity and diversity of mouse tissue macrophages. Nat Immunol 2012;13:1118–1128.

20 Rogler G, Hausmann M, Vogl D, et al: Isolation and phenotypic characterization of colonic macrophages. Clin Exp Immunol 1998;112:205–215.

21 Smythies LE, Shen R, Bimczok D, et al: Inflammation anergy in human intestinal macrophages is due to Smad-induced IkappaBalpha expression and NF-kappaB inactivation. J Biol Chem 2010;285:19593–19604.

22 MacDonald KP, Palmer JS, Cronau S, et al: An antibody against the colony-stimulating factor 1 receptor depletes the resident subset of monocytes and tissue- and tumor-associated macrophages but does not inhibit inflammation. Blood 2010;116:3955–3963.

23 Cerovic V, Houston SA, Scott CL, et al: Intestinal CD103(−) dendritic cells migrate in lymph and prime effector T cells. Mucosal Immunol 2013;6:104–113.

24 Schulz O, Jaensson E, Persson EK, et al: Intestinal CD103+, but not CX3CR1+, antigen sampling cells migrate in lymph and serve classical dendritic cell functions. J Exp Med 2009;206:3101–3114.

25 Smith PD, Ochsenbauer-Jambor C, Smythies LE: Intestinal macrophages: unique effector cells of the innate immune system. Immunol Rev 2005;206:149–159.

26 Ma TY, Iwamoto GK, Hoa NT, et al: TNF-alpha-induced increase in intestinal epithelial tight junction permeability requires NF-kappa B activation. Am J Physiol Gastrointest Liver Physiol 2004; 286:G367–G376.
27 Pender SL, Quinn JJ, Sanderson IR, et al: Butyrate upregulates stromelysin-1 production by intestinal mesenchymal cells. Am J Physiol Gastrointest Liver Physiol 2000;279:G918–G924.
28 Muller AJ, Kaiser P, Dittmar KE, et al: Salmonella gut invasion involves TTSS-2-dependent epithelial traversal, basolateral exit, and uptake by epithelium-sampling lamina propria phagocytes. Cell Host Microbe 2012;11:19–32.
29 Nagashima R, Maeda K, Imai Y, et al: Lamina propria macrophages in the human gastrointestinal mucosa: their distribution, immunohistological phenotype, and function. J Histochem Cytochem 1996;44:721–731.
30 Pull SL, Doherty JM, Mills JC, et al: Activated macrophages are an adaptive element of the colonic epithelial progenitor niche necessary for regenerative responses to injury. Proc Natl Acad Sci U S A 2005;102:99–104.
31 Rani R, Smulian AG, Greaves DR, et al: TGF-beta limits IL-33 production and promotes the resolution of colitis through regulation of macrophage function. Eur J Immunol 2011;41:2000–2009.
32 Smythies LE, Sellers M, Clements RH, et al: Human intestinal macrophages display profound inflammatory anergy despite avid phagocytic and bacteriocidal activity. J Clin Invest 2005;115:66–75.
33 Bain CC, Bravo-Blas A, Scott CL, et al: Constant replenishment from circulating monocytes maintains the macrophage pool in the intestine of adult mice. Nat Immunol 2014;15:929–937.
34 Fahlman C, Jacobsen FW, Veiby OP, et al: Tumor necrosis factor-alpha (TNF-alpha) potently enhances in vitro macrophage production from primitive murine hematopoietic progenitor cells in combination with stem cell factor and interleukin-7:novel stimulatory role of p55 TNF receptors. Blood 1994;84: 1528–1533.
35 Witsell AL, Schook LB: Tumor necrosis factor alpha is an autocrine growth regulator during macrophage differentiation. Proc Natl Acad Sci U S A 1992;89: 4754–4758.
36 Caux C, Saeland S, Favre C, et al: Tumor necrosis factor-alpha strongly potentiates interleukin-3 and granulocyte-macrophage colony-stimulating factor-induced proliferation of human CD34+ hematopoietic progenitor cells. Blood 1990;75:2292–2298.
37 Caux C, Dezutter-Dambuyant C, Schmitt D, et al: GM-CSF and TNF-alpha cooperate in the generation of dendritic Langerhans cells. Nature 1992; 360:258–261.
38 Zhang Y, Mukaida N, Wang J, et al: Induction of dendritic cell differentiation by granulocyte-macrophage colony-stimulating factor, stem cell factor, and tumor necrosis factor alpha in vitro from lineage phenotypes-negative c-kit+ murine hematopoietic progenitor cells. Blood 1997;90:4842–4853.
39 Collins T, Read MA, Neish AS, et al: Transcriptional regulation of endothelial cell adhesion molecules: NF-kappa B and cytokine-inducible enhancers. FASEB J 1995;9:899–909.
40 Zigmond E, Varol C, Farache J, et al: Ly6C hi monocytes in the inflamed colon give rise to proinflammatory effector cells and migratory antigen-presenting cells. Immunity 2012;37:1076–1090.
41 Chomarat P, Dantin C, Bennett L, et al: TNF skews monocyte differentiation from macrophages to dendritic cells. J Immunol 2003;171:2262–2269.
42 Ostrand-Rosenberg S, Sinha P: Myeloid-derived suppressor cells: linking inflammation and cancer. J Immunol 2009; 182:4499–4506.
43 Gabrilovich DI, Ostrand-Rosenberg S, Bronte V: Coordinated regulation of myeloid cells by tumours. Nat Rev Immunol 2012;12:253–268.
44 Hu X, Li B, Li X, et al: Transmembrane TNF-alpha promotes suppressive activities of myeloid-derived suppressor cells via TNFR2. J Immunol 2014;192:1320–1331.
45 Vos AC, Wildenberg ME, Arijs I, et al: Regulatory macrophages induced by infliximab are involved in healing in vivo and in vitro. Inflamm Bowel Dis 2012;18:401–408.
46 Turnbull EL, Yrlid U, Jenkins CD, et al: Intestinal dendritic cell subsets: differential effects of systemic TLR4 stimulation on migratory fate and activation in vivo. J Immunol 2005;174:1374–1384.
47 Steinman RM, Hawiger D, Liu K, et al: Dendritic cell function in vivo during the steady state: a role in peripheral tolerance. Ann N Y Acad Sci 2003;987:15–25.
48 Yrlid U, Milling SW, Miller JL, et al: Regulation of intestinal dendritic cell migration and activation by plasmacytoid dendritic cells, TNF-alpha and type 1 IFNs after feeding a TLR7/8 ligand. J Immunol 2006;176:5205–5212.
49 Banchereau J, Steinman RM: Dendritic cells and the control of immunity. Nature 1998;392:245–252.
50 Cella M, Engering A, Pinet V, et al: Inflammatory stimuli induce accumulation of MHC class II complexes on dendritic cells. Nature 1997;388:782–787.
51 Pierre P, Turley SJ, Gatti E, et al: Developmental regulation of MHC class II transport in mouse dendritic cells. Nature 1997;388:787–792.
52 Sallusto F, Cella M, Danieli C, et al: Dendritic cells use macropinocytosis and the mannose receptor to concentrate macromolecules in the major histocompatibility complex class II compartment: downregulation by cytokines and bacterial products. J Exp Med 1995;182:389–400.
53 Baldwin HM, Ito-Ihara T, Isaacs JD, et al: Tumour necrosis factor alpha blockade impairs dendritic cell survival and function in rheumatoid arthritis. Ann Rheum Dis 2010;69:1200–1207.
54 Abe K, Yarovinsky FO, Murakami T, et al: Distinct contributions of TNF and LT cytokines to the development of dendritic cells in vitro and their recruitment in vivo. Blood 2003;101:1477–1483.
55 Ritter U, Meissner A, Ott J, et al: Analysis of the maturation process of dendritic cells deficient for TNF and lymphotoxin-alpha reveals an essential role for TNF. J Leukoc Biol 2003;74:216–222.
56 Winzler C, Rovere P, Rescigno M, et al: Maturation stages of mouse dendritic cells in growth factor-dependent long-term cultures. J Exp Med 1997;185:317–328.

57 Ding X, Yang W, Shi X, et al: TNF receptor 1 mediates dendritic cell maturation and CD8 T cell response through two distinct mechanisms. J Immunol 2011; 187:1184–1191.
58 Sato K, Nagayama H, Tadokoro K, et al: Extracellular signal-regulated kinase, stress-activated protein kinase/c-Jun N-terminal kinase, and p38mapk are involved in IL-10-mediated selective repression of TNF-alpha-induced activation and maturation of human peripheral blood monocyte-derived dendritic cells. J Immunol 1999;162: 3865–3872.
59 Bhattacharyya S, Sen P, Wallet M, et al: Immunoregulation of dendritic cells by IL-10 is mediated through suppression of the PI3K/Akt pathway and of IkappaB kinase activity. Blood 2004;104:1100–1109.
60 Colonna M, Trinchieri G, Liu YJ: Plasmacytoid dendritic cells in immunity. Nat Immunol 2004;5:1219–1226.
61 Geissmann F, Dieu-Nosjean MC, Dezutter C, et al: Accumulation of immature Langerhans cells in human lymph nodes draining chronically inflamed skin. J Exp Med 2002;196:417–430.
62 Keeton R, Allie N, Dambuza I, et al: Soluble TNFRp75 regulates host protective immunity against Mycobacterium tuberculosis. J Clin Invest 2014;124:1537–1551.
63 Gottlieb AB, Chamian F, Masud S, et al: TNF inhibition rapidly down-regulates multiple proinflammatory pathways in psoriasis plaques. J Immunol 2005;175: 2721–2729.
64 Sheikh SZ, Plevy SE: The role of the macrophage in sentinel responses in intestinal immunity. Curr Opin Gastroenterol 2010;26:578–582.
65 Harris J, Keane J: How tumour necrosis factor blockers interfere with tuberculosis immunity. Clin Exp Immunol 2010; 161:1–9.
66 Kirchner S, Holler E, Haffner S, et al: Effect of different tumor necrosis factor (TNF) reactive agents on reverse signaling of membrane integrated TNF in monocytes. Cytokine 2004;28:67–74.
67 Shen C, Assche GV, Colpaert S, et al: Adalimumab induces apoptosis of human monocytes: a comparative study with infliximab and etanercept. Aliment Pharmacol Ther 2005;21:251–258.
68 Friedmann E, Hauben E, Maylandt K, et al: SPPL2a and SPPL2b promote intramembrane proteolysis of TNFalpha in activated dendritic cells to trigger IL-12 production. Nat Cell Biol 2006;8:843–848.
69 Xin L, Wang J, Zhang H, et al: Dual regulation of soluble tumor necrosis factor-alpha induced activation of human monocytic cells via modulating transmembrane TNF-alpha-mediated 'reverse signaling'. Int J Mol Med 2006;18: 885–892.
70 Hedl M, Li J, Cho JH, Abraham C: Chronic stimulation of Nod2 mediates tolerance to bacterial products. Proc Natl Acad Sci U S A 2007;104:19440–19445.
71 Roberts PJ, Riley GP, Morgan K, et al: The physiological expression of inducible nitric oxide synthase (iNOS) in the human colon. J Clin Pathol 2001;54: 293–297.
72 Rugtveit J, Haraldsen G, Hogasen AK, et al: Respiratory burst of intestinal macrophages in inflammatory bowel disease is mainly caused by CD14+L1+ monocyte derived cells. Gut 1995;37:367–373.
73 Chen X, Baumel M, Mannel DN, et al: Interaction of TNF with TNF receptor type 2 promotes expansion and function of mouse CD4+CD25+ T regulatory cells. J Immunol 2007;179:154–161.
74 Valencia X, Stephens G, Goldbach-Mansky R, et al: TNF downmodulates the function of human CD4+CD25hi T-regulatory cells. Blood 2006;108:253–261.
75 Thompson CB: Apoptosis in the pathogenesis and treatment of disease. Science 1995;267:1456–1462.
76 Lombardo E, Alvarez-Barrientos A, Maroto B, et al: TLR4-mediated survival of macrophages is MyD88 dependent and requires TNF-alpha autocrine signalling. J Immunol 2007;178:3731–3739.
77 Pirtskhalaishvili G, Shurin GV, Esche C, et al: TNF-alpha protects dendritic cells from prostate cancer-induced apoptosis. Prostate Cancer Prostatic Dis 2001;4: 221–227.
78 Ludewig B, Graf D, Gelderblom HR, et al: Spontaneous apoptosis of dendritic cells is efficiently inhibited by TRAP (CD40-ligand) and TNF-alpha, but strongly enhanced by interleukin-10. Eur J Immunol 1995;25:1943–1950.
79 Lugering A, Schmidt M, Lugering N, et al: Infliximab induces apoptosis in monocytes from patients with chronic active Crohn's disease by using a caspase-dependent pathway. Gastroenterology 2001;121:1145–1157.
80 Atreya R, Zimmer M, Bartsch B, et al: Antibodies against tumor necrosis factor (TNF) induce T-cell apoptosis in patients with inflammatory bowel diseases via TNF receptor 2 and intestinal CD14(+) macrophages. Gastroenterology 2011;141:2026–2038.
81 Waetzig GH, Rosenstiel P, Arlt A, et al: Soluble tumor necrosis factor (TNF) receptor-1 induces apoptosis via reverse TNF signaling and autocrine transforming growth factor-beta1. FASEB J 2005; 19:91–93.
82 Elson CO, Cong Y, McCracken VJ, et al: Experimental models of inflammatory bowel disease reveal innate, adaptive, and regulatory mechanisms of host dialogue with the microbiota. Immunol Rev 2005;206:260–276.
83 Grimm MC, Pullman WE, Bennett GM, et al: Direct evidence of monocyte recruitment to inflammatory bowel disease mucosa. J Gastroenterol Hepatol 1995;10:387–395.
84 Kamada N, Hisamatsu T, Okamoto S, et al: Unique CD14 intestinal macrophages contribute to the pathogenesis of Crohn disease via IL-23/IFN-gamma axis. J Clin Invest 2008;118:2269–2280.
85 Schenk M, Bouchon A, Seibold F, et al: TREM-1–expressing intestinal macrophages crucially amplify chronic inflammation in experimental colitis and inflammatory bowel diseases. J Clin Invest 2007;117:3097–3106.
86 Platt AM, Bain CC, Bordon Y, et al: An independent subset of TLR expressing CCR2-dependent macrophages promotes colonic inflammation. J Immunol 2010;184:6843–6854.
87 Takada Y, Hisamatsu T, Kamada N, et al: Monocyte chemoattractant protein-1 contributes to gut homeostasis and intestinal inflammation by composition of IL-10-producing regulatory macrophage subset. J Immunol 2010;184:2671–2676.
88 Weber B, Saurer L, Schenk M, et al: CX3CR1 defines functionally distinct intestinal mononuclear phagocyte subsets which maintain their respective functions during homeostatic and inflammatory conditions. Eur J Immunol 2011;41:773–779.
89 Maini RN, Elliott MJ, Brennan FM, et al: Beneficial effects of tumour necrosis factor-alpha (TNF-alpha) blockade in rheumatoid arthritis (RA). Clin Exp Immunol 1995;101:207–212.

90 Mueller C: Tumour necrosis factor in mouse models of chronic intestinal inflammation. Immunology 2002;105: 1–8.
91 Garrett WS, Gallini CA, Yatsunenko T, et al: Enterobacteriaceae act in concert with the gut microbiota to induce spontaneous and maternally transmitted colitis. Cell Host Microbe 2010;8:292–300.
92 Neurath MF, Finotto S, Glimcher LH: The role of Th1/Th2 polarization in mucosal immunity. Nat Med 2002;8:567–573.
93 Nagar M, Jacob-Hirsch J, Vernitsky H, et al: TNF activates a NF-kappaB-regulated cellular program in human CD45RA-regulatory T cells that modulates their suppressive function. J Immunol 2010; 184:3570–3581.
94 Christen U, Von Herrath MG: IP-10 and type 1 diabetes: a question of time and location. Autoimmunity 2004;37:273–282.
95 Yang XD, Tisch R, Singer SM, et al: Effect of tumor necrosis factor alpha on insulin-dependent diabetes mellitus in NOD mice. I. The early development of autoimmunity and the diabetogenic process. J Exp Med 1994;180:995–1004.
96 Ehrenstein MR, Evans JG, Singh A, et al: Compromised function of regulatory T cells in rheumatoid arthritis and reversal by anti-TNFalpha therapy. J Exp Med 2004;200:277–285.
97 Kim EY, Teh HS: TNF type 2 receptor (p75) lowers the threshold of T cell activation. J Immunol 2001;167:6812–6820.
98 Rolhion N, Darfeuille-Michaud A: Adherent-invasive Escherichia coli in inflammatory bowel disease. Inflamm Bowel Dis 2007;13:1277–1283.
99 Mueller T, Podolsky DK: Nucleotide-binding-oligomerization domain proteins and toll-like receptors: sensors of the inflammatory bowel diseases' microbial environment. Curr Opin Gastroenterol 2005;21:419–425.
100 Kuhn R, Lohler J, Rennick D, et al: Interleukin-10-deficient mice develop chronic enterocolitis. Cell 1993;75: 263–274.
101 Takeda K, Clausen BE, Kaisho T, et al: Enhanced Th1 activity and development of chronic enterocolitis in mice devoid of Stat3 in macrophages and neutrophils. Immunity 1999;10:39–49.
102 Hirotani T, Lee PY, Kuwata H, et al: The nuclear IkappaB protein IkappaBNS selectively inhibits lipopolysaccharide-induced IL-6 production in macrophages of the colonic lamina propria. J Immunol 2005;174:3650–3657.
103 Hoshi N, Schenten D, Nish SA, et al: MyD88 signalling in colonic mononuclear phagocytes drives colitis in IL-10-deficient mice. Nat Commun 2012; 3:1120.
104 Ueda Y, Kayama H, Jeon SG, et al: Commensal microbiota induce LPS hyporesponsiveness in colonic macrophages via the production of IL-10. Int Immunol 2010;22:953–962.
105 Glocker EO, Kotlarz D, Boztug K, et al: Inflammatory bowel disease and mutations affecting the interleukin-10 receptor. N Engl J Med 2009;361:2033–2045.
106 Murugan D, Albert MH, Langemeier J, et al: Very early onset inflammatory bowel disease associated with aberrant trafficking of IL-10R1 and cure by T cell replete haploidentical bone marrow transplantation. J Clin Immunol 2014;34:331–339.
107 Zigmond E, Bernshtein B, Friedlander G, et al: Macrophage-restricted interleukin-10 receptor deficiency, but not IL-10 deficiency, causes severe spontaneous colitis. Immunity 2014;40:720–733.
108 Shouval DS, Biswas A, Goettel JA, et al: Interleukin-10 receptor signaling in innate immune cells regulates mucosal immune tolerance and anti-inflammatory macrophage function. Immunity 2014;40:706–719.
109 Kontoyiannis D, Kotlyarov A, Carballo E, et al: Interleukin-10 targets p38 MAPK to modulate ARE-dependent TNF mRNA translation and limit intestinal pathology. EMBO J 2001;20:3760–3770.
110 Kontoyiannis D, Pasparakis M, Pizarro TT, et al: Impaired on/off regulation of TNF biosynthesis in mice lacking TNF AU-rich elements: implications for joint and gut-associated immunopathologies. Immunity 1999;10:387–398.
111 Celada A, Maki RA: IFN-gamma induces the expression of the genes for MHC class II I-A beta and tumor necrosis factor through a protein kinase C-independent pathway. J Immunol 1991;146:114–120.
112 Collart MA, Belin D, Vassalli JD, et al: Gamma interferon enhances macrophage transcription of the tumor necrosis factor/cachectin, interleukin 1, and urokinase genes, which are controlled by short-lived repressors. J Exp Med 1986;164:2113–2118.
113 Vila-del Sol V, Punzon C, Fresno M: IFN-gamma-induced TNF-alpha expression is regulated by interferon regulatory factors 1 and 8 in mouse macrophages. J Immunol 2008;181: 4461–4470.
114 Corazza N, Eichenberger S, Eugster HP, et al: Nonlymphocyte-derived tumor necrosis factor is required for induction of colitis in recombination activating gene (RAG)2(–/–) mice upon transfer of CD4(+)CD45RB(hi) T cells. J Exp Med 1999;190:1479–1492.
115 Garrett WS, Lord GM, Punit S, et al: Communicable ulcerative colitis induced by T-bet deficiency in the innate immune system. Cell 2007;131:33–45.
116 Powell N, Walker AW, Stolarczyk E, et al: The transcription factor T-bet regulates intestinal inflammation mediated by interleukin-7 receptor+ innate lymphoid cells. Immunity 2012;37:674–684.
117 Mowat AM, Agace WW: Regional specialization within the intestinal immune system. Nat Rev Immunol 2014; 14:667–685.

Aymeric Rivollier
Section of Immunology and Vaccinology
National Veterinary Institute, Technical University of Denmark
Frederiksberg (Denmark)
E-Mail ayri@vet.dtu.dk

Rogler G, Herfarth H, Hibi T, Nielsen OH (eds): Anti-Tumor Necrosis Factor Therapy in Inflammatory Bowel Disease.
Front Gastrointest Res. Basel, Karger, 2015, vol 34, pp 27–34 (DOI: 10.1159/000381382)

Physiological Role of TNF in Mucosal Immunology: Regulation of T-Cell Function

Michael Scharl

Division of Gastroenterology and Hepatology, University Hospital Zurich, Zurich, and Zurich Center for Integrative Human Physiology, University of Zurich, Zurich, Switzerland

Abstract

T-cells are the key players in the adaptive immune system. In the healthy individual, the components of the adaptive immune system cooperate with each other as well as with the innate immune system to establish a sufficient immune response. After antigen presentation, T-lymphocytes become activated and differentiate into effector T-cells that finally initiate and control the adaptive immune response. To prevent pathologic immune responses against the body, lymphocytes undergo a strict maturation process in the thymus, and the activation and the proliferation of peripheral lymphocytes remain tightly controlled. TNF, which is a pleiotropic cytokine produced by many cell types upon different stimuli under various physiological and pathological conditions, plays a key role in the maturation, proliferation, differentiation and survival of T-lymphocytes. A large number of studies demonstrated that TNF and its receptors, TNF receptor 1 and 2, control T-lymphocyte biology, and the correct function of the TNF signaling network is critical for proper T-lymphocyte development and function.

Introduction

The adaptive immune system represents a highly specific, specialized, long-lasting and adaptable network of cells and processes that aims to prevent or eliminate infections with pathogens. The adaptive immune response is activated when pathogens generate a certain threshold level of antigens or danger signals that is sufficient to activate dendritic cells (DCs). The most important functions of the adaptive immune system include the recognition and discrimination of self from nonself antigens during antigen presentation, the initiation of processes that eliminate specific pathogens or pathogen-infected cells and the development of an immunological memory, in which each pathogen is recalled by specific signature antibodies or T-cell receptors [1].

The key players in the adaptive immune system are T-cells. In the healthy individual, the components of the adaptive immune system cooperate with each other as well as with the innate immune system to establish a sufficient immune response. After antigen presentation, T-lymphocytes become activated and differentiate into effector T-cells that finally initiate and control the adaptive immune response. To prevent pathologic immune responses against the body, lymphocytes undergo a strict maturation process in the thymus, and the activation and the proliferation of peripheral lymphocytes remain tightly controlled [1].

TNF plays a key role in the maturation, proliferation, differentiation and survival of T-lymphocytes. A large number of studies demonstrated that TNF and its receptors, TNF receptor (TNF-R)1 and TNF-R2, control T-lymphocyte biology, and the correct function of the TNF signaling network is critical for proper T-lymphocyte development and function [2].

Main Points

The Role of TNF in Thymic T-Cell Development

The development of T-cells takes place in the thymus. It has been well documented that the thymic microenvironment directs not only the differentiation but also the positive and negative selection of immature T-cells. Lymphoid progenitor cells originating from the bone marrow migrate to the thymus to complete their antigen-independent maturation into functional T-cells. In the thymus, T-cells finally develop their specific T-cell markers, including T-cell receptor (TCR), cluster of differentiation (CD)3, CD4 or CD8, and CD2 [1].

CD4/CD8 double-positive TCR^{low} cells must successfully undergo thymic education through positive and negative selection before they can leave the thymus. Cells that have successfully rearranged their TCR will die in the thymus cortex if they do not bind to self major histocompatibility complexes (MHCs) within 3–4 days. Positive selection occurs when double-positive T-cells bind to cortical thymic epithelial cells that express MHC class I or II and self peptides at a high enough affinity to generate a survival signal. Positive selection is the process that enables the TCR to recognize peptides that are bound to MHC molecules. Without this, T-cells might be distracted by binding to soluble antigens, the job for which B cells are specialized. At the end of this positive selection, the surviving T-cells are mature T-cells, which are CD3 (TCR) high, single-positive for either CD4 or CD8, and can exit into the periphery. In contrast, negative selection occurs when double-positive T-cells bind to bone marrow-derived antigen presenting cells, namely macrophages or DCs that express MHC class I or II and self peptides, at a high enough affinity to generate an apoptosis signal. Of note, this selection mechanism occurs on self peptides since MHC molecules present self peptides in the absence of pathogens [3, 4].

It has been well documented that TNF is expressed in the developing thymus of mice and humans [5–7]. TNF can also be synthesized in thymocytes of adult mice [8]. In the thymus, TNF mRNA is localized to the subcortical regions of the thymic medulla. This region has been associated with the thymocytic T-cell selection processes [9]. A large number of studies suggest that TNF is critically involved in regulating T-cell lineage commitment and early thymocyte development. On the one hand, the role of TNF might consist of promoting the differentiation and the proliferation of T-cells. For that purpose, membrane-bound TNF seems to be responsible. Further, TNF seems to be involved in the apoptosis of immature thymocytes [9, 10]. Using irradiated non-obese diabetic/severe combined immunodeficient mice, there is also evidence for a role of TNF in augmenting human T-cell lymphopoiesis [11]. These findings suggest that thymic TNF plays an important role in thymocyte production by providing positive as well as negative signals at early stages of T-cell differentiation [12]. Using mouse models, it has been verified that the overproduction of TNF after lipopolysaccharide injection results in apoptosis of double-positive thymocytes, which is completely abrogated when TNF function is inhibited by co-administration of anti-

TNF antibodies [13]. This indicates that TNF has a strong impact on thymocyte homeostasis under stressful conditions.

In contrast, the exact role of TNF in the negative selection of T-cells is less obvious. Some studies using TNF-R-knockout (KO) mice or fetal thymic organ cultures suggested a possible role of TNF in promoting negative selection [14, 15]. However, experiments using class I- and class II-restricted TCR-transgenic (TCR-tg) mice failed to demonstrate a direct role of TNF in mediating thymocyte negative selection [16, 17]. This discrepancy might be because those artificial experimental settings do not completely reflect the physiological negative selection events and processes. Further, the recognized death of double-positive T-cells could be due to molecules, such as cytokines or steroids, that have been induced by activated peripheral T-cells. A further possibility is that a number of co-receptors is cooperatively involved in the negative selection process and that blocking only one of these co-receptors results in insignificant defects [15, 18]. At this point, it must also be mentioned that TNF function in the thymus affects T-cell tolerance via not only the modulation of negative selection but also the regulation of the production of regulatory T-cells (Tregs) [19]. However, at present, the exact mechanisms are still controversial, and there seems to be a striking difference in the effects of TNF depending on whether natural Tregs or inducible Tregs are present [20, 21].

In contrast to thymocytes that are single-positive for either CD4 or CD8, one hallmark of naive T-cells in secondary lymphoid organs is their unique ability to produce TNF rapidly after activation and prior to acquiring other effector functions. It has been demonstrated that the ability of T-cells to produce TNF increases progressively with time in the periphery as a function of their maturation state, indicating that the expression of TNF in naive T-cells is regulated via a gradual regulatory process that requires functional maturation in peripheral lymphoid organs [22].

Physiological Role of TNF in T-Cell Responses

Role of TNF in Regulating T-Cell Proliferation and Activation

The selection and maturation of T-cells represents only the first part of their life. After leaving the thymus, mature T-cells are ready to disseminate into the periphery and to take on their role in the immune system. Studies with human T-lymphocytes provided the first evidence that TNF plays a critical role in not only T-cell maturation and selection but also T-cell differentiation and, finally, T-cell-mediated immune responses. The immunoregulatory activity of TNF has been demonstrated using recombinant human TNF. This molecule was able to amplify T-cell proliferation in response to a variety of stimuli, such as IL-2, anti-CD3, alloantigen or phorbol esters [23–26]. Additionally, recombinant human TNF was implicated in the upregulation of MHC molecules, IFN-γ production, and high-affinity IL-2R and TNF-R2 expression [23, 26–28]. Interestingly, these effects have been well attributed to optimal TNF-induced activation of NF-κB and the NF-κB family member c-Rel [26, 28].

Notably, in studies using human T-cells, the regulation of TCR-mediated T-cell activation was dependent on TNF-R2, highlighting a role of TNF-R2, but not TNF-R1, in delivering co-stimulatory signals that are distinct from CD28 [27]. The role of TNF-R2 as a T-cell co-stimulatory molecule was subsequently confirmed in mouse models using TNF-R2-KO mice. Here, the loss of TNF-R2 resulted in a reduction in the proliferative capacity of CD4 and CD8 T-cells and restricted IFN-γ, TNF and IL-2 expression in response to anti-CD3 crosslinking or antigenic stimulation. This finally lowers the threshold of T-cell activation [29, 30]. TNF-R2 also plays a critical role as a co-stimulator in IL-2 induction and T-cell survival. TNF-R2 signaling modulates AKT activity and NF-κB activation; however, neither of these defects can be rescued by CD28 co-ligation [31]. In addition to those functions, TNF-R2 is important for the survival of T-cells during their proliferative response. This effects seems to be associated with the upregulation of Bcl-xL, Bcl-2 and survivin expression [29, 30].

Further studies revealed an essential role of TNF in modulating the thresholds for CD8 T-cell survival, activation, and tolerance. Using TNF-KO mice that had been crossed with TCR-tg animals, TNF-deficient CD8 T-cells were generated. These cells exhibited an abnormally high TCR signal threshold for T-cell responses. Interestingly, in co-culture experiments, this event was fully restored when TNF from activated wild-type cells was applied [32]. Of note, TNF does not only play an important role as a co-stimulatory ligand in the responses of naive T-cells to antigens. It must be noted that TNF also has a serious impact on T-cell tolerance. The loss of TNF in T-cells causes defective anergy induction and clonal deletion. This could be the result of altered signaling thresholds in response to self antigen recognition. Further, endogenous TNF is critically involved in maintaining the homeostasis of naive CD8 T-cells. Interestingly, rapid production of TNF following TCR engagement of naive CD8 T-cells has been observed [33]. Using TCR-tg TNF-deficient naive CD8 T-cells, it has been demonstrated that naive CD8 T-cells exhibit a survival defect compared to their TNF-deficient counterparts. After transfer to lymphopenic recipients, naive TCR-tg or polyclonal CD8 TNF-deficient T-cells undergo impaired homeostatic expansion. This process finally induces TNF-R2 expression on T-cells [32].

Wiede et al. reported that the age-dependent polyclonal hyperactivation of T-cells is reduced in TNF-negative gld/gld mice. This is in good accordance with the observed role of endogenous TNF in the activation of T-cells. The TNF-negative gld/gld mice exhibited an attenuated course of generalized lymphoproliferative disorder. This observation was associated with a decrease in peripheral T-cell activation and reduced serum IFN-γ levels [34]. TNF also limits the duration of the CD8 T-lymphocyte effector phase and CD8 T-cell memory magnitude, and TNF-TNF-R2 interactions are critical for the optimal initiation of CD8 T-cell function [35, 36]. Additionally, TNF is involved in CD8 cytotoxic T-lymphocyte-mediated lysis [37].

A number of studies also suggest a difference in TNF-related effects on T-cell homeostasis depending on the duration of the respective TNF exposure to T-cells. On the one hand, a relatively brief exposure to TNF seems to exert a co-stimulatory effect on T-cells. In contrast, the effects of prolonged TNF exposure to T-cells appear to be quite different. Chronic exposure to TNF alters T-cell responses by attenuating TCR signaling and impairs the activation of T-cells through the TCR/CD3 complex. This finally results in impaired production of cytokines such as IL-2, IFN-γ, IL-4, IL-10, TNF and LT by T-cells from both humans and TCR-tg mice in response to recombinant TNF. These effects could be reversed by the administration of anti-TNF antibodies to patients with rheumatoid arthritis in vivo [38, 39]. The observed attenuation of T-cell activation in response to chronic TNF exposure was associated with defective Ca^{2+} responses and, at least in part, with reduced surface expression of CD3ζ, attenuated LAT and PLCγ tyrosine phosphorylation, and CD28 downregulation [40, 41]. These findings are of particular importance since they suggest that intact proximal TCR signaling can be disrupted by chronic TNF-R signaling. Of note, the inhibitory effect of chronic TNF exposure on human T-cell activation and TCR signaling in particular seems to be dependent on TNF-R2 but not TNF-R1 [42]. This observation contrasts with the findings in mouse or Jurkat T-cells. Here, TNF-R1 downregulates proximal TCR signaling by activating sphingomyelinase and impairing store-operated Ca^{2+} influx [43].

Role of TNF in T-Cell Survival

Using T lymphoblasts, the cytotoxic effect of the TNF/TNF-R pathway on T-cells was initially demonstrated. Here, TNF caused the apoptosis of human and mouse T-cell blasts in a Fas-independent manner [44]. In line with this finding, TNF induced the apoptosis of lymphocytes, as well as naive and memory CD8 T-cells, in aged humans. This effect resulted from changes in TNF-R expression and in the activation of caspases, finally resulting in enhanced activation-induced T-cell death [45, 46]. In contrast to these observations, in two studies using TNF-KO/TCR-tg mice, the downregulation of the immune response and the peripheral deletion (death) of CD8 T-cells did not require TNF-R-ligand interactions, in particular those involving TNF-R1, after lymphocytic choriomeningitis virus infection [47, 48]. Accordingly, in TCR-tg mice, the in vivo neutralization of TNF appeared to have no impact on CD4 T-cell apoptosis in the absence of a Fas pathway defect [49]. In contrast, the in vivo neutralization of TNF in another TCR-tg mouse model showed that TNF is responsible for controlling the intrahepatic apoptosis of activated T-cells, thereby regulating peripheral T-cell numbers [50].

Interestingly, the cytotoxic effect of TNF on activated T-cells can be mediated by both TNF-R1 and TNF R2 [45]. Using TNF-R1- and TNF-R2-KO mice, the role of both TNF-Rs in mediating T-cell death was directly assessed and further defined. These experiments revealed that TNF mediates the activation-induced death of CD8 T-cells, but not CD4 T-cells, via TNF-R2 signaling. Notably, TNF-R2-deficient CD8 T-cells were resistant to Fas/Fas ligand-induced cell death in these models [51, 52]. However, in vitro experiments with TNF-R2-deficient CD8 T-cells demonstrated that TNF-R2 in fact transmits survival signals during TCR stimulation. This seems likely to be due the upregulation of Bcl-xL and the activation of NF-κB [31]. NF-κB has already been shown to suppress TNF-induced apoptosis and, therefore, to protect from TNF-induced cell death [53]. Using TCR-tg TNF-R2-KO mice, these results were confirmed in vivo. After infection with *Listeria monocytogenes*, these mice exhibited increased CD8 T-cell apoptosis, which was accompanied by reduced expression of Bcl-2 and survivin [29]. In contrast, using TCR-tg/TNF-R1-KO mice, no role of TNF-R1 in the death of activated CD8 T-cells was demonstrated after infecting these animals with lymphocytic choriomeningitis virus [47, 48]. Nevertheless, TNF-R1 and CD95 (Fas) contributed to peptide-induced deletion under certain conditions [48]. A further study revealed that TNF-R1 mediates the deletion of peripheral cytotoxic T-lymphocytes in vivo. Here, using TCR-tg/TNF-R1-KO mice, it was shown that TNF-R1 plays a critical role in the activation-induced death of CD8 T-cells. However, this might only be the case after challenge with low antigen concentrations, as after challenge with high antigen concentrations, the numbers of both TNF-R1-KO and wild-type CD8 T-cells diminished with similar kinetics [54].

In humans, T-cells might be highly susceptible to TNF-induced cell death depending on the respective underlying pathological condition. In particular, only T-cells from HIV-infected patients were sensitive to either TNF-R1- or TNF-R2-mediated apoptosis. However, this observation was not associated with alterations in the expression levels of the TNF-Rs. TNF-R-mediated T-cell apoptosis in HIV patients was associated with progressive disease, while it was clearly reduced in patients who were receiving treatment with antiretroviral agents. Interestingly, T-cells from HIV patients exhibited a lack of protection from apoptotic cell death, which was caused by reduced levels of Bcl-2 but enhanced levels of active caspases 3 and 8 [55]. In addition to apoptosis, HIV-infected CD4 T-cells undergo a nonapoptotic form of necrotic programmed cell death named necroptosis. In this study, altered TNF levels due to HIV-1 infection were shown to play a key role in inducing necroptosis [56].

An interesting observation was made using TNF or TNF-R2 agonistic antibodies. These molecules were able to selectively kill activated CD8 T-lymphocytes in type I diabetes patients. Of great interest was the fact that TNF-R2-mediated apoptosis was only induced in antigen-specific autoreactive CD8 T-cells but not in other activated T-cell subsets [57]. However, a membrane-bound form of TNF presented by exosomes actually delays T-cell activation-induced cell death [58]. These findings demonstrate that the TNF/TNF-R pathways play a critical role in the apoptotic death of T-lymphocytes, particularly CD8 T-cells. However, the role of TNF is mainly important in settings of low antigenic stimulation. In contrast, in the setting of T-cell activation due to high antigen concentrations and/or fully mature DCs, the model becomes much more complex, and the involvement of several additional pathways might be able to compensate for the absence of intact TNF-R pathways [2].

Conclusions and Future Directions

TNF and its receptors play a crucial role in T-cell maturation, proliferation, activation and survival, and the tight control of T-cell biology is essential for sufficient immune responses. It is already evident that subtle alterations in this complex signaling network might result in severe dysfunction of the adaptive immune system. Dysregulated TNF signaling might cause aberrant immune T-cell function and survival, finally resulting in the onset of (chronic) inflammatory diseases. E.g., this can observed in inflammatory bowel disease, in which TNF and aberrant T-cell responses have been well demonstrated to play an essential pathophysiological role. Though a lot is already known about T-cell biology, a deeper and even more detailed understanding of T-cell biology and its connection to TNF and TNF-Rs is needed in order to establish new treatment modalities for TNF- and/or T-cell-associated diseases.

Funding

This research was supported by research grants from the Swiss National Science Foundation to MS (Grant No. 314730–146204 & CRSII3_154488/1) and the Swiss IBD Cohort (Grant No. 3347CO-108792).

References

1 Brownlie RJ, Zamoyska R: T cell receptor signalling networks: branched, diversified and bounded. Nat Rev Immunol 2013;13:257–269.
2 Chatzidakis I, Mamalaki C: T cells as sources and targets of TNF: implications for immunity and autoimmunity. Curr Dir Autoimmun 2010;11:105–118.
3 Alberola-Ila J, Hogquist KA, Swan KA, et al: Positive and negative selection invoke distinct signaling pathways. J Exp Med 1996;184:9–18.
4 Ashton-Rickardt PG, Bandeira A, Delaney JR, et al: Evidence for a differential avidity model of T cell selection in the thymus. Cell 1994;76:651–663.
5 Ohsawa T, Natori S: Expression of tumor necrosis factor at a specific developmental stage of mouse embryos. Dev Biol 1989;135:459–461.
6 Deman J, Martin MT, Delvenne P, et al: Analysis by in situ hybridization of cells expressing mRNA for tumor-necrosis factor in the developing thymus of mice. Dev Immunol 1992;2:103–109.
7 Krangel MS, Yssel H, Brocklehurst C, et al: A distinct wave of human T cell receptor gamma/delta lymphocytes in the early fetal thymus: evidence for controlled gene rearrangement and cytokine production. J Exp Med 1990;172:847–859.
8 Giroir BP, Brown T, Beutler B: Constitutive synthesis of tumor necrosis factor in the thymus. Proc Natl Acad Sci U S A 1992;89:4864–4868.
9 Baseta JG, Stutman O: TNF regulates thymocyte production by apoptosis and proliferation of the triple negative (CD3-CD4-CD8-) subset. J Immunol 2000;165:5621–5630.
10 Zuniga-Pflucker JC, Jiang D, Lenardo MJ: Requirement for TNF-alpha and IL-1 alpha in fetal thymocyte commitment and differentiation. Science 1995;268:1906–1909.
11 Samira S, Ferrand C, Peled A, et al: Tumor necrosis factor promotes human T-cell development in nonobese diabetic/severe combined immunodeficient mice. Stem Cells 2004;22:1085–1100.
12 Croft M: The TNF family in T cell differentiation and function–unanswered questions and future directions. Semin Immunol 2014;26:183–190.
13 Kato Y, Morikawa A, Sugiyama T, et al: Role of tumor necrosis factor-alpha and glucocorticoid on lipopolysaccharide (LPS)-induced apoptosis of thymocytes. FEMS Immunol Med Microbiol 1995;12:195–204.

14 Page DM, Roberts EM, Peschon JJ, et al: TNF receptor-deficient mice reveal striking differences between several models of thymocyte negative selection. J Immunol 1998;160:120–133.
15 Page DM: Cutting edge: thymic selection and autoreactivity are regulated by multiple coreceptors involved in T cell activation. J Immunol 1999;163:3577–3581.
16 Jondal M, Okret S, McConkey D: Killing of immature CD4+ CD8+ thymocytes in vivo by anti-CD3 or 5′-(N-ethyl)-carboxamide adenosine is blocked by glucocorticoid receptor antagonist RU-486. Eur J Immunol 1993;23:1246–1250.
17 Martin S, Bevan MJ: Antigen-specific and nonspecific deletion of immature cortical thymocytes caused by antigen injection. Eur J Immunol 1997;27:2726–2736.
18 Kishimoto H, Sprent J: Several different cell surface molecules control negative selection of medullary thymocytes. J Exp Med 1999;190:65–73.
19 Wu AJ, Hua H, Munson SH, et al: Tumor necrosis factor-alpha regulation of CD4+CD25+ T cell levels in NOD mice. Proc Natl Acad Sci U S A 2002;99: 12287–12292.
20 Housley WJ, Adams CO, Nichols FC, et al: Natural but not inducible regulatory T cells require TNF-alpha signaling for in vivo function. J Immunol 2011;186: 6779–6787.
21 Bilate AM, Lafaille JJ: Can TNF-alpha boost regulatory T cells? J Clin Invest 2010;120:4190–4192.
22 Priyadharshini B, Welsh RM, Greiner DL, et al: Maturation-dependent licensing of naive T cells for rapid TNF production. PLoS One 2010;5:e15038.
23 Scheurich P, Thoma B, Ucer U, et al: Immunoregulatory activity of recombinant human tumor necrosis factor (TNF)-alpha: induction of TNF receptors on human T cells and TNF-alpha-mediated enhancement of T cell responses. J Immunol 1987;138: 1786–1790.
24 Yokota S, Geppert TD, Lipsky PE: Enhancement of antigen- and mitogen-induced human T lymphocyte proliferation by tumor necrosis factor-alpha. J Immunol 1988;140:531–536.
25 Shalaby MR, Espevik T, Rice GC, et al: The involvement of human tumor necrosis factors-alpha and -beta in the mixed lymphocyte reaction. J Immunol 1988;141:499–503.
26 Pimentel-Muinos FX, Munoz-Fernandez MA, Fresno M: Control of T lymphocyte activation and IL-2 receptor expression by endogenously secreted lymphokines. J Immunol 1994;152:5714–5722.
27 Aspalter RM, Eibl MM, Wolf HM: Regulation of TCR-mediated T cell activation by TNF-RII. J Leukoc Biol 2003;74:572–582.
28 Banerjee D, Liou HC, Sen R: c-Rel-dependent priming of naive T cells by inflammatory cytokines. Immunity 2005; 23:445–458.
29 Kim EY, Priatel JJ, Teh SJ, et al: TNF receptor type 2 (p75) functions as a costimulator for antigen-driven T cell responses in vivo. J Immunol 2006;176: 1026–1035.
30 Kim EY, Teh HS: TNF type 2 receptor (p75) lowers the threshold of T cell activation. J Immunol 2001;167:6812–6820.
31 Kim EY, Teh HS: Critical role of TNF receptor type-2 (p75) as a costimulator for IL-2 induction and T cell survival: a functional link to CD28. J Immunol 2004;173:4500–4509.
32 Chatzidakis I, Fousteri G, Tsoukatou D, et al: An essential role for TNF in modulating thresholds for survival, activation, and tolerance of CD8+ T cells. J Immunol 2007;178:6735–6745.
33 Brehm MA, Daniels KA, Welsh RM: Rapid production of TNF-alpha following TCR engagement of naive CD8 T cells. J Immunol 2005;175:5043–5049.
34 Wiede F, Roomberg A, Cretney E, et al: Age-dependent, polyclonal hyperactivation of T cells is reduced in TNF-negative gld/gld mice. J Leukoc Biol 2009;85: 108–116.
35 Singh A, Suresh M: A role for TNF in limiting the duration of CTL effector phase and magnitude of CD8 T cell memory. J Leukoc Biol 2007;82:1201–1211.
36 Kafrouni MI, Brown GR, Thiele DL: The role of TNF-TNFR2 interactions in generation of CTL responses and clearance of hepatic adenovirus infection. J Leukoc Biol 2003;74:564–571.
37 Ratner A, Clark WR: Role of TNF-alpha in CD8+ cytotoxic T lymphocyte-mediated lysis. J Immunol 1993;150:4303–4314.
38 Cope AP, Liblau RS, Yang XD, et al: Chronic tumor necrosis factor alters T cell responses by attenuating T cell receptor signaling. J Exp Med 1997;185: 1573–1584.
39 Cope AP, Londei M, Chu NR, et al: Chronic exposure to tumor necrosis factor (TNF) in vitro impairs the activation of T cells through the T cell receptor/CD3 complex; reversal in vivo by anti-TNF antibodies in patients with rheumatoid arthritis. J Clin Invest 1994; 94:749–760.
40 Isomaki P, Panesar M, Annenkov A, et al: Prolonged exposure of T cells to TNF down-regulates TCR zeta and expression of the TCR/CD3 complex at the cell surface. J Immunol 2001;166:5495–5507.
41 Bryl E, Vallejo AN, Weyand CM, et al: Down-regulation of CD28 expression by TNF-alpha. J Immunol 2001;167:3231–3238.
42 Aspalter RM, Wolf HM, Eibl MM: Chronic TNF-alpha exposure impairs TCR-signaling via TNF-RII but not TNF-RI. Cell Immunol 2005;237:55–67.
43 Church LD, Hessler G, Goodall JE, et al: TNFR1-induced sphingomyelinase activation modulates TCR signaling by impairing store-operated Ca2+ influx. J Leukoc Biol 2005;78:266–278.
44 Sarin A, Conan-Cibotti M, Henkart PA: Cytotoxic effect of TNF and lymphotoxin on T lymphoblasts. J Immunol 1995; 155:3716–3718.
45 Aggarwal S, Gollapudi S, Gupta S: Increased TNF alpha induced apoptosis in lymphocytes from aged humans: changes in TNF-alpha receptor expression and activation of caspases. J Immunol 1999; 162:2154–2161.
46 Gupta S, Gollapudi S: TNF-alpha-induced apoptosis in human naive and memory CD8+ T cells in aged humans. Exp Gerontol 2006;41:69–77.
47 Reich A, Korner H, Sedgwick JD, et al: Immune down-regulation and peripheral deletion of CD8 T cells does not require TNF receptor-ligand interactions nor CD95 (Fas, APO-1). Eur J Immunol 2000;30:678–682.
48 Nguyen LT, McKall-Faienza K, Zakarian A, et al: TNF receptor 1 (TNFR1) and CD95 are not required for T cell deletion after virus infection but contribute to peptide-induced deletion under limited conditions. Eur J Immunol 2000;30: 683–688.
49 Sytwu HK, Liblau RS, McDevitt HO: The roles of Fas/APO-1 (CD95) and TNF in antigen-induced programmed cell death in T cell receptor transgenic mice. Immunity 1996;5:17–30.

50 Murray DA, Crispe IN: TNF-alpha controls intrahepatic T cell apoptosis and peripheral T cell numbers. J Immunol 2004;173:2402–2409.
51 Zheng L, Fisher G, Miller RE, et al: Induction of apoptosis in mature T cells by tumour necrosis factor. Nature 1995; 377:348–351.
52 Teh HS, Seebaran A, Teh SJ: TNF receptor 2-deficient CD8 T cells are resistant to Fas/Fas ligand-induced cell death. J Immunol 2000;165:4814–4821.
53 Van Antwerp DJ, Martin SJ, Kafri T, et al: Suppression of TNF-alpha-induced apoptosis by NF-kappaB. Science 1996; 274:787–789.
54 Speiser DE, Sebzda E, Ohteki T, et al: Tumor necrosis factor receptor p55 mediates deletion of peripheral cytotoxic T lymphocytes in vivo. Eur J Immunol 1996;26:3055–3060.
55 de Oliveira Pinto LM, Garcia S, Lecoeur H, et al: Increased sensitivity of T lymphocytes to tumor necrosis factor receptor 1 (TNFR1)- and TNFR2-mediated apoptosis in HIV infection: relation to expression of Bcl-2 and active caspase-8 and caspase-3. Blood 2002;99:1666–1675.
56 Pan T, Wu S, He X, et al: Necroptosis takes place in human immunodeficiency virus type-1 (HIV-1)-infected CD4+ T lymphocytes. PLoS One 2014;9:e93944.
57 Ban L, Zhang J, Wang L, et al: Selective death of autoreactive T cells in human diabetes by TNF or TNF receptor 2 agonism. Proc Natl Acad Sci U S A 2008; 105:13644–13649.
58 Zhang HG, Liu C, Su K, et al: A membrane form of TNF-alpha presented by exosomes delays T cell activation-induced cell death. J Immunol 2006;176: 7385–7393.

PD Dr. Med. Michael Scharl
Division of Gastroenterology and Hepatology, University Hospital Zurich
Rämistrasse 100
CH–8091 Zurich (Switzerland)
E-Mail michael.scharl@usz.ch

Rogler G, Herfarth H, Hibi T, Nielsen OH (eds): Anti-Tumor Necrosis Factor Therapy in Inflammatory Bowel Disease.
Front Gastrointest Res. Basel, Karger, 2015, vol 34, pp 35–48 (DOI: 10.1159/000381386)

Pathophysiological Role of TNF in Inflammatory Bowel Disease: TNF and Its Impact on Barrier Function

Michael Schumann · Aline Kühnel

Medizinische Klinik m.S. Gastroenterologie, Rheumatologie und Infektiologie, Campus Benjamin Franklin, Charité – Universitätsmedizin Berlin, Berlin, Germany

Abstract

The mucosal barrier needs to maintain a discrete balance between the absorption of nutrients and antigens to educate the immune system on the one hand and the restriction of massive antigenic or microbial transfer from the luminal intestinal compartment on the other hand. It is a complex system composed of very morphologically disparate components, including (i) the mucus layer, (ii) antimicrobial peptides, (iii) a paracellular epithelial cell barrier, and (iv) a transcellular epithelial cell barrier, which synergize to perform a barrier function. The proinflammatory cytokine TNF-α is involved in the integrity of each of these components. This review focuses on the physiology of these components and sheds light on their relevance to TNF-associated inflammation.

The Intestinal Mucosal Barrier

The intestinal mucosa is versatile. Aside from the assimilation of nutritional components, the mucosa imposes a barrier function, which is defined as a restriction of the free passage of water, ions, and larger solutes including antigenic material [1]. Thereby, it guarantees controlled contact with the intestinal microflora, allowing for distinct contact with bacterial antigens to form immunologic competence. This highly regulated process includes (i) dosing of the barrier-passing antigen and (ii) the processing of antigenic molecules. Various components contribute to the mucosal barrier: the mucus layer and the epithelial barrier, which is separated into the paracellular and transcellular epithelial barriers. Polarity-associated mechanisms that organize the epithelial barrier will be explained thereafter.

The Mucus

Aside from water, components of the mucus include ions (chloride, bicarbonate, and sodium). Specifically, *bicarbonate* is believed to not only directly protect the mucosa against the acidic pH of luminal content but also support mucus secretion and mucin unfolding [2–4]. Bicarbonate is secreted by intestinal epithelial cells (IECs) either directly via the cystic fibrosis transmembrane regulator or – also in a cystic fibrosis transmembrane regulator-dependent manner – via the anion exchanger solute carrier family-26 (also known as downregulated in adenoma). Interestingly, the latter process appears to be regulated in inflammation [4].

The major protein components of mucus are *mucins,* which are large proteins (*Muc2*: ~5,200 amino acids) that are posttranslationally glycosylated in the Golgi apparatus and which play a pivotal role in mucus generation, as *Muc2* knockout mice do not form a mucus layer [5, 6]. The core of their protein backbone consists of repeats of proline, serine and threonine (so-called PTS sequences), which enable the anchoring of carbohydrates such as N-acetyl-galactosamine to the peptide backbone via the OH-groups on serine and threonine. Secondary to this biochemical structure, a gel-like consistency of the mucus develops, since these glycans bind to large amounts of water.

Elegant research has revealed how *Muc2*, the prevalent mucin in the small and the large intestine, forms regular 6-sided mucin networks via N-terminal homotrimerization and C-terminal homodimerization. On the one hand, these large networks need to be densely packed within goblet cell vesicles and, on the other hand, need to be very rapidly unfolded and expanded within milliseconds when secreted [7]. This is achieved by intramolecular interactions that strongly depend on a high calcium concentration and a pH of 6 in goblet cell vesicles as opposed to the low calcium concentration and the higher pH of the milieu once the mucins are secreted. As mentioned above, the latter conditions are probably guaranteed by bicarbonate. After secretion, *Muc2* networks quickly spread out to form a flat, netlike structure that expands by >1,000-fold in volume and that has the inherent tendency to spontaneously form sheets [8]. Interestingly, only the colon mucus forms laminar mucus sheets in its inner layer, which remains anchored to the epithelial cells, thus preventing its aspiration and precluding the penetration of bacteria [9] (fig. 1). In the healthy colon mucosa, this inner mucus layer is therefore free of bacteria, in contrast to the loosened outer mucus layer, which is a habitat of the commensal flora. How can this difference in biophysical properties between these two layers be explained? Apparently, distinct proteases, like the epithelial cell-anchored metalloprotease meprin-β, cleave *Muc2*, thereby contributing to the loosening of the mucus of the outer layer in the colon, as well as the mucus in the small intestine [10]. Small intestinal mucus is only one-layered and (opposed to the colon inner mucus layer) is easy to aspirate [9]. Since small intestinal mucus is much more permeable to macromolecules as well as bacteria-sized particles, it is assumed that this difference in mucus composition reflects distinct functions of the small intestine (absorption of nutritional components) compared to the colon (barrier to microflora).

The main mucus-secreting cell is the goblet cell. Goblet cells are born in the crypt and follow – as enterocytes – an upward migratory flow, but these cells differentiate secondary to the expression of the transcription factor *Math1* into a secretory cell type rather than an absorptive cell type (such as the enterocyte) [11].

Antimicrobial Peptides

Antimicrobial peptides (AMPs) are a well-preserved component of the innate response within metazoans. Within humans, cathelicidin *LL-37* and defensins have been identified as functionally important. Their main biochemical features include their relatively short peptide sequence (~30 amino acids) and their cationic nature, which, together with their ~50% hydrophobic residues, results in an amphipathic tertiary structure [12]. The sequence homology to the protease inhibitor cathelin, a characteristic double-leucine at the C-terminal end and a length of 37 amino acids of the processed polypeptide gave rise to the name *cathelicidin LL-37.* It is secreted by epithelial cells and is antimicrobially active against a wide variety of Gram-negative and Gram-positive bacteria, as well as fungi and viruses [13]. Exogenous

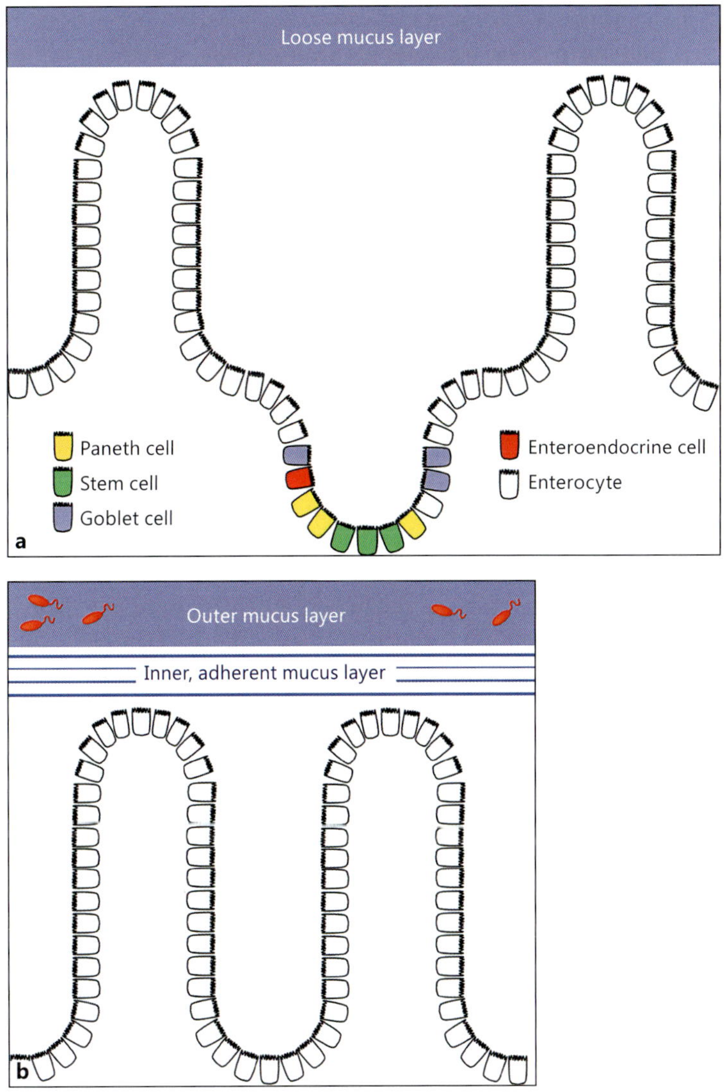

Fig. 1. Mucus layer in the small intestine (**a**) and the colon (**b**). ©1972 Friend and Gilula. Journal of Cell Biology. 53:758–776. doi:10.1083/jcb.53.3.758.

administration of murine cathelicidin to the mouse colon was effective in the treatment of *Clostridium difficile* colitis, confirming antibacterial activity in the gut mucosa [14]. The best studied AMPs are *defensins*, which have been thought to disrupt microbial membranes by forming membrane pores. However, recent work has instead suggested that defensins interact with Lipid II and thereby interrupt bacterial cell wall synthesis [15]. Depending on their intramolecular disulfide bonding pattern, defensins present in the gut are subdivided into α- and β-defensins [16]. Of the six α-defensins identified in Paneth cells so far, human defensin-5 *(HD5)* and human defensin-6 *(HD6)* are of particular importance for the small intestinal immune system. Contrary to α-defensins, β-defensins are primarily expressed in epithelial cells. While human β-defensin *(HBD)-1* is expressed constitutively, the expression of *HBD-2* and *HBD-3* is induced by proinflammatory cytokines or by the presence of microorganisms. Interestingly, the antimicrobial activity of *HBD-1* is strictly dependent on its redox state, as it is highly active only when the intramolecular disulfide bridges are opened, either under reducing conditions or by the epithelial thioredoxin system [17, 18].

Paracellular Epithelial Barrier

Aside from the epithelial cell body, which imposes a barrier by itself that can be lost in the context of epithelial apoptosis, the essential structure of the paracellular barrier is the apical junctional complex. It is localized to the apical half of the lateral membrane of the epithelial cell and is composed of tight junctions (TJs) and adherens junctions (AJs). While AJs (and, to some extent, desmosomes) are considered to maintain a mechanical linkage between adjacent cells, TJs are instead responsible for sealing the intercellular space to a variety of particles, thereby regulating selective paracellular solute transport [19] (fig. 2a).

Adherens Junctions

AJs consist of two functional subunits, which are the 'core adhesive' cadherin/catenin complex and the nectin/afadin interaction [20]. *Cadherins* are type I transmembrane proteins that – through their extracellular N-terminus – form homotypic, Ca^{++}-dependent interactions with identical molecules on adjacent cells (i.e. interaction *'in trans'*). The intracellular C-terminus is protected from proteolysis by its association to *β-catenin* and connects to the actomyosin network supported by α-catenin (thus its name, from the *Latin catena*, chain) and epithelial protein lost in neoplasm, allowing G-actin monomers to polymerize into fibrillar F-actin [21, 22]. Another member of this complex, p120-catenin, further stabilizes the complex by suppressing its immediate endocytosis. *Nectins* are calcium-independent single-transmembrane proteins of the IgG superfamily that possess three extracellular immunoglobulin-like loops for heterophilic rather than homophilic interactions *in trans*. The intracellular domain can interact with the scaffolding protein AF6/afadin, which, in turn, interacts with the actin cytoskeleton and the small GTPase Rap1 [23].

Tight Junctions

A definitive description of TJs was given by the famous researcher Jared Diamond with his beer-can model of epithelia, in which barrel-shaped epithelial cells resemble beer-cans within a six-pack. Here, the space between the cans corresponds to the lateral intercellular spaces, and the plastic of the six-pack corresponds to the TJs, which are designed as hoops that encircle the apical membrane of each cell [24]. These hoops separate the luminal compartment from the basolateral compartment, constituting the *gate function* of TJs, which describes their control of paracellular transport as proven by their ability to stop the diffusion of the 139 Da-molecule lanthanum (as shown by transmission electron microscopy, fig. 2b, c) [25]. However, there is a second, distinct function of TJs, namely, the *fence function,* which relates to their ability to restrict the lateral diffusion of membrane proteins and lipids to either the apical or the basolateral compartment (fig. 2d) [26, 27]. Freeze-fracture electron microscopy revealed TJs to be built up as a meshwork of strands that reveal differing degrees of complexity and strand continuity in a tissue- and inflammation-dependent manner [28]. On the molecular level, TJs are composed of integral membrane proteins and associated proteins. *Integral TJ proteins* include single-transmembrane proteins (JAM-A, CAR) and four-transmembrane proteins, such as those from the claudin family and TAMPs (i.e. occludin and tricellulin) [26] (table 1). The claudin family appears to regulate TJ ion selectivity and thus includes not only proteins that convey a barrier function against solutes (e.g. claudin-1, -4, -5 and -8) but also others that form a pore. This paracellular pore (or, synonymously, channel) is considered to be a high-capacity size- and charge-selective route for ions (Na^+, K^+: claudin-2 and -15;

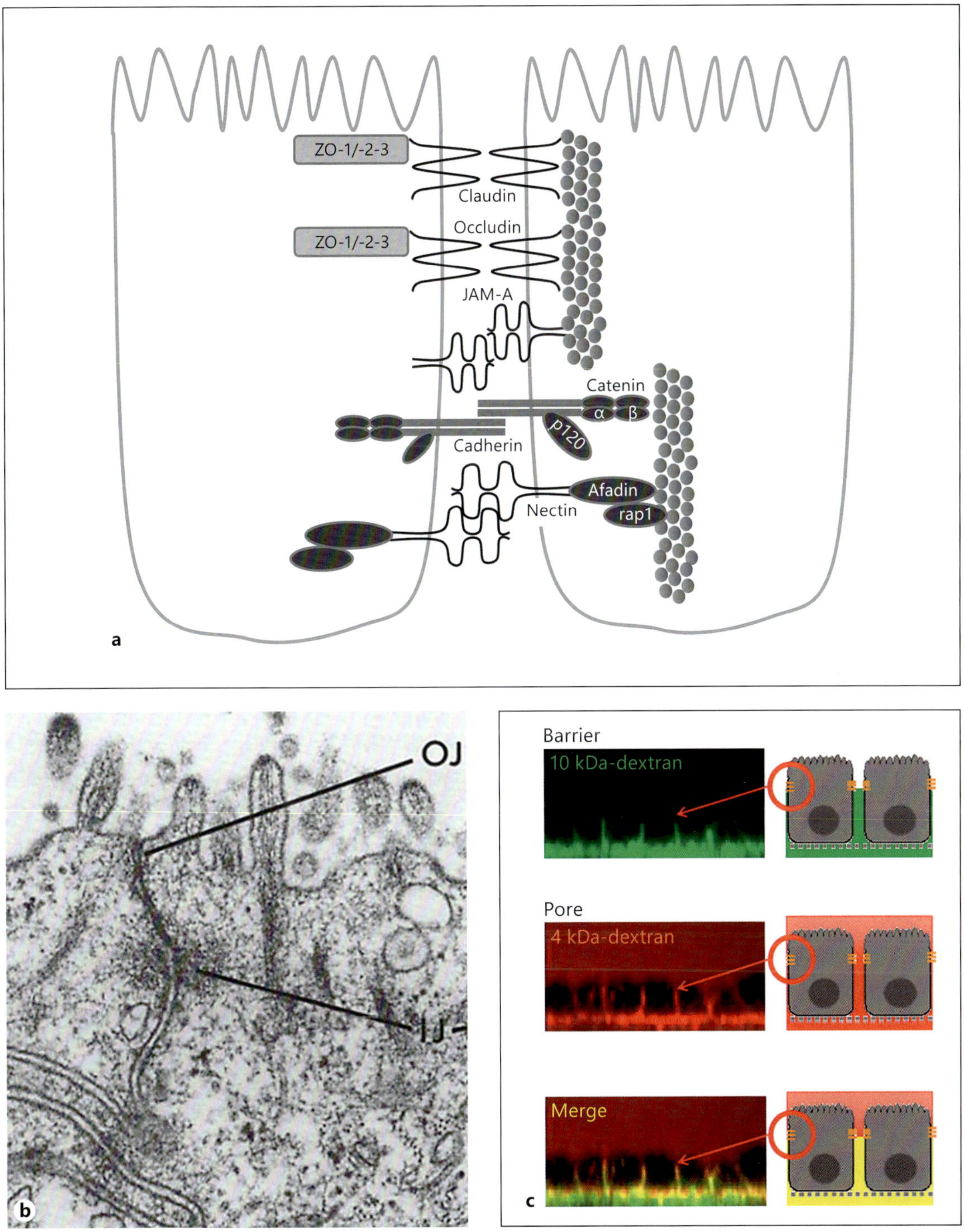

Fig. 2. Apical junctional complex. **a** Protein composition. **b** Tight junction (TJ) on transmission electron microscopy: lanthanum (139 Da) stops at the height of the TJ, which is designated as a 'kissing point'; see arrow. Lu, lumen *(from Friend and Gilula* [107]*, with permission)*. **c** Gate function of TJs *(***c** *and* **d** *from Günzel and Fromm* [26]*, with permission)*.

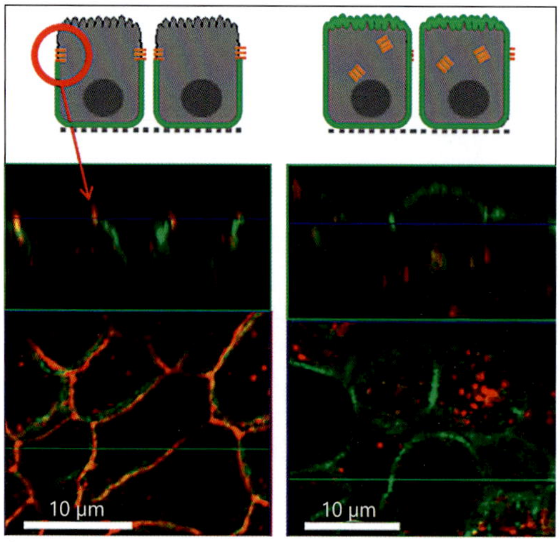

Fig. 2. Apical junctional complex. **d** Fence function of TJs (*c and **d** from Günzel and Fromm* [26], *with permission*).

Table 1. Integral TJ proteins

	Member	TM domains	Function[1]
JAM-A	Junctional adhesion molecule-A	1	B
CAR	Coxsackievirus and adenovirus receptor	1	B
Claudins	*24 members*		
	Claudin-1	4	B
	Claudin-2	4	C^+
	Claudin-4	4	B
	Claudin-5	4	B
	Claudin-8	4	B
	Claudin-15	4	C^+
	Claudin-17	4	A^-
TAMPs[2]	Occludin	4	B
	Tricellulin	4	B
	MarvelD3	4	B

[1] Function of the respective protein: B = barrier-forming; C^+ = cation pore-forming claudin; A^- = anion pore-forming claudin. [2] TAMPs = Tight junction-associated MARVEL proteins.

Cl^-: claudin-17) or water (claudin-2) [29, 30]. The TAMP occludin was the first integral TJ protein to be discovered [31]. It is not an irreplaceable component of the TJ backbone, since the lack of occludin leaves TJs morphologically intact and does not cause any obvious defect in their gate or fence function [32, 33]. On the other hand, roles for occludin in the dynamic reorganization of TJs have been discovered, including the coordination of wound healing, the extrusion of apoptotic IECs from the epithelial layer, the interaction of IECs with intraepithelial lymphocytes and the cytokine-induced reconstruction of TJs [33–36]. The name of another TAMP, tricellulin, refers to its preferred expression in tricellular junctions. Interestingly, tricellulin expression regulates macromolecular permeability rather than the paracellular passage of ions. Thereby, it contributes to another paracellular route of transport, a low-capacity leak pathway that is permeable to larger macromolecules but that is not ion selective and that possibly regulates the passage of small antigens to the lamina propria [1, 37].

Integral TJ proteins interact with one or more of *TJ scaffolding/adapter proteins*, presumably to assign the place where the polymerization of integral TJ proteins should start. Thus, epithelial cells cannot form TJs after zonula occludens (ZO) proteins are knocked down [38]. This interaction primarily depends on the binding of a C-terminal claudin motif to PDZ domains, which are found in most nonintegral TJ-associated proteins (table 2) [26]. Interestingly, ZO adaptor proteins might also fix the TJ localization relative to the AJ, since the SH3 and GUK domains of the ZO-1 protein interact with the AJ-associated factors α-catenin and afadin [38].

Another important, but so far ill-defined, aspect of TJ physiology is their presumed localization within lipid microdomains, so-called rafts, emphasized by a rapid loss of TJ-associated barrier function under cholesterol-reduced conditions [39, 40]. This implicates distinct modes of regulation, e.g. their endocytosis by caveolins.

Table 2. TJ scaffolding/adapter proteins

	Member	PDZ domains
ZO-1 to -3	Zonula occludens protein-1 to -3	3
MAGI-1 to -3	Membrane-associated guanylate kinase, WW and PDZ domain-containing protein 1	6
MUPP-1	Multiple PDZ domain protein	13
Par3	Partition defective-3	3
Par6	Partition defective-6	1
Cingulin	Cingulin	0
PATJ	Pals1-associated TJ protein	10

The *regulation of the barrier properties mediated by TJs* is based on several mechanisms, including (i) transcriptional regulation, (ii) phosphorylation and (iii) endocytosis of TJ components. Transcriptional regulation is pivotal for claudin-2 expression, which is found solely at the crypt level of the colon mucosa under physiological conditions. Analysis of the promoter region and functional studies uncovered that its expression is regulated by several transcription factors, including CDX2, HNF-1α, and GATA-4, on the one hand and the Wnt-activated LEF-1/β-catenin-pathway on the other hand [41, 42]. Similarly, the expression of claudin-4 strongly depends on the transcription factor Grhl2, which is differentially expressed in gastrointestinal epithelia [43] (and own observations).

Studying apical Na^+/glucose co-transport revealed the importance of the myosin light chain kinase (MLCK) pathway as a pivotal regulator of TJ permeability, presumably by the reversible contraction of the apical actomyosin ring [44]. It was subsequently shown that phosphorylation of the myosin light chain increases permeability after various physiological and pathophysiological stimuli [45, 46]. The third mode of TJ regulation, endocytosis of integral TJ proteins, can also be secondary to MLCK activation and has been reported to make use of the caveolin, clathrin and micropinocytotic endocytosis pathways [45, 47, 48].

Transcellular Epithelial Barrier

Ion conductance across the intestinal mucosa as a measure of paracellular ion permeability and the permeation of macromolecules (e.g. inert sugars or polypeptides) are not linearly correlated. More importantly, their degree of correlation is reduced with increasing molecular size of the solute, suggesting that the passage of ions and macromolecules occurs via two distinct pathways [49]. Aside from the paracellular low-capacity leak pathway (see above), the transcellular pathway is pivotal to macromolecular permeability. This process involves a mechanism of apical endocytosis, intracellular trafficking and processing followed by basolateral release [50]. Dependent on the cell type and the stimuli, uptake might involve various endocytosis mechanisms (fig. 3). In celiac disease, duodenal IECs transcytose gliadin fragments from the luminal compartment to the subepithelial compartment, a process involving SIgA-gliadin complexes that specifically bind to the CD71 receptor on IECs and involving the apical endosome [51, 52].

On the other hand, M cells located in the follicle-associated epithelium (FAE) of Peyer's patches are particularly involved in the transcytosis of bacteria [53, 54]. Since the FAE layer produces less mucus, luminal antigens have better access to the transcytotically active cells of the FAE. Interestingly, M cells, which are competent to take up various bacteria, as shown for *Yersinia*,

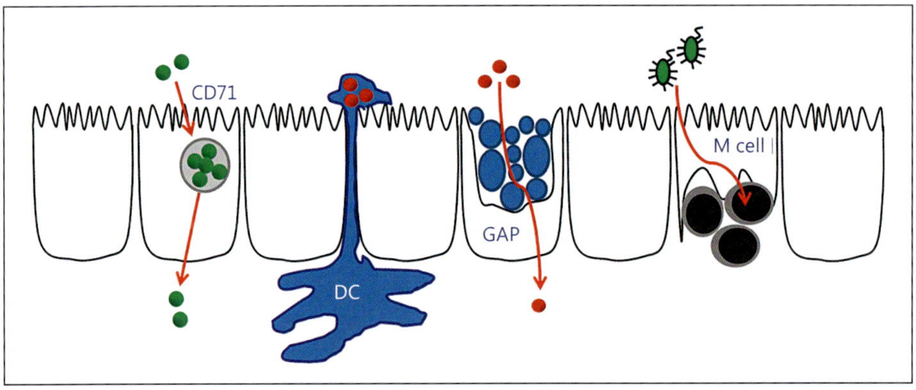

Fig. 3. Mechanisms of transcytotic antigen passage. CD71 = CD71-dependent transcytosis of gliadin; DC = dendritic cell; GAP = goblet cell-associated antigen passage.

Salmonella and *Listeria* species, are situated in the human terminal ileum only centimeters proximal to the colon, the compartment with the highest bacterial load. Other cells that take up luminal antigens include subepithelial CX3CR1^{+} dendritic cells in the villous mucosa and lysozyme^{+} dendritic cells in the FAE, which 'capture' contents using long dendrites that protrude either paracellularly or transcellularly through M cell pores into the intestinal lumen [55, 56]. Recently, goblet cell-associated antigen passage has been implicated as a new transcellular antigen route, implying the uptake of large amounts of antigen by goblet cells [57].

Alterations of the Intestinal Barrier in Inflammatory Bowel Disease and the Function of TNF

In the intestinal mucosa, TNF-α is synthesized by various lamina propria cells, including macrophages and T cells, and by IECs themselves. To generate soluble TNF, membrane-bound TNF is cleaved off by the metalloprotease ADAM17, formerly called TNF α-converting enzyme [58, 59]. TNF targets within the intestinal mucosa include IECs and intestinal myofibroblasts. IECs express both TNF receptors (TNF-Rs), TNF-R1 and TNF-R2. The activation of TNF-R1, which is more extensively studied than TNF-R2, results in the formation of a membrane-bound protein complex that includes TNF-R-associated death domain, receptor-interacting serine/threonine kinase-1 and TNF-R-associated factor 2. TNF-R-associated factor 2 further activates c-Jun N-terminal kinase, thereby increasing its transcriptional activity [60]. On the other hand, receptor-interacting serine/threonine kinase-1 contributes to the activation of the NF-κB pathway. NF-κB is normally retained in the cytoplasm by IκB and translocates to the nucleus to induce the transcription of target genes once the coordinated degradation of IκB is induced by TNF. Third, TNF-R-associated death domain binds to Fas-associated death domain and interacts with caspase-8, thereby inducing IEC death via either apoptosis or necroptosis [61].

The important role of TNF-α in intestinal inflammation was highlighted by TNF^{ARE} mice, which spontaneously and upon lipopolysaccharide stimulation secrete higher levels of TNF-α and which develop spontaneous terminal ileitis resembling Crohn's disease (CD) [62], by the observation of inflammatory bowel disease (IBD)-like pathologies in individuals carrying mutations in genes associated with the TNF-pathway, such as NEMO and ADAM17 [63], and, of course, by the successful introduction of antibodies targeting TNF as a treatment option for IBD [64].

TNF-α in the Regulation of Intestinal Mucus
Evidence for a role of the integrity of the intestinal mucus layer in intestinal inflammation was found in mice lacking Muc2, which spontaneously develop colitis with commensals that directly contact the IEC layer and with profound alterations in the architecture of the colon mucosa [5, 6]. Accordingly, when dextran sodium sulfate is administered to mice *per os* to induce IBD-like colitis, the mucus becomes more penetrable for bacteria, contributing to the pathogenesis of colitis in this model [65]. Increased levels of TNF-α lead to significant alterations of the mucus composition by reducing mucin-producing goblet cells and by increasing the Muc2 mRNA levels, presumably via a MAP kinase-dependent pathway [66–68]. On the other hand, the lack of Muc2 induces the expression of TNF-α [6]. Furthermore, bicarbonate secretion is shown to be reduced by downregulated in adenoma, an important component in mucus secretion [69].

TNF-α and Antimicrobial Peptides
AMPs are differentially expressed in IBD. Paneth cell α-defensins were shown to be decreased in ileal CD – a finding that was connected to mutations in the *NOD2* gene [70, 71]. Furthermore, the Wnt signaling effectors Tcf-1 and Tcf-4 were found to be reduced, resulting in reduced transcription of *HD5* and *HD6* [72, 73]. In contrast, *HD5* and *HD6* were found to be increased in ulcerative colitis, which was explained by the appearance of metaplastic Paneth cells in the inflamed colon [74].

With respect to β-defensins, *HBD1* is constitutively expressed. In contrast, the expression of *HBD2-4* is inducible, e.g. by active colitis (ulcerative colitis rather than CD) or by the probiotic strain *E. coli Nissle* via NF-κB [75–77]. Some reports suggested that this expression is stimulated by T helper 17 cell-related cytokines IL-17 or IL-22 rather than by TNF-α [78, 79]. However, mice lacking functional NF-κB signaling express reduced levels of *HBD3*, suggesting that *HBD3* might be regulated by TNF-α, as well [80].

The complex results in AMP research posed the question of whether AMP regulation is a causative factor for IBD development or is secondary to chronic inflammation. This was tackled by a study that examined the expression of 81 AMP genes before and after anti-TNF treatment, revealing that with the exception of very few genes, including *HD5* and *HBD1,* the majority of AMP genes that were significantly dysregulated in inflammation could be brought back to a normal level by infliximab therapy. These results suggested that the regulation of most AMPs in IBD occurs secondary to inflammation, and this result implicates AMP dysregulation as a reaction of the mucosal immune system to inflammation rather than a primary event [81]. Even if these findings hold true, AMPs might still be interesting for designing specific diagnostics or even as therapeutic targets in IBD.

Epithelial Cell Death Induced by TNF-α
There was some debate regarding whether epithelial cell death imposes a defect in barrier dysfunction or whether neighboring cells can immediately close cell gaps without even transient relevant loss of barrier function [82]. Finally, the existence of transient leaks imposed on an otherwise healthy layer was proven by revealing locally increased electrical conductivity [83]. In line with this finding, barrier defects imposed by inducers of apoptosis were eliminated by apoptosis inhibitors [84]. Interestingly, TNF-α was capable of causing barrier defects via the induction of IEC apoptosis [85], which had implications for the barrier defect found in CD, since this was at least partially based on IEC apoptosis, which was significantly reduced by anti-TNF treatment [86, 87]. The existence of TNF-induced IEC death

was confirmed in vivo and was proven to be signaled via TNF-R1 [80, 88]. Further cell death signaling is complex and involves either the canonical caspase-8 and caspase-3-dependent pathway of extrinsically-activated apoptosis or a more recently discovered RIP3-dependent pathway that leads to necroptosis [61]. Furthermore, once epithelial NF-κB signaling is impaired, TNF-dependent IEC apoptosis rises sharply, leading to severe barrier defects in vivo, along with subsequent bacterial translocation into the mucosa [80]. The latter finding was of particular importance, since an IEC-targeted defect of the NF-κB pathway induced a primary barrier defect sufficient to induce colitis. In accordance with these findings, a co-culture model examining the impact of nonpolarized monocytes or M1-polarized macrophages on IEC barrier function revealed TNF-dependent IEC apoptosis as a major pathway driving the impairment of barrier function [89].

The Apical Junctional Complex and TNF-α

TNF-α synergizes with interferon-γ (IFN-γ) to substantially reduce transepithelial resistance, a measure of epithelial barrier function, which might be secondary to TNF-R regulation by IFN-γ and to synergistic effects on occludin expression [85, 90–92]. This is paralleled by a reduction in the number of TJ strands and by the endocytosis of TJ proteins such as occludin, claudin-1, JAM-A and ZO-1 [93].

Corresponding to these cell culture results, TJ strand discontinuities and complex changes in TJ protein composition, including the downregulation of occludin and claudin-1 and the upregulation of the pore-forming claudin-2, were found in the colon mucosa of CD patients and were normalized when anti-TNF treatment was imposed [86, 87]. Interestingly, profound functional defects in the TJ barrier were also found in other autoimmune intestinal diseases including ulcerative colitis and celiac disease [94, 95]. However, these were rather related to IL-13 and IFN-γ.

As pointed out earlier, the phosphorylation of myosin light chain by MLCK regulates TJ permeability by the reversible contraction of the apical actomyosin ring [44], a process also activated by TNF-α [91, 96]. MLCK activity not only imposes TJ permeability by inducing the endocytosis of TJ proteins but also inhibits apical Na^+/H^+ exchanger-3. This coordinated inhibition of epithelial Na^+/H^+ exchanger-3 and barrier function results in TNF-mediated diarrhea in vivo [97, 98]. Interestingly, increased expression of the barrier-active long form of MLCK was found in patients with IBD secondary to NF-κB regulation [99, 100].

TNF-α and Transcytosis

Since luminal bacterial antigen is a driving force for inducing or maintaining intestinal inflammation in IBD, transcytosis as a route that accomplishes transepithelial transport of macromolecular bacterial components is putatively pivotal. However, published data on this topic are scarce. In general, transcytosis of model antigens such as horseradish peroxidase or β-lactoglobulin is elevated not only in the ileal mucosa of CD patients but also in the jejunum of children with cow′s milk allergy, and anti-TNF has been shown to abrogate the accompanying barrier defect in the allergic jejunum [101, 102]. On the other hand, horseradish peroxidase transcytosis in CD mucosae was not only associated with increased TNF-expression but also induced by TNF-α in a cell culture model of IEC transcytosis. With regard to bacteria, adherent invasive *E. coli* were shown to transcytose FAE in CD via M cells by interacting with their long polar fimbriae [103]. Interestingly, this process depends on the expression of CEACAM6 by ileal IECs upon their strong induction by TNF-α [104]. Last but not least, bacteria that are capable of invading the epithelial layer, such as adherent invasive *E. coli*, survive secondary to a defective autophagy machinery in CD ileal lesions, inducing the secretion of high levels of TNF-α, which further deteriorates the intestinal barrier [105, 106].

Conclusion

It is currently clear that intestinal inflammation goes along with barrier defects involving all of the aforementioned components of the mucosal barrier system. Moreover, most models of IBD pathogenesis assign an important role of the barrier defect in disease development. However, in more specific aspects of barrier function, the *chicken-or-egg* question remains to be answered. The principal results – including the IEC-targeted knockout model of the NF-κB pathway and primary MLCK activation – confirm that barrier dysfunction is a decisive step in chronic intestinal inflammation.

References

1 Shen L, Weber CR, Raleigh DR, et al: Tight junction pore and leak pathways: a dynamic duo. Annu Rev Physiol 2011;73:283–309.
2 Garcia MA, Yang N, Quinton PM: Normal mouse intestinal mucus release requires cystic fibrosis transmembrane regulator-dependent bicarbonate secretion. J Clin Invest 2009;119:2613–2622.
3 Gustafsson JK, Ermund A, Ambort D, et al: Bicarbonate and functional CFTR channel are required for proper mucin secretion and link cystic fibrosis with its mucus phenotype. J Exp Med 2012;209:1263–1272.
4 Seidler UE: Gastrointestinal HCO3- transport and epithelial protection in the gut: new techniques, transport pathways and regulatory pathways. Curr Opin Pharmacol 2013;13:900–908.
5 Johansson ME, Phillipson M, Petersson J, et al: The inner of the two Muc2 mucin-dependent mucus layers in colon is devoid of bacteria. Proc Natl Acad Sci U S A 2008;105: 15064–15069.
6 Van der Sluis M, De Koning BA, De Bruijn AC, et al: Muc2-deficient mice spontaneously develop colitis, indicating that MUC2 is critical for colonic protection. Gastroenterology 2006;131.117–129.
7 Ambort D, Johansson ME, Gustafsson JK, et al: Calcium and pH-dependent packing and release of the gel-forming MUC2 mucin. Proc Natl Acad Sci U S A 2012;109:5645–5650.
8 Ambort D, Johansson ME, Gustafsson JK, et al: Perspectives on mucus properties and formation–lessons from the biochemical world. Cold Spring Harb Perspect Med 2012;2.
9 Johansson ME, Sjovall H, Hansson GC: The gastrointestinal mucus system in health and disease. Nat Rev Gastroenterol Hepatol 2013;10:352–361.
10 Schutte A, Ermund A, Becker-Pauly C, et al: Microbial-induced meprin beta cleavage in MUC2 mucin and a functional CFTR channel are required to release anchored small intestinal mucus. Proc Natl Acad Sci U S A 2014;111:12396–12401.
11 Clevers H, Batlle E: SnapShot: the intestinal crypt. Cell 2013;152:1198–1198.e2.
12 Cederlund A, Gudmundsson GH, Agerberth B: Antimicrobial peptides important in innate immunity. FEBS J 2011;278:3942–3951.
13 Kai-Larsen Y, Agerberth B: The role of the multifunctional peptide LL-37 in host defense. Front Biosci 2008;13: 3760–3767.
14 Hing TC, Ho S, Shih DQ, et al: The antimicrobial peptide cathelicidin modulates Clostridium difficile-associated colitis and toxin A-mediated enteritis in mice. Gut 2013;62:1295–1305.
15 Sass V, Schneider T, Wilmes M, et al: Human beta-defensin 3 inhibits cell wall biosynthesis in Staphylococci. Infect Immun 2010;78:2793–2800.
16 Ostaff MJ, Stange EF, Wehkamp J: Antimicrobial peptides and gut microbiota in homeostasis and pathology. EMBO Mol Med 2013;5:1465–1483.
17 Jaeger SU, Schroeder BO, Meyer-Hoffert U, et al: Cell-mediated reduction of human beta-defensin 1:a major role for mucosal thioredoxin. Mucosal Immunol 2013;6:1179–1190.
18 Schroeder BO, Wu Z, Nuding S, et al: Reduction of disulphide bonds unmasks potent antimicrobial activity of human beta-defensin 1. Nature 2011;469:419–423.
19 Quiros M, Nusrat A: RhoGTPases, actomyosin signaling and regulation of the epithelial Apical Junctional Complex. Semin Cell Dev Biol 2014; 36C:194–203.
20 Niessen CM, Gottardi CJ: Molecular components of the adherens junction. Biochim Biophys Acta 2008; 1778:562–571.
21 Abe K, Takeichi M: EPLIN mediates linkage of the cadherin catenin complex to F-actin and stabilizes the circumferential actin belt. Proc Natl Acad Sci U S A 2008;105:13–19.
22 Vasioukhin V, Bauer C, Yin M, et al: Directed actin polymerization is the driving force for epithelial cell-cell adhesion. Cell 2000;100:209–219.
23 Ogita H, Rikitake Y, Miyoshi J, et al: Cell adhesion molecules nectins and associating proteins: Implications for physiology and pathology. Proc Jpn Acad Ser B Phys Biol Sci 2010;86: 621–629.
24 Diamond JM: Twenty-first Bowditch lecture. The epithelial junction: bridge, gate, and fence. Physiologist 1977;20:10–18.
25 Farquhar MG, Palade GE: Junctional complexes in various epithelia. J Cell Biol 1963;17:375–412.
26 Gunzel D, Fromm M: Claudins and other tight junction proteins. Compr Physiol 2012;2:1819–1852. John Wiley & Sons, Inc. Copyright © 2012 American Physiological Society. All rights reserved.

27 van Meer G, Simons K: The function of tight junctions in maintaining differences in lipid composition between the apical and the basolateral cell surface domains of MDCK cells. EMBO J 1986;5:1455–1464.
28 Schulzke JD, Bentzel CJ, Schulzke I, et al: Epithelial tight junction structure in the jejunum of children with acute and treated celiac sprue. Pediatr Res 1998;43:435–441.
29 Krug SM, Gunzel D, Conrad MP, et al: Claudin-17 forms tight junction channels with distinct anion selectivity. Cell Mol Life Sci 2012;69:2765–2778.
30 Rosenthal R, Milatz S, Krug SM, et al: Claudin-2, a component of the tight junction, forms a paracellular water channel. J Cell Sci 2010;123:1913–1921.
31 Furuse M, Hirase T, Itoh M, et al: Occludin: a novel integral membrane protein localizing at tight junctions. J Cell Biol 1993;123:1777–1788.
32 Saitou M, Furuse M, Sasaki H, et al: Complex phenotype of mice lacking occludin, a component of tight junction strands. Mol Biol Cell 2000;11: 4131–4142.
33 Yu AS, McCarthy KM, Francis SA, et al: Knockdown of occludin expression leads to diverse phenotypic alterations in epithelial cells. Am J Physiol Cell Physiol 2005;288: C1231–C1241.
34 Du D, Xu F, Yu L, et al: The tight junction protein, occludin, regulates the directional migration of epithelial cells. Dev Cell 2010;18:52–63.
35 Edelblum KL, Shen L, Weber CR, et al: Dynamic migration of gammadelta intraepithelial lymphocytes requires occludin. Proc Natl Acad Sci U S A 2012;109:7097–7102.
36 Van Itallie CM, Fanning AS, Holmes J, et al: Occludin is required for cytokine-induced regulation of tight junction barriers. J Cell Sci 2010;123: 2844–2852.
37 Krug SM, Amasheh S, Richter JF, et al: Tricellulin forms a barrier to macromolecules in tricellular tight junctions without affecting ion permeability. Mol Biol Cell 2009;20: 3713–3724.
38 Umeda K, Ikenouchi J, Katahira-Tayama S, et al: ZO-1 and ZO-2 independently determine where claudins are polymerized in tight-junction strand formation. Cell 2006;126:741–754.
39 Lambert D, O'Neill CA, Padfield PJ: Depletion of Caco-2 cell cholesterol disrupts barrier function by altering the detergent solubility and distribution of specific tight-junction proteins. Biochem J 2005;387:553–560.
40 Nusrat A, Parkos CA, Verkade P, et al: Tight junctions are membrane microdomains. J Cell Sci 2000;113: 1771–1781.
41 Escaffit F, Boudreau F, Beaulieu JF: Differential expression of claudin-2 along the human intestine: Implication of GATA-4 in the maintenance of claudin-2 in differentiating cells. J Cell Physiol 2005;203:15–26.
42 Mankertz J, Hillenbrand B, Tavalali S, et al: Functional crosstalk between Wnt signaling and Cdx-related transcriptional activation in the regulation of the claudin-2 promoter activity. Biochem Biophys Res Commun 2004;314:1001–1007.
43 Werth M, Walentin K, Aue A, et al: The transcription factor grainyhead-like 2 regulates the molecular composition of the epithelial apical junctional complex. Development 2010; 137:3835–3845.
44 Turner JR, Rill BK, Carlson SL, et al: Physiological regulation of epithelial tight junctions is associated with myosin light-chain phosphorylation. Am J Physiol 1997;273:C1378–C1385.
45 Marchiando AM, Graham WV, Turner JR: Epithelial barriers in homeostasis and disease. Annu Rev Pathol 2010;5:119–144.
46 Yuhan R, Koutsouris A, Savkovic SD, et al: Enteropathogenic *Escherichia coli*-induced myosin light chain phosphorylation alters intestinal epithelial permeability. Gastroenterology 1997;113:1873–1882.
47 Bruewer M, Utech M, Ivanov AI, et al: Interferon-gamma induces internalization of epithelial tight junction proteins via a macropinocytosis-like process. FASEB J 2005;19:923–933.
48 Ikari A, Takiguchi A, Atomi K, et al: Epidermal growth factor increases clathrin-dependent endocytosis and degradation of claudin-2 protein in MDCK II cells. J Cell Physiol 2011; 226:2448–2456.
49 Madara JL, Dharmsathaphorn K: Occluding junction structure-function relationships in a cultured epithelial monolayer. J Cell Biol 1985;101: 2124–2133.
50 Heyman M, Desjeux JF: Cytokine-induced alteration of the epithelial barrier to food antigens in disease. Ann N Y Acad Sci 2000;915:304–311.
51 Matysiak-Budnik T, Moura IC, Arcos-Fajardo M, et al: Secretory IgA mediates retrotranscytosis of intact gliadin peptides via the transferrin receptor in celiac disease. J Exp Med 2008;205:143–154.
52 Schumann M, Richter JF, Wedell I, et al: Mechanisms of epithelial translocation of the {alpha}2-gliadin-33mer in celiac sprue. Gut 2008;57: 747–754.
53 Keita AV, Gullberg E, Ericson AC, et al: Characterization of antigen and bacterial transport in the follicle-associated epithelium of human ileum. Lab Invest 2006;86:504–516.
54 Keita AV, Salim SY, Jiang T, et al: Increased uptake of non-pathogenic E. coli via the follicle-associated epithelium in longstanding ileal Crohn's disease. J Pathol 2008;215: 135–144.
55 Lelouard H, Henri S, De Bovis B, et al: Pathogenic bacteria and dead cells are internalized by a unique subset of Peyer's patch dendritic cells that express lysozyme. Gastroenterology 2010;138:173–184.e1–e3.
56 Rescigno M, Urbano M, Valzasina B, et al: Dendritic cells express tight junction proteins and penetrate gut epithelial monolayers to sample bacteria. Nat Immunol 2001;2:361–367.
57 McDole JR, Wheeler LW, McDonald KG, et al: Goblet cells deliver luminal antigen to CD103+ dendritic cells in the small intestine. Nature 2012;483: 345–349.
58 Black RA, Rauch CT, Kozlosky CJ, et al: A metalloproteinase disintegrin that releases tumour-necrosis factor-alpha from cells. Nature 1997;385: 729–733.
59 Roulis M, Armaka M, Manoloukos M, et al: Intestinal epithelial cells as producers but not targets of chronic TNF suffice to cause murine Crohn-like pathology. Proc Natl Acad Sci U S A 2011;108:5396–5401.
60 Chen G, Goeddel DV: TNF-R1 signaling: a beautiful pathway. Science 2002;296:1634–1635.

61 Gunther C, Martini E, Wittkopf N, et al: Caspase-8 regulates TNF-alpha-induced epithelial necroptosis and terminal ileitis. Nature 2011;477: 335–339.

62 Kontoyiannis D, Pasparakis M, Pizarro TT, et al: Impaired on/off regulation of TNF biosynthesis in mice lacking TNF AU-rich elements: implications for joint and gut-associated immunopathologies. Immunity 1999;10:387–398.

63 Uhlig HH: Monogenic diseases associated with intestinal inflammation: implications for the understanding of inflammatory bowel disease. Gut 2013;62:1795–1805.

64 Rutgeerts P, Vermeire S, Van Assche G: Biological therapies for inflammatory bowel diseases. Gastroenterology 2009;136:1182–1197.

65 Johansson ME, Gustafsson JK, Sjoberg KE, et al: Bacteria penetrate the inner mucus layer before inflammation in the dextran sulfate colitis model. PloS One 2010;5:e12238.

66 Dharmani P, Leung P, Chadee K: Tumor necrosis factor-alpha and Muc2 mucin play major roles in disease onset and progression in dextran sodium sulphate-induced colitis. PloS One 2011;6:e25058.

67 Iwashita J, Sato Y, Sugaya H, et al: mRNA of MUC2 is stimulated by IL-4, IL-13 or TNF-alpha through a mitogen-activated protein kinase pathway in human colon cancer cells. Immunol Cell Biol 2003;81: 275–282.

68 McElroy SJ, Prince LS, Weitkamp JH, et al: Tumor necrosis factor receptor 1-dependent depletion of mucus in immature small intestine: a potential role in neonatal necrotizing enterocolitis. Am J Physiol Gastrointest Liver Physiol 2011;301:G656–G666.

69 Xiao F, Juric M, Li J, et al: Loss of downregulated in adenoma (DRA) impairs mucosal HCO3(–) secretion in murine ileocolonic inflammation. Inflamm Bowel Dis 2012;18:101–111.

70 Wehkamp J, Harder J, Weichenthal M, et al: NOD2 (CARD15) mutations in Crohn's disease are associated with diminished mucosal alpha-defensin expression. Gut 2004;53: 1658–1664.

71 Wehkamp J, Salzman NH, Porter E, et al: Reduced Paneth cell alpha-defensins in ileal Crohn's disease. Proc Natl Acad Sci U S A 2005;102: 18129–18134.

72 Beisner J, Teltschik Z, Ostaff MJ, et al: TCF-1-mediated Wnt signaling regulates Paneth cell innate immune defense effectors HD-5 and -6: implications for Crohn's disease. Am J Physiol Gastrointest Liver Physiol 2014;307:G487–G498.

73 Wehkamp J, Wang G, Kubler I, et al: The Paneth cell alpha-defensin deficiency of ileal Crohn's disease is linked to Wnt/Tcf-4. J Immunol 2007;179:3109–3118.

74 Noble CL, Abbas AR, Cornelius J, et al: Regional variation in gene expression in the healthy colon is dysregulated in ulcerative colitis. Gut 2008; 57:1398–1405.

75 Fahlgren A, Hammarstrom S, Danielsson A, et al: beta-Defensin-3 and -4 in intestinal epithelial cells display increased mRNA expression in ulcerative colitis. Clin Exp Immunol 2004;137:379–385.

76 Wehkamp J, Harder J, Wehkamp K, et al: NF-kappaB- and AP-1-mediated induction of human beta defensin-2 in intestinal epithelial cells by *Escherichia coli* Nissle 1917: a novel effect of a probiotic bacterium. Infect Immun 2004;72:5750–5758.

77 Wehkamp J, Harder J, Weichenthal M, et al: Inducible and constitutive beta-defensins are differentially expressed in Crohn's disease and ulcerative colitis. Inflamm Bowel Dis 2003;9:215–223.

78 Brand S, Beigel F, Olszak T, et al: IL-22 is increased in active Crohn's disease and promotes proinflammatory gene expression and intestinal epithelial cell migration. Am J Physiol Gastrointest Liver Physiol 2006; 290:G827–G838.

79 Rahman A, Fahlgren A, Sundstedt C, et al: Chronic colitis induces expression of beta-defensins in murine intestinal epithelial cells. Clin Exp Immunol 2011;163:123–130.

80 Nenci A, Becker C, Wullaert A, et al: Epithelial NEMO links innate immunity to chronic intestinal inflammation. Nature 2007;446:557–561.

81 Arijs I, De Hertogh G, Lemaire K, et al: Mucosal gene expression of antimicrobial peptides in inflammatory bowel disease before and after first infliximab treatment. PloS One 2009; 4:e7984.

82 Madara JL: Maintenance of the macromolecular barrier at cell extrusion sites in intestinal epithelium: physiological rearrangement of tight junctions. J Membr Biol 1990;116:177–184.

83 Bojarski C, Weiske J, Schoneberg T, et al: The specific fates of tight junction proteins in apoptotic epithelial cells. J Cell Sci 2004;117: 2097–2107.

84 Gitter AH, Bendfeldt K, Schulzke JD, et al: Leaks in the epithelial barrier caused by spontaneous and TNF-alpha-induced single-cell apoptosis. FASEB J 2000;14:1749–1753.

85 Schmitz H, Fromm M, Bentzel CJ, et al: Tumor necrosis factor-alpha (TNFalpha) regulates the epithelial barrier in the human intestinal cell line HT-29/B6. J Cell Sci 1999;112: 137–146.

86 Zeissig S, Bojarski C, Buergel N, et al: Downregulation of epithelial apoptosis and barrier repair in active Crohn's disease by tumour necrosis factor alpha antibody treatment. Gut 2004;53:1295–1302.

87 Zeissig S, Burgel N, Gunzel D, et al: Changes in expression and distribution of claudin 2, 5 and 8 lead to discontinuous tight junctions and barrier dysfunction in active Crohn's disease. Gut 2007;56:61–72.

88 Piguet PF, Vesin C, Guo J, et al: TNF-induced enterocyte apoptosis in mice is mediated by the TNF receptor 1 and does not require p53. Eur J Immunol 1998;28:3499–3505.

89 Lissner D, Schumann M, Batra A, et al: Monocyte and M1 macrophage-induced barrier defect contributes to chronic intestinal inflammation in IBD. Inflamm Bowel Dis 2015, in press.

90 Mankertz J, Tavalali S, Schmitz H, et al: Expression from the human occludin promoter is affected by tumor necrosis factor alpha and interferon gamma. J Cell Sci 2000;113:2085–2090.

91 Wang F, Graham WV, Wang Y, et al: Interferon-gamma and tumor necrosis factor-alpha synergize to induce intestinal epithelial barrier dysfunction by up-regulating myosin light chain kinase expression. Am J Pathol 2005;166:409–419.

92 Wang F, Schwarz BT, Graham WV, et al: IFN-gamma-induced TNFR2 expression is required for TNF-dependent intestinal epithelial barrier dysfunction. Gastroenterology 2006; 131:1153–1163.

93 Bruewer M, Luegering A, Kucharzik T, et al: Proinflammatory cytokines disrupt epithelial barrier function by apoptosis-independent mechanisms. J Immunol 2003;171: 6164–6172.

94 Heller F, Florian P, Bojarski C, et al: Interleukin-13 is the key effector Th2 cytokine in ulcerative colitis that affects epithelial tight junctions, apoptosis, and cell restitution. Gastroenterology 2005;129:550–564.

95 Schumann M, Gunzel D, Buergel N, et al: Cell polarity-determining proteins Par-3 and PP-1 are involved in epithelial tight junction defects in coeliac disease. Gut 2012;61:220–228.

96 Zolotarevsky Y, Hecht G, Koutsouris A, et al: A membrane-permeant peptide that inhibits MLC kinase restores barrier function in in vitro models of intestinal disease. Gastroenterology 2002;123:163–172.

97 Clayburgh DR, Barrett TA, Tang Y, et al: Epithelial myosin light chain kinase-dependent barrier dysfunction mediates T cell activation-induced diarrhea in vivo. J Clin Invest 2005;115:2702–2715.

98 Clayburgh DR, Musch MW, Leitges M, et al: Coordinated epithelial NHE3 inhibition and barrier dysfunction are required for TNF-mediated diarrhea in vivo. J Clin Invest 2006;116:2682–2694.

99 Blair SA, Kane SV, Clayburgh DR, et al: Epithelial myosin light chain kinase expression and activity are upregulated in inflammatory bowel disease. Lab Invest 2006;86:191–201.

100 Graham WV, Wang F, Clayburgh DR, et al: Tumor necrosis factor-induced long myosin light chain kinase transcription is regulated by differentiation-dependent signaling events. Characterization of the human long myosin light chain kinase promoter. J Biol Chem 2006;281: 26205–26215.

101 Heyman M, Grasset E, Ducroc R, et al: Antigen absorption by the jejunal epithelium of children with cow's milk allergy. Pediatr Res 1988;24:197–202.

102 Soderholm JD, Streutker C, Yang PC, et al: Increased epithelial uptake of protein antigens in the ileum of Crohn's disease mediated by tumour necrosis factor alpha. Gut 2004;53:1817–1824.

103 Chassaing B, Rolhion N, de Vallee A, et al: Crohn disease – associated adherent-invasive *E. coli* bacteria target mouse and human Peyer's patches via long polar fimbriae. J Clin Invest 2011;121:966–975.

104 Barnich N, Carvalho FA, Glasser AL, et al: CEACAM6 acts as a receptor for adherent-invasive E. coli, supporting ileal mucosa colonization in Crohn disease. J Clin Invest 2007;117:1566–1574.

105 Scharl M, Rogler G: Inflammatory bowel disease: dysfunction of autophagy? Dig Dis 2012;30(suppl 3): 12–19.

106 Scharl M, Wojtal KA, Becker HM, et al: Protein tyrosine phosphatase nonreceptor type 2 regulates autophagosome formation in human intestinal cells. Inflamm Bowel Dis 2012;18:1287–1302.

107 Friend DS, Gilula NB: Variations in tight and gap junctions in mammalian tissues. J Cell Biol 1972;53:758–776.

Dr. Michael Schumann
Medizinische Klinik m.S. Gastroenterologie, Rheumatologie und Infektiologie
Campus Benjamin Franklin der Charité – Universitätsmedizin
Berlin Hindenburgdamm 30, DE–12200 Berlin (Germany)
E-Mail michael.schumann@charite.de

Rogler G, Herfarth H, Hibi T, Nielsen OH (eds): Anti-Tumor Necrosis Factor Therapy in Inflammatory Bowel Disease.
Front Gastrointest Res. Basel, Karger, 2015, vol 34, pp 49–55 (DOI: 10.1159/000381409)

Pathophysiological Role of TNF in Inflammatory Bowel Disease: TNF and Its Effect on Innate Immune Defense

Michael Scharl

Division of Gastroenterology and Hepatology, University Hospital Zurich, Zurich, and Zurich Center for Integrative Human Physiology, University of Zurich, Zurich, Switzerland

Abstract

A characteristic feature of active inflammatory bowel disease is the infiltration of innate and adaptive immune cells into the intestinal lamina propria. This complex mixture of a broad variety of cells should ensure that inflammatory responses to invading pathogens are sufficient and tightly controlled. TNF plays a crucial role in the regulation of innate immune responses. By inducing its signaling cascades, TNF activates a number of molecular mechanisms that have been clearly associated with the pathogenesis of chronic intestinal inflammation. TNF orchestrates the secretion of inflammatory mediators and controls the recognition and initial handling of invading bacteria. Of particular importance, TNF may be involved in not only the activation and the function of innate intestinal immune cells, particularly intestinal macrophages, but also the proliferation, survival and differentiation of these macrophages. All in all, though a lot is already known about the role of TNF in regulating innate immune responses, a deeper and even more detailed understanding of these mechanisms is needed in order to provide even better care to outpatients.

Introduction

A characteristic feature of active inflammatory bowel disease (IBD) is the infiltration of innate and adaptive immune cells into the intestinal lamina propria. This complex mixture of a broad variety of cells should ensure that inflammatory responses to invading pathogens are sufficient and tightly controlled. In the healthy intestine, this co-existence of immune cells maintains the balance between immune tolerance to luminal microbiota and the need to defend the body against pathogens and/or the excessive entry of luminal pathogens. However, in IBD patients, this balance is out of control, which finally results in intestinal inflammation [1].

Cytokines that are secreted by immune cells play a critical role in maintaining or disrupting this balance. These cytokines represent key signals in the intestinal immune system. They have been well documented to participate in the disruption of the normal extent of inflammation, which is always occurring, at least to some extent; this inflammation represents so-called physiological inflammation present in the gut [2]. TNF, which is mainly secreted by monocytes and T-cells, has been shown to play a pivotal role in the pathogenesis of IBD. It was first identified in 1975 as an endotoxin-induced serum factor that causes the necrosis of tumors [3]. Since then, TNF has been demonstrated to exert a variety of biological functions that are mainly related to inflammation, cell proliferation, cell differentiation and cancer growth. Consequently, TNF has been associated with a broad range of inflammatory, infectious and malignant conditions. For all these pathologies, the regulation of the innate immune responses by TNF is crucial.

Main Points

TNF Biology and Signaling Pathways

TNF exists in two forms, as a transmembrane protein and as a soluble molecule that is processed by proteolytic cleavage from the transmembrane TNF by the metalloproteinase TNF-converting enzyme (also referred to as ADAM17). With respect to IBD, membrane-bound TNF rather than soluble TNF seems to play a major role in driving intestinal inflammation [2]. This observation is supported by the fact that the neutralization of membrane-bound TNF induces T-cell apoptosis and suppresses experimental colitis in mice but that the activation of TNF receptor (TNF-R)2 (which is only induced by membrane-bound TNF) on T-cells aggravates murine colitis [4, 5].

After binding to its receptors TNF-R1 and TNF-R2, TNF causes a broad range of pro-inflammatory events via receptor-mediated activation of the transcription factor nuclear factor κB (NF-κB). From a functional perspective, TNF-R1 is associated with most of the cellular effects caused by TNF, such as cytotoxicity, cell growth, NF-κB activation and adhesion molecule and cytokine induction). However, in some cell types, TNF-R2 has also been demonstrated to play an important role in cytotoxicity and NF-κB activation, in addition to its effect on lymphocyte proliferation [6].

The TNF-TNF-R interaction results in the induction of intracellular signaling without receptor-complex internalization, causing the phosphorylation of IκBα and the activation of the NF-κB (p50–p65) heterotrimer. NF-κB finally induces the expression of many cytokines, enzymes, and adhesion molecules. The activation of NF-κB-dependent pathways by TNF also contributes to the prolongation of inflammatory processes, which causes further ulceration and degradation of the inflamed intestinal mucosa by the release and activation of matrix metalloproteinases [2]. This fits well with the observation that in lamina propria mononuclear cells from both Crohn's disease (CD) and ulcerative colitis (UC) patients, elevated expression levels of TNF and enhanced nuclear translocation and, consequently, activation of NF-κB have been detected [7, 8].

TNF in the Intestine of Inflammatory Bowel Disease Patients and TNF-Induced Effects

In the intestine of IBD patients, the synthesis of membrane-bound and soluble TNF is clearly enhanced in lamina propria mononuclear cells, particularly $CD14^+$ macrophages, adipocytes, fibroblasts and T-cells [9–11]. In UC patients TNF is mostly located in subepithelial macrophages, whereas in CD intestinal tissue, TNF-positive cells can also be detected in the lamina propria and the submucosa [12]. The transcription of the TNF gene in activated monocytes, macrophages, platelets, adipocytes and T-cells finally results in the secretion of TNF [13]. The soluble and circulating TNF molecules can bind to the two described TNF-Rs, which finally results in the induction of multiple biological effects, including the activation of macrophages, the augmentation of T-cell responses, the expression of leukocyte adhesion molecules, such as E-selectin, intercellular adhesion molecule-1 and vascular cell adhesion molecule-1, the recruitment of neutrophils to sites of inflammation and the formation of granulomas [14]. All of these mechanisms have been demonstrated to play a crucial role in IBD pathogenesis

[15]. TNF also enhances vascular permeability, which promotes the transendothelial passage of fluid and macromolecules, resulting in edema development [16]. TNF has also been demonstrated to be highly inducible in response to cell contact with bacterial lipopolysaccharide (LPS) in humans and mice [17], and recently, LPS-induced TNF factor, a transcription factor that enhances the TNF expression levels in human macrophages, was detected in colonic tissue and macrophages from CD and UC patients [18].

In the end, TNF-induced signaling results in a broad range of pro-inflammatory events that critically contribute to IBD pathogenesis. Among them are enhanced angiogenesis and the activation of endothelial cells by the upregulation of adhesion molecules, the induction of necroptotic Paneth cell death, the production of matrix metalloproteinases by myofibroblasts, which contributes to further tissue damage, and the secretion of cytokines and chemokines from endothelial, epithelial and mucosal mononuclear cells. These latter events result in the TNF-induced upregulation of pro-inflammatory cytokines such as IL-6 and IL-1β, thereby enhancing the early inflammatory response cascade as well as the recruitment of inflammatory cells to the epithelium and the submucosa. Additionally, TNF activates effector T-cells, causes direct damage to intestinal epithelial cells, and impairs intestinal epithelial barrier function via the activation of myosin light chain kinase [2]. Further, TNF-induced TNF-R1 signaling promotes cell death via the activation of receptor-interacting protein kinase 1 and pro-apoptotic caspase-3 [11, 19–21].

Intestinal Macrophages: A Special Innate Immune Cell Population in Inflammatory Bowel Disease Patients

Macrophages are innate immune cells that form the line of first defense and that represent a major defense system against the invasion of the host by microorganisms such as bacteria, viruses, fungi and protozoa. They play a crucial role in tissue homeostasis, adaptive immune response coordination, inflammation and tissue repair, as well as the recognition, phagocytosis, and destruction of invading organisms. Further, macrophages play an essential role in antigen presentation to cells of the adaptive immune system and are responsible for the secretion of a broad range of molecules, such as cytokines, chemokines, complement components and arachidonic acid intermediates [2]. Of note, macrophages not only secrete these molecules but also respond to them in an autocrine and/or paracrine manner, which finally enhances the inflammatory response [6].

Interestingly, in the intestine exists a special population of myeloid immune cells, intestinal macrophages (iMACs) and dendritic cells, that – in contrast to macrophages/dendritic cells in other tissues – display a hyporesponsive, tolerance-inducing phenotype [22]. In particular, iMACs from CD patients exhibit significantly higher expression of the surface molecules CD14, CD16, HLA-DR, CD11b and CD11c. This indicates that these iMACs represent an additional macrophage population in the inflamed mucosa, reflecting either the recruitment of new cells from the blood or a phenotypic change to resident cells [23, 24]. The specialty of these iMACs is that they eliminate intracellular bacteria without provoking an immune reaction [25]. However, in CD patients exists a special macrophage population displaying high expression of T-cell co-stimulatory molecules that are presumably responsible for the perpetuation of the immune response [26]. Interestingly, this special population of iMACs in the inflamed mucosa in CD exhibits enhanced activation of NF-κB [7], which might be, at least in part, due to increased levels of TNF.

TNF and Intestinal Macrophages

Given the importance of TNF for proper function of the intestinal immune system, a large number of studies have clearly addressed the role of TNF in macrophage biology. It has become evident that TNF represents a very powerful pro-inflammatory agent and regulates many aspects of macrophage function [6]. TNF secretion is rapidly induced after infection with pathogens, tissue damage due to trauma or contact with bacterial LPS. This makes TNF one of the most important, most abundant and earliest pro-inflammatory mediators in inflamed or injured tissue [27]. One of its most important functions in the early innate immune response is to orchestrate the initiation and the execution of the pro-inflammatory cytokine signaling cascade. Among its various functions is its pivotal role in orchestrating the production of a pro-inflammatory 'master regulator' of pro-inflammatory cytokine responses [28]. By inducing this cytokine network, TNF is closely associated with the functional properties of iMACs at the functional level. Further, TNF is involved in not only the regulation of cytokine secretion but also the induction of lipid signal transduction mediators such as prostaglandins [29]. These observations suggest that TNF is an absolutely critical molecule for the activation of inflammatory cells and for the recruitment of these cells to sites of inflammation [30].

TNF and Pattern Recognition Receptors

Toll-like receptors (TLRs) represent a certain subtype of pattern recognition receptors (PRRs). PRRs display cellular molecules that act as receptors of the innate immune system for so-called pathogen-associated molecular patterns, which are structural motifs or molecules that are characteristic and highly conserved within a specific class of microbes [31]. Interestingly, TLRs have been demonstrated to induce the secretion of TNF from macrophages. This, in turn, results in the activation of macrophages, in addition to certain co-factors [6]. However, in contrast, exogenously added TNF is only able to activate macrophages after they are primed with interferon (IFN)γ. This is because TNF and IFNγ cross-talk at the level of TNF-R1 to induce macrophage activation. Of note, TNF displays an enhanced ability to induce NF-κB when IFNγ is present. This might be because IFNγ induces the nuclear translocalization of signal transducer and activator of transcription 1α. This event prevents the recruitment of signal transducer and activator of transcription 1α to TNF-R1, which allows for elevated activation of NF-κB in response to TNF [32]. Notably, similar to its effect on TLRs, TNF has also been demonstrated to induce the expression of another PRR that is the most prominent CD risk gene, nucleotide oligomerization domain 2 (NOD2), via NF-κB [33]. NOD2, in turn, has been demonstrated to regulate TNF secretion in immune cells as well as to play a critical role in the intestinal immune response to bacteria [34]. Additionally, in macrophages, TNF is involved in the expression of IL-1β, which, together with IL-18, acts as the main functional effector molecule of two additional PRRs, NACHT, LRR and PYD domains-containing protein (NALP)3 and NALP6. Again, IL-1β is also able to induce TNF expression in human macrophages [35].

These effects of TNF on the regulation of PRR function and expression might display one of the key mechanisms underlying the important role of TNF in IBD pathogenesis. It has been demonstrated that iMACs from CD patients exhibit increased expression of TLR2 and TLR4, which might contribute to their enhanced activity in response to pathogen-associated molecular patterns. The absence of TLRs abolishes the ability of mucosal macrophages to react to bacterial wall products, while the presence of TLRs supports inflammatory processes [36]. Similarly, the dysfunction of NOD2 in iMACs is associated with defective bacterial clearance, prolonged bacterial infection and immune system hyperactivation, which contribute to the enhanced secretion of pro-inflammatory cytokines, e.g. TNF, and a further activation of the immune system [37–39]. NALP3 and NALP6 form multiprotein complexes, so-called inflammasomes, which process pro-IL-1β into its mature form by proteolytic cleavage [40]. Low-level inflammasome activity seems to be essential for wound healing and tissue repair in the intestine

[40], and physiologic NALP3 and NALP6 activity have been demonstrated to be involved in shaping the intestinal microbiota composition [41, 42]. However, uncontrolled inflammasome activity results in even more severe inflammation [40].

TNF, Autophagy and Endoplasmic Reticulum Stress

NOD2 has also been critically linked to the correct function of the autophagosome. Autophagy is a cellular mechanism that is critical for the handling of invading bacteria, the presentation of antigens, and the induction of antigen-specific CD4 T-cell responses. Intestinal innate immune cells from CD patients carrying either the CD-associated ATG16L1 or NOD2 variation exhibit a defect in autophagosome formation, bacterial trafficking and antigen presentation [43, 44]. The presence of the CD-associated ATG16L1 variant has also been demonstrated to cause enhanced inflammasome activation and pro-inflammatory cytokine secretion [45, 46]. Interestingly, some studies have suggested a role of TNF in the induction of autophagy [47, 48], and autophagy seems to play a role in the long-term control of TNF-induced NF-κB activity [49], finally suggesting a feedback loop between TNF activity and autophagy. A further mechanism that has been associated with the development of IBD as well as with autophagy is endoplasmic reticulum (ER) stress. Polymorphisms within ER stress response genes, such as XBP1, have been associated with elevated susceptibility for IBD. Enhanced ER stress can be detected in the intestinal epithelium of IBD patients, and pro-inflammatory conditions and cytokines, including TNF, are able to exacerbate ER stress [50, 51].

Activation, Proliferation, Survival and Differentiation of Macrophages

Upon activation, macrophages not only secrete immunomodulatory molecules but also migrate to sites of inflammation to face and finally destroy invading pathogens. This process is accompanied by the enhanced production of toxic reactive oxygen species, including nitric oxide, and the enhanced expression of inducible nitric oxide synthase [52]. Further, TNF induces the prolonged activation of macrophages via an autocrine loop that is dependent on low and sustained production of IFNβ. IFNβ acts synergistically with canonical TNF to induce the prolonged expression of pro-inflammatory molecules and the delayed expression of genes encoding IFN response molecules. By these molecules, macrophages are finally primed for elevated responses to a subsequent challenge with microbial products or cytokines. It is thought that this feedforward loop plays a critical role in inflammatory response prolongation [53].

Further, autocrine TNF signaling is required for the long-term survival of macrophages [54], and TNF is associated with macrophage differentiation. If TNF is absent from differentiating macrophages, the cells follow a proliferative program instead of a differentiation program. These results suggest that 'autocrine' TNF effects are important in promoting macrophage differentiation [55]. Lastly, TNF mediates the removal of dying neutrophils by macrophages and, therefore, might also play an important in the resolution of inflammation [56].

Conclusions and Future Directions

TNF plays a crucial role in the regulation of innate immune responses. During intestinal inflammation, increased levels of TNF can be detected in the intestinal tissue of IBD patients. By inducing its signaling cascades, TNF activates a number of molecular mechanisms that have been clearly associated with the pathogenesis of chronic intestinal inflammation. TNF orchestrates the secretion of inflammatory mediators and controls the recognition and initial handling of invading bacteria. Of particular importance might be that TNF is involved in not only the activation and the function of innate intestinal immune cells, particularly iMACs, but also the proliferation, survival and differentiation of these macrophages. All in all, though a lot is already known about the role of TNF in regulating innate immune responses, a deeper and even more detailed understanding of these mechanisms is needed in order to provide even better care to outpatients.

Funding

This research was supported by research grants from the Swiss National Science Foundation to MS (Grant No. 314730–146204 & CRSII3_154488/1) and the Swiss IBD Cohort (Grant No. 3347CO-108792).

References

1 Kaser A, Zeissig S, Blumberg RS: Inflammatory bowel disease. Annu Rev Immunol 2010;28:573–621.
2 Neurath MF: Cytokines in inflammatory bowel disease. Nat Rev Immunol 2014; 14:329–342.
3 Carswell EA, Old LJ, Kassel RL, et al: An endotoxin-induced serum factor that causes necrosis of tumors. Proc Natl Acad Sci U S A 1975;72:3666–3670.
4 Holtmann MH, Douni E, Schutz M, et al: Tumor necrosis factor-receptor 2 is upregulated on lamina propria T cells in Crohn's disease and promotes experimental colitis in vivo. Eur J Immunol 2002;32:3142–3151.
5 Perrier C, de Hertogh G, Cremer J, et al: Neutralization of membrane TNF, but not soluble TNF, is crucial for the treatment of experimental colitis. Inflamm Bowel Dis 2013;19:246–253.
6 Parameswaran N, Patial S: Tumor necrosis factor-alpha signaling in macrophages. Crit Rev Eukaryot Gene Expr 2010;20:87–103.
7 Rogler G, Brand K, Vogl D, et al: Nuclear factor kappaB is activated in macrophages and epithelial cells of inflamed intestinal mucosa. Gastroenterology 1998;115:357–369.
8 van Heel DA, Udalova IA, De Silva AP, et al: Inflammatory bowel disease is associated with a TNF polymorphism that affects an interaction between the OCT1 and NF(-kappa)B transcription factors. Hum Mol Genet 2002;11:1281–1289.
9 Strober W, Fuss IJ, Blumberg RS: The immunology of mucosal models of inflammation. Annu Rev Immunol 2002; 20:495–549.
10 Kamada N, Hisamatsu T, Okamoto S, et al: Unique CD14 intestinal macrophages contribute to the pathogenesis of Crohn disease via IL-23/IFN-gamma axis. J Clin Invest 2008;118:2269–2280.
11 Atreya R, Zimmer M, Bartsch B, et al: Antibodies against tumor necrosis factor (TNF) induce T-cell apoptosis in patients with inflammatory bowel diseases via TNF receptor 2 and intestinal CD14(+) macrophages. Gastroenterology 2011;141:2026–2038.
12 Murch SH, Braegger CP, Walker-Smith JA, et al: Location of tumour necrosis factor alpha by immunohistochemistry in chronic inflammatory bowel disease. Gut 1993;34:1705–1709.
13 Podolsky DK: The current future understanding of inflammatory bowel disease. Best Pract Res Clin Gastroenterol 2002; 16:933–943.
14 Sands BE, Kaplan GG: The role of TNFalpha in ulcerative colitis. J Clin Pharmacol 2007;47:930–941.
15 Targan SR, Hanauer SB, van Deventer SJ, et al: A short-term study of chimeric monoclonal antibody cA2 to tumor necrosis factor alpha for Crohn's disease. Crohn's Disease cA2 Study Group. N Engl J Med 1997;337:1029–1035.
16 Bevilacqua MP, Pober JS, Majeau GR, et al: Recombinant tumor necrosis factor induces procoagulant activity in cultured human vascular endothelium: characterization and comparison with the actions of interleukin 1. Proc Natl Acad Sci U S A 1986;83:4533–4537.
17 Mukhopadhyay S, Hoidal JR, Mukherjee TK: Role of TNFalpha in pulmonary pathophysiology. Respir Res 2006;7:125.
18 Stucchi A, Reed K, O'Brien M, et al: A new transcription factor that regulates TNF-alpha gene expression, LITAF, is increased in intestinal tissues from patients with CD and UC. Inflamm Bowel Dis 2006;12:581–587.
19 Su L, Nalle SC, Shen L, et al: TNFR2 activates MLCK-dependent tight junction dysregulation to cause apoptosis-mediated barrier loss and experimental colitis. Gastroenterology 2013;145:407–415.
20 Gunther C, Martini E, Wittkopf N, et al: Caspase-8 regulates TNF-alpha-induced epithelial necroptosis and terminal ileitis. Nature 2011;477:335–339.
21 Meijer MJ, Mieremet-Ooms MA, van Duijn W, et al: Effect of the anti-tumor necrosis factor-alpha antibody infliximab on the ex vivo mucosal matrix metalloproteinase-proteolytic phenotype in inflammatory bowel disease. Inflamm Bowel Dis 2007;13:200–210.
22 Mowat AM: Anatomical basis of tolerance and immunity to intestinal antigens. Nat Rev Immunol 2003;3:331–341.
23 Rogler G, Andus T, Aschenbrenner E, et al: Alterations of the phenotype of colonic macrophages in inflammatory bowel disease. Eur J Gastroenterol Hepatol 1997;9:893–899.
24 Rogler G, Hausmann M, Vogl D, et al: Isolation and phenotypic characterization of colonic macrophages. Clin Exp Immunol 1998;112:205–215.
25 Bilsborough J, Viney JL: Gastrointestinal dendritic cells play a role in immunity, tolerance, and disease. Gastroenterology 2004;127:300–309.
26 Rogler G, Hausmann M, Spottl T, et al: T-cell co-stimulatory molecules are upregulated on intestinal macrophages from inflammatory bowel disease mucosa. Eur J Gastroenterol Hepatol 1999; 11:1105–1111.
27 Feldmann M, Brennan FM, Elliott M, et al: TNF alpha as a therapeutic target in rheumatoid arthritis. Circ Shock 1994; 43:179–184.
28 Maini RN, Elliott MJ, Brennan FM, et al: Beneficial effects of tumour necrosis factor-alpha (TNF-alpha) blockade in rheumatoid arthritis (RA). Clin Exp Immunol 1995;101:207–212.
29 Vassalli P: The pathophysiology of tumor necrosis factors. Annu Rev Immunol 1992;10:411–452.

30 Clark IA: How TNF was recognized as a key mechanism of disease. Cytokine Growth Factor Rev 2007;18:335–343.
31 Ausubel FM: Are innate immune signaling pathways in plants and animals conserved? Nat Immunol 2005;6:973–979.
32 Wesemann DR, Benveniste EN: STAT-1 alpha and IFN-gamma as modulators of TNF-alpha signaling in macrophages: regulation and functional implications of the TNF receptor 1:STAT-1 alpha complex. J Immunol 2003;171:5313–5319.
33 Gutierrez O, Pipaon C, Inohara N, et al: Induction of Nod2 in myelomonocytic and intestinal epithelial cells via nuclear factor-kappa B activation. J Biol Chem 2002;277:41701–41705.
34 Kobayashi KS, Chamaillard M, Ogura Y, et al: Nod2-dependent regulation of innate and adaptive immunity in the intestinal tract. Science 2005;307:731–734.
35 Puren AJ, Fantuzzi G, Gu Y, et al: Interleukin-18 (IFNgamma-inducing factor) induces IL-8 and IL-1beta via TNFalpha production from non-CD14+ human blood mononuclear cells. J Clin Invest 1998;101:711–721.
36 Hausmann M, Kiessling S, Mestermann S, et al: Toll-like receptors 2 and 4 are up-regulated during intestinal inflammation. Gastroenterology 2002;122:1987–2000.
37 Kosovac K, Brenmoehl J, Holler E, et al: Association of the NOD2 genotype with bacterial translocation via altered cell-cell contacts in Crohn's disease patients. Inflamm Bowel Dis 2010;16:1311–1321.
38 Biswas A, Petnicki-Ocwieja T, Kobayashi KS: Nod2: a key regulator linking microbiota to intestinal mucosal immunity. J Mol Med 2012;90:15–24.
39 Kim YG, Kamada N, Shaw MH, et al: The Nod2 sensor promotes intestinal pathogen eradication via the chemokine CCL2-dependent recruitment of inflammatory monocytes. Immunity 2011;34:769–780.
40 Zaki MH, Boyd KL, Vogel P, et al: The NLRP3 inflammasome protects against loss of epithelial integrity and mortality during experimental colitis. Immunity 2010;32:379–391.
41 Elinav E, Strowig T, Kau AL, et al: NLRP6 inflammasome regulates colonic microbial ecology and risk for colitis. Cell 2011;145:745–757.
42 Hirota SA, Ng J, Lueng A, et al: NLRP3 inflammasome plays a key role in the regulation of intestinal homeostasis. Inflamm Bowel Dis 2011;17:1359–1372.
43 Cooney R, Baker J, Brain O, et al: NOD2 stimulation induces autophagy in dendritic cells influencing bacterial handling and antigen presentation. Nat Med 2010;16:90–97.
44 Travassos LH, Carneiro LA, Ramjeet M, et al: Nod1 and Nod2 direct autophagy by recruiting ATG16L1 to the plasma membrane at the site of bacterial entry. Nat Immunol 2010;11:55–62.
45 Saitoh T, Fujita N, Jang MH, et al: Loss of the autophagy protein Atg16L1 enhances endotoxin-induced IL-1beta production. Nature 2008;456:264–268.
46 Plantinga TS, Crisan TO, Oosting M, et al: Crohn's disease-associated ATG16L1 polymorphism modulates pro-inflammatory cytokine responses selectively upon activation of NOD2. Gut 2011;60:1229–1235.
47 Scharl M, Wojtal KA, Becker HM, et al: Protein tyrosine phosphatase nonreceptor type 2 regulates autophagosome formation in human intestinal cells. Inflamm Bowel Dis 2012;18:1287–1302.
48 Yu L, Alva A, Su H, et al: Regulation of an ATG7-beclin 1 program of autophagic cell death by caspase-8. Science 2004;304:1500–1502.
49 Colleran A, Ryan A, O'Gorman A, et al: Autophagosomal IkappaB alpha degradation plays a role in the long term control of tumor necrosis factor-alpha-induced nuclear factor-kappaB (NF-kappaB) activity. J Biol Chem 2011;286:22886–22893.
50 Kaser A, Lee AH, Franke A, et al: XBP1 links ER stress to intestinal inflammation and confers genetic risk for human inflammatory bowel disease. Cell 2008;134:743–756.
51 Adolph TE, Tomczak MF, Niederreiter L, et al: Paneth cells as a site of origin for intestinal inflammation. Nature 2013;503:272–276.
52 Salkowski CA, Detore G, McNally R, et al: Regulation of inducible nitric oxide synthase messenger RNA expression and nitric oxide production by lipopolysaccharide in vivo: the roles of macrophages, endogenous IFN-gamma, and TNF receptor-1-mediated signaling. J Immunol 1997;158:905–912.
53 Yarilina A, Park-Min KH, Antoniv T, et al: TNF activates an IRF1-dependent autocrine loop leading to sustained expression of chemokines and STAT1-dependent type I interferon-response genes. Nat Immunol 2008;9:378–387.
54 Lombardo E, Alvarez-Barrientos A, Maroto B, et al: TLR4-mediated survival of macrophages is MyD88 dependent and requires TNF-alpha autocrine signalling. J Immunol 2007;178:3731–3739.
55 Witsell AL, Schook LB: Tumor necrosis factor alpha is an autocrine growth regulator during macrophage differentiation. Proc Natl Acad Sci U S A 1992;89:4754–4758.
56 Michlewska S, Dransfield I, Megson IL, et al: Macrophage phagocytosis of apoptotic neutrophils is critically regulated by the opposing actions of pro-inflammatory and anti-inflammatory agents: key role for TNF-alpha. FASEB J 2009;23:844–854.

PD Dr. Med. Michael Scharl
Division of Gastroenterology and Hepatology, University Hospital Zurich
Rämistrasse 100
CH–8091 Zurich (Switzerland)
E-Mail michael.scharl@usz.ch

Rogler G, Herfarth H, Hibi T, Nielsen OH (eds): Anti-Tumor Necrosis Factor Therapy in Inflammatory Bowel Disease.
Front Gastrointest Res. Basel, Karger, 2015, vol 34, pp 56–61 (DOI: 10.1159/000381410)

TNF and Its Impact on Adaptive Immune Mechanisms and Chronic Inflammation

Britta Siegmund

Medical Department (Gastroenterology, Infectious Diseases, Rheumatology), Charité – Universitätsmedizin Berlin, Campus Benjamin Franklin, Berlin, Germany

Abstract

Anti-TNFα strategies were introduced into the field of inflammatory bowel disease treatment over a decade ago. Still, the precise mechanism of action is a matter of debate. Here, the focus will be on the role of TNFα in the adaptive immune system and the anti-inflammatory effects resulting from neutralizing TNFα. The mechanisms involved indicate a tight network between the adaptive and the innate immune systems since activation of either arm results in stimulation of the other. In the subpopulation of patients responding to anti-TNFα therapy, this strategy mostly results in a significant improvement in life quality. However, ultimately, we hope to identify the initial event leading to intestinal inflammation, which will hopefully indicate a more specific therapeutic approach that will allow for better life quality for more than just a subpopulation.

Introduction

The introduction of anti-TNFα therapy first for rheumatoid arthritis and later for inflammatory bowel disease challenged established therapeutic options and improved quality of life for a substantial proportion of patients. Still, the mode of action has not been completely deciphered. Besides IL-1, TNFα is one of the central cytokines involved in multiple mechanisms of immune defense as well as maintenance of an inflammatory condition. While monocytes, macrophages and dendritic cells represent the key sources of TNFα production, other cell populations, including B and T cells, have been demonstrated to produce equal amounts of TNFα. In fact, the absence of TNFα in these cellular compartments is accompanied by structural changes in secondary lymphoid organs, as outlined below, thus indicating the fundamental role of TNFα not only as an indispensable molecule for the function of the immune system but also as a crucial mediator between the innate and the adaptive immune systems. In this chapter, the particular role of TNFα with regard to the adaptive immune system will be described. This includes a description of additional modes of action besides apoptosis induction.

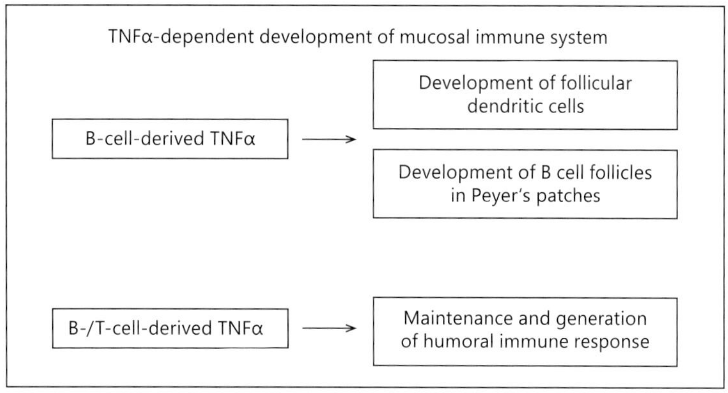

Fig. 1. TNFα-dependent development of the mucosal immune system. B-cell-derived TNFα is indispensable for the development of follicular dendritic cells as well as B cell follicles in the Peyer's patches. B- and T-cell-derived TNFα is crucial for the generation and maintenance of the humoral immune response.

Main Points

Mechanisms Mediating the Anti-Inflammatory Effect of Anti-TNF Therapy

As discussed in other chapters in this book, the induction of apoptosis in T cells [1] as well as in peripheral blood monocytes [2] has been considered as the central mechanism mediating the anti-inflammatory effect observed in inflammatory bowel diseases. In vivo analysis indicated that locally occurring apoptosis correlated with the clinical benefit of anti-TNF therapy [3]. While these studies support the 'apoptosis theory', relevant clinical and basic research data are in conflict with this theory, as outlined below, hence suggesting that apoptosis is not the exclusive mode of action.

Infliximab and adalimumab, both with known clinical efficacy in inflammatory bowel diseases, have been shown to induce apoptosis in multiple in vitro and in vivo assays [4]. However, certolizumab, despite its clinical efficacy in Crohn's disease, does not induce apoptosis [5]. Strikingly, onercept (a soluble p55 TNF receptor) does induce apoptosis but still exerts no clinical efficacy in Crohn's disease [6]. These findings strongly suggest that other mechanisms contribute to the anti-inflammatory effect of anti-TNF therapy.

In the following section, the impact of TNF on the adaptive immune system will be discussed, and a possible yet not completely proven mechanism will be suggested.

Evidence of TNFα Being Significant for the Adaptive Immune System

Structural Considerations

TNFα is not only central for the maintenance of inflammatory conditions but also indispensable for the structural development of the mucosal immune system. Secondary lymphoid organs provide a unique microenvironment for generation of immune responses. By using a cell-type-specific conditional knockout approach, the Nedospasov group dissected the contribution of TNFα produced by either B or T cells. B-cell-derived TNFα controlled the development of follicular dendritic cells and B cell follicles in Peyer's patches. In lymph nodes, cooperation between TNFα expressed by B and TNFα expressed by T cells was required for the generation and maintenance of an efficient humoral immune response. Thus, this work indicates that the maintenance of each type of secondary lymphoid organ is orchestrated by the distinct contributions of membrane-bound and soluble TNFα produced by B and T lymphocytes [7] (fig. 1).

Linking TNFα and the Adaptive Immune System

Initial evidence that TNFα plays a significant role in the adaptive arm of the immune system derives from early work in the transfer model of colitis. In this model, originally described by Fiona Powrie, colitis is induced by transferring naïve T cells into immunodeficient *Scid or Rag2*$^{-/-}$ mice. The severity of intestinal inflammation could be reduced by continuous neutralization of TNFα, suggesting that either neutralization of TNFα directly affects T cell activation or that the secondary activation mediated by T cells is abrogated [8]. A subsequent study provided evidence supporting the latter. Here, the transfer of either naïve TNFα-deficient or wildtype T cells resulted in comparable colitis severity. In contrast, the transfer of naïve T cells into TNFα$^{-/-}$ Rag2$^{-/-}$ mice failed to induce colitis, indicating that T-cell-mediated activation of non-T cells is crucial for the TNFα-driven pro-inflammatory effect [9]. These data indicate the tightly regulated interaction of the innate and the adaptive immune systems. In humans, in vitro-cultured colonic T cells exhibited higher levels of IFNγ and TNFα in cells derived from Crohn's disease patients when compared to controls. Neutralization of TNFα by coincubation with infliximab resulted in inhibition of IFNγ expression, hence indicating a direct effect of infliximab on the secretion of pro-inflammatory cytokines by intestinal T cells [10].

Indirect evidence that TNFα strongly affects the T helper cell response derives from the major complication of anti-TNFα therapy, namely, reactivation of latent tuberculosis. Early data from the tuberculosis research field indicated that a proper T helper cell type 1 response is indispensable for the development of an appropriate immune response, including the formation of granulomas [11]. In the absence of TNFα, mice could not control tuberculosis infection [12]. Looking back, it is not surprising that after the introduction of anti-TNFα therapy first for rheumatoid arthritis and later for inflammatory bowel diseases, cases of miliary tuberculosis were observed [13]. This resulted in national and international guidelines for screening for the presence of latent tuberculosis in patients receiving treatment with anti-TNFα [14] (fig. 2a).

To define the interaction of T cells with antigen-presenting cells in more depth, one has to consider the process of antigen presentation and the signals involved. Dendritic cells in the lamina propria continuously capture antigens, process them and migrate to the draining lymph nodes. During this process, dendritic cells up-regulate cell surface expression of molecules required for the activation of naïve T cells [15]. For the activation of naïve T cells, three signals are required: (i) The first signal is the antigen itself, expressed on the surface of the dendritic cell by human leukocyte antigen class II molecules. (ii) The second signal is provided by so-called costimulatory molecules, such as CD40 and CD80/86, which are recognized by CD40L and CD28, respectively, on T cells. (iii) The third signal depends on the local cytokine milieu that is produced by the dendritic cell as well as on the surrounding environment. The quantity and quality of the three signals determines whether immune tolerance or an immune response is induced. Not surprisingly, in patients with active Crohn's disease, CD40 is up-regulated in various cell types, including microvascular endothelial cells as well as lamina propria T cells and platelets, with levels of the soluble form being increased in the serum of patients with inflammatory bowel disease [16]. In line with these findings, Hart et al. revealed high expression of CD40 on intestinal dendritic cells isolated from the inflamed mucosa of patients with Crohn's disease when compared to cells from Crohn's disease patients with noninflamed mucosa or from healthy controls. More importantly, CD40 expression on dendritic cells was profoundly decreased after infliximab treatment, independent of resolution of inflammation [17]. These data indicate that the CD40/CD40L pathway plays a central role in intestinal inflammation and is regulated by TNFα (fig. 2b).

TNFα and Regulatory T Cells

T cell priming by antigen-presenting cells can result in a variety of T cell subpopulations, depending on the costimulatory molecules as well as the milieu (signals 2 and 3). One T cell subpopulation

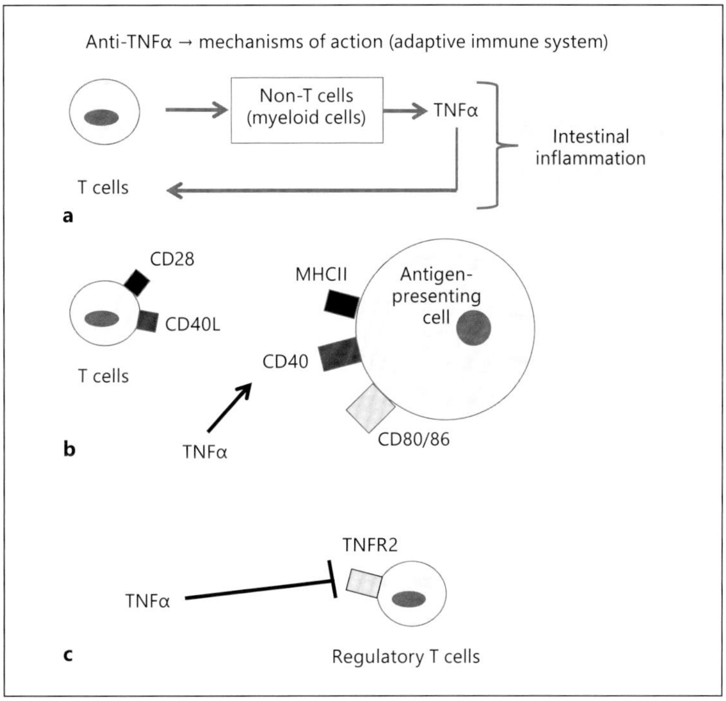

Fig. 2. The anti-inflammatory effects of anti-TNFα on the adaptive immune system. **a** Activated T cells stimulate non-T cells (myeloid cells, epithelial cells) to produce TNFα. TNFα activates T cells (required for distinct infections such as tuberculosis) and, in parallel, promotes the inflammatory process. Anti-TNFα can abrogate this vicious circle. **b** TNFα up-regulates costimulatory molecules on antigen-presenting cells, thus resulting in maintenance and even worsening of the inflammatory process. Neutralization of TNFα can suppress this process. **c** TNFα inhibits the function of regulatory T cells via TNFR2. Anti-TNFα strategies result not only in functioning regulatory T cells but also in an increased frequency of these cells.

is the so-called regulatory T cells, which can be divided into several subgroups. The absence of functional regulatory T cells that occurs in immunodysregulation, polyendocrinopathy and enteropathy, X-linked syndrome results in a syndrome comprising several autoimmune diseases that ultimately results in death unless bone marrow transplantation is performed [18]. The immune dysfunction or absence in this syndrome is induced by a mutation in *Foxp3*, the key transcription factor for the development of regulatory T cells. As indicated by the phenotype of the syndrome, the presence of regulatory T cells is detrimental to the maintenance of self-tolerance and the prevention of autoimmune disease. This is true even though *Foxp3* does not represent the exclusive marker for regulatory T cells [19]. How does TNFα influence regulatory T cells? Data from patients with rheumatoid arthritis suggest that TNFα inhibits the suppressor function of regulatory T cells through TNFR2. Infliximab treatment not only restored the capacity of regulatory T cells to inhibit cytokine production but also conferred a suppressive phenotype upon conventional T cells. In addition, infliximab treatment was followed by a significant rise in the number of T cells with a regulatory phenotype in rheumatoid arthritis patients responding to the treatment, correlating with a decrease in the inflammatory marker C-reactive protein [20]. A study by Nadkarni et al. further indicated that infliximab treatment is followed by the induction of a specific population of regulatory T cells whose suppressor function is exerted through the anti-inflammatory cytokines TGFβ and IL-10. These regulatory cells lack the expression of CD62L, hence distinguishing them from the natural regulatory T cells present in healthy individuals and in patients with active rheumatoid arthritis [21] (fig. 2c).

A recent study provided further evidence linking the innate and the adaptive immune systems. Here, the immunosuppressive effect of different anti-TNFα therapies on activated T cells in vitro was investigated [22]. The data provide evidence that neutralization of TNFα results in inhibition of T cell proliferation. For this inhibitory function to be exerted, binding of the compound to membrane-bound TNFα was required. While infliximab as well as adalimumab did bind to membrane-bound TNFα, certolizumab only showed intermediate binding, while etanercept and control IgG did not bind at all. In addition, the compound must possess an Fc region to interact with the Fc receptor on antigen-presenting cells. Binding of the respective anti-TNFα compound to the antigen-presenting cell induces the formation of a distinct macrophage subset with an immunosuppressive phenotype. These macrophages are characterized by a regulatory phenotype and associated expression of the mannose receptor CD206, production of anti-inflammatory cytokines and consequent inhibition of T cell proliferation.

These results are in line with a recently developed concept in macrophage biology. The lamina propria consists of resident regulatory macrophages, and in the case of inflammation, monocytes will be recruited and will subsequently polarize into either inflammatory or regulatory macrophages, depending on the local milieu. This concept has been proven by showing that mice with IL-10-deficient macrophages did not develop colitis, whereas mice with IL-10R-deficient macrophages developed colitis, indicate that the local milieu determined the effector function of this cell population [23]. Thus, by neutralizing TNFα in the lamina propria, the milieu is strongly shifted toward a rather regulatory milieu, allowing for regeneration of the mucosal balance.

Conclusions and Future Directions

Not surprisingly considering the central role of TNFα within inflammatory mechanisms, targeting TNFα affects the innate (as outlined in other chapters in this book) as well as the adaptive immune systems. From this, one could conclude that each patient with inflammatory bowel disease and inflammatory activity should, in theory, respond to anti-TNFα strategies. Since this is definitely not the case, a more detailed understanding of the interaction of the blockade, the innate and the adaptive immune systems and the potential specific role of the microbiota in this network has to be achieved, with the ultimate goal of improving treatment options as well as the life quality of our patients.

References

1 ten Hove T, van Montfrans C, Peppelenbosch MP, van Deventer SJ: Infliximab treatment induces apoptosis of lamina propria T lymphocytes in Crohn's disease. Gut 2002;50:206–211.

2 Lugering A, Schmidt M, Lugering N, Pauels HG, Domschke W, Kucharzik T: Infliximab induces apoptosis in monocytes from patients with chronic active Crohn's disease by using a caspase-dependent pathway. Gastroenterology 2001;121:1145–1157.

3 Van den Brande JM, Koehler TC, Zelinkova Z, Bennink RJ, te Velde AA, ten Cate FJ, van Deventer SJ, Peppelenbosch MP, Hommes DW: Prediction of antitumour necrosis factor clinical efficacy by real-time visualisation of apoptosis in patients with Crohn's disease. Gut 2007; 56:509–517.

4 Shen C, Assche GV, Colpaert S, Maerten P, Geboes K, Rutgeerts P, Ceuppens JL: Adalimumab induces apoptosis of human monocytes: a comparative study with infliximab and etanercept. Aliment Pharmacol Ther 2005;21:251–258.

5 Nesbitt A, Fossati G, Bergin M, Stephens P, Stephens S, Foulkes R, Brown D, Robinson M, Bourne T: Mechanism of action of certolizumab pegol (cdp870): in vitro comparison with other anti-tumor necrosis factor alpha agents. Inflamm Bowel Dis 2007;13:1323–1332.

6 Peake ST, Bernardo D, Mann ER, Al-Hassi HO, Knight SC, Hart AL: Mechanisms of action of anti-tumor necrosis factor alpha agents in Crohn's disease. Inflamm Bowel Dis 2013;19:1546–1555.

7 Tumanov AV, Grivennikov SI, Kruglov AA, Shebzukhov YV, Koroleva EP, Piao Y, Cui CY, Kuprash DV, Nedospasov SA: Cellular source and molecular form of tnf specify its distinct functions in organization of secondary lymphoid organs. Blood 2010;116:3456–3464.

8 Powrie F, Leach MW, Mauze S, Menon S, Caddle LB, Coffman RL: Inhibition of th1 responses prevents inflammatory bowel disease in scid mice reconstituted with cd45rbhi cd4+ t cells. Immunity 1994;1:553–562.

9 Corazza N, Eichenberger S, Eugster HP, Mueller C: Nonlymphocyte-derived tumor necrosis factor is required for induction of colitis in recombination activating gene (rag)2(–/–) mice upon transfer of cd4(+)cd45rb(hi) t cells. J Exp Med 1999;190:1479–1492.

10 Agnholt J, Kaltoft K: Infliximab downregulates interferon-gamma production in activated gut t-lymphocytes from patients with Crohn's disease. Cytokine 2001;15:212–222.

11 Singh IG, Mukherjee R, Talwar GP, Kaufmann SH: In vitro characterization of t cells from mycobacterium w-vaccinated mice. Infect Immun 1992;60:257–263.

12 Kindler V, Sappino AP, Grau GE, Piguet PF, Vassalli P: The inducing role of tumor necrosis factor in the development of bactericidal granulomas during BCG infection. Cell 1989;56:731–740.

13 Rovere Querini P, Vecellio M, Sabbadini MG, Ciboddo G: Miliary tuberculosis after biological therapy for rheumatoid arthritis. Rheumatology (Oxford) 2002; 41:231.

14 Rahier JF, Magro F, Abreu C, Armuzzi A, Ben-Horin S, Chowers Y, Cottone M, de Ridder L, Doherty G, Ehehalt R, Esteve M, Katsanos K, Lees CW, Macmahon E, Moreels T, Reinisch W, Tilg H, Tremblay L, Veereman-Wauters G, Viget N, Yazdanpanah Y, Eliakim R, Colombel JF: Second European evidence-based consensus on the prevention, diagnosis and management of opportunistic infections in inflammatory bowel disease. J Crohns Colitis 2014;8:443–468.

15 Banchereau J, Steinman RM: Dendritic cells and the control of immunity. Nature 1998;392:245–252.

16 Danese S, Sans M, Scaldaferri F, Sgambato A, Rutella S, Cittadini A, Pique JM, Panes J, Katz JA, Gasbarrini A, Fiocchi C: TNF-alpha blockade down-regulates the cd40/cd40l pathway in the mucosal microcirculation: A novel anti-inflammatory mechanism of infliximab in Crohn's disease. J Immunol 2006;176: 2617–2624.

17 Hart AL, Al-Hassi HO, Rigby RJ, Bell SJ, Emmanuel AV, Knight SC, Kamm MA, Stagg AJ: Characteristics of intestinal dendritic cells in inflammatory bowel diseases. Gastroenterology 2005;129: 50–65.

18 Baud O, Goulet O, Canioni D, Le Deist F, Radford I, Rieu D, Dupuis-Girod S, Cerf-Bensussan N, Cavazzana-Calvo M, Brousse N, Fischer A, Casanova JL: Treatment of the immune dysregulation, polyendocrinopathy, enteropathy, x-linked syndrome (ipex) by allogeneic bone marrow transplantation. N Engl J Med 2001;344:1758–1762.

19 Bernardo D, Al-Hassi HO, Mann ER, Tee CT, Murugananthan AU, Peake ST, Hart AL, Knight SC: T-cell proliferation and forkhead box p3 expression in human t cells are dependent on t-cell density: physics of a confined space? Hum Immunol 2012;73:223–231.

20 Ehrenstein MR, Evans JG, Singh A, Moore S, Warnes G, Isenberg DA, Mauri C: Compromised function of regulatory t cells in rheumatoid arthritis and reversal by anti-TNFalpha therapy. J Exp Med 2004;200:277–285.

21 Nadkarni S, Mauri C, Ehrenstein MR: Anti-TNF-alpha therapy induces a distinct regulatory t cell population in patients with rheumatoid arthritis via TGF-beta. J Exp Med 2007;204:33–39.

22 Vos AC, Wildenberg ME, Arijs I, Duijvestein M, Verhaar AP, de Hertogh G, Vermeire S, Rutgeerts P, van den Brink GR, Hommes DW: Regulatory macrophages induced by infliximab are involved in healing in vivo and in vitro. Inflamm Bowel Dis 2012;18:401–408.

23 Zigmond E, Bernshtein B, Friedlander G, Walker CR, Yona S, Kim KW, Brenner O, Krauthgamer R, Varol C, Muller W, Jung S: Macrophage-restricted interleukin-10 receptor deficiency, but not il-10 deficiency, causes severe spontaneous colitis. Immunity 2014;40: 720–733.

Britta Siegmund
Medical Department (Gastroenterology, Infectious Diseases, Rheumatology)
Charité – Universitätsmedizin Berlin, Campus Benjamin Franklin
Hindenburgdamm 30
DE–12200 Berlin (Germany)
E-Mail britta.siegmund@charite.de

Rogler G, Herfarth H, Hibi T, Nielsen OH (eds): Anti-Tumor Necrosis Factor Therapy in Inflammatory Bowel Disease.
Front Gastrointest Res. Basel, Karger, 2015, vol 34, pp 62–72 (DOI: 10.1159/000381411)

Binding of Membrane-Bound TNF

Raja Atreya · Ulrike Billmeier · Timo Rath · Helmut Neumann · Markus F. Neurath

Medical Clinic 1, Friedrich-Alexander University Erlangen-Nürnberg, Erlangen, Germany

Abstract

The efficacy of anti-TNF antibodies in inflammatory bowel diseases (IBD) has been attributed to multiple effects, but the precise molecular mechanism of action has still not been thoroughly characterized. It has been shown that the available anti-TNF agents are able to block soluble TNF in vitro. However, mere neutralization of soluble TNF cannot be the only therapeutic modality of therapeutically efficient anti-TNF agents, as accumulating evidence indicates that effector cells expressing membrane-bound TNF are critically involved in the induction and perpetuation of chronic mucosal inflammation. Transmembrane TNF (mTNF) is characterized by a unique bipolar function in the inflammatory reaction, as it not only can act as a ligand but also mediates reverse signaling into mTNF-expressing cells. Accordingly, it was demonstrated that anti-TNF antibodies exert their main therapeutic properties by binding to mTNF. The anti-TNF antibodies that are therapeutically effective in IBD are able to form more stable immune complexes, with greater avidity in binding to mTNF, than the anti-TNF agent etanercept, which failed to show a therapeutic effect in Crohn's disease patients. Apart from complement-dependent and antibody-dependent cell-mediated cytotoxicity, the induction of apoptosis is regarded as the major therapeutic effect of anti-TNF antibodies in regard to their binding to mTNF-expressing mucosal cells. The distinct mechanisms leading to the induction of programmed cell death include outside-to-inside signaling, resulting in direct induction of apoptosis in mTNF-bearing intestinal cells, and also inhibition of the interaction between mTNF-expressing macrophages and TNFR2-expressing T cells, leading to indirect induction of mucosal T-cell apoptosis. Altogether, current data suggest that mTNF regulation in antigen-presenting cells, rather than in T cells, seems to be the main therapeutic effect of anti-TNF agents in IBD. The decisive role of mTNF in the molecular mechanism of action of anti-TNF antibodies is underscored by the predictive capacity of in vivo mucosal mTNF expression concerning the therapeutic response to subsequent anti-TNF treatment in Crohn's disease patients. Growing understanding of both the pathogenic role of mTNF-expressing mucosal cells in IBD and the interaction of mTNF with anti-TNF antibodies will further contribute to the prediction of therapeutic efficacy, the characterization of molecular targets for forthcoming novel therapies and the development of new anti-TNF agents.

Introduction

Inflammatory bowel diseases (IBD) are defined as relapsing inflammation of the gastrointestinal tract not due to specific pathogens [1]. Although the precise etiology of IBD is still unclear, aberrant activation of the mucosal immune system, with excessive CD4+ T-cell activation and uncontrolled production of pro-inflammatory cytokines, is regarded as the central pathogenic mechanism involved in the initiation and perpetuation of the inflammatory process [2].

In this setting, TNF-α is believed to be a decisive mediator in the initiation and amplification of the mucosal inflammatory cascade in IBD and therefore plays a pivotal role in disease pathogenesis [3]. Accordingly, several studies have demonstrated that TNF production is elevated in the intestinal mucosa and serum of IBD patients [4–6]. TNF has been shown to be involved in T-cell activation and proliferation; cytokine and chemokine secretion; cell recruitment; angiogenesis; extracellular matrix degradation; and, most importantly, heightened resistance to apoptosis among mucosal T cells in IBD [7, 8].

Accordingly, the TNF-neutralizing antibodies infliximab (chimeric IgG1 monoclonal antibody), adalimumab (fully human IgG1 monoclonal antibody) and certolizumab pegol (pegylated humanized Fab' fragment monoclonal antibody) have been approved for the treatment of Crohn's disease [9–11], while infliximab, adalimumab and golimumab (fully human IgG1 monoclonal antibody) are effectively used in ulcerative colitis [12–14].

The therapeutic efficacy of these clinically effective anti-TNF antibodies has been attributed to multiple effects, but the main molecular mechanism of action is still not well understood. Accumulating evidence suggests that mere neutralization of only soluble TNF (sTNF) does not sufficiently explain the therapeutic potency of anti-TNF agents, as this effect is also achieved by etanercept (a TNFR2 fusion protein), which failed to show any therapeutic efficacy in a trial with Crohn's disease patients [15].

Recent data have indicated that the precursor form of sTNF, transmembrane TNF (mTNF), is critically involved in the process of intestinal inflammation [16, 17]. Correspondingly growing attention has been paid to the differential effects induced by the binding of TNF antagonists to mTNF-expressing mucosal cells in IBD. In this regard, the direct and indirect induction of apoptosis in mucosal CD4+ T cells due to the binding of anti-TNF antibodies to mTNF+ cells has been regarded as the central molecular mechanism of action of these agents in IBD [17].

In the following sections, we would like to give an overview regarding the biological functions of mTNF in the immunopathogenesis of IBD and to characterize the binding and neutralizing activities of anti-TNF antibodies toward mTNF-bearing cells to elucidate the mechanistic effects of these agents in IBD.

Main Points

TNF Biology

The pro-inflammatory cytokine TNF is initially translated as a transmembrane precursor protein (mTNF) that is expressed as a 26-kilodalton cell surface type II polypeptide on activated monocytes, macrophages and lymphocytes as well as on other cell types [18, 19]. The soluble 17-kilodalton form is yielded via proteolytic cleavage by the metalloproteinase TNF-α-converting enzyme (TACE) [20]. It was shown that TACE activity is increased in ulcerative colitis, but not in Crohn's disease patients [21]. The TNF ligands exert their biological functions via interaction with two distinct cell surface receptors of the TNFR family [22]. While TNFR1 is constitutively expressed in most tissues, the expression of TNFR2 is tightly regulated and preferentially occurs in lymphocytes and endothelial cells [18]. Ligation of TNFR1 is associated with NF-κB activation, cytotoxicity, induction of pro-inflammatory cytokines and pro- or anti-apoptotic signals. TNFR2 activation has been associated with T-cell activation and proliferation, production of pro-inflammatory cytokines and pro- or anti-apoptotic signals [18].

These two isoforms not only can be found on the membrane of cells but also can be detected as soluble receptors circulating in the serum. Although sTNF and mTNF have comparable bioactivities in activating TNFR1, sTNF preferentially binds to TNFR1 owing to a 30-fold faster dissociation rate from TNFR2 than from TNFR1 [23]. This observation has led to a ligand-passing hypothesis in which sTNF bound to TNFR2 is quickly passed to TNFR1. Therefore, most of the biological activities of sTNF are mediated through TNFR1 [23]. In contrast, mTNF preferentially binds to TNFR2, which is only then fully activated, playing an important role in inflammatory processes during cell-cell interaction [19]. Surface TNFRs are also able to ligate mTNF on an opposing cell, subsequently transmitting outside-to-inside (reverse) signals into mTNF-bearing cells. The cellular pathways involved include activation of the p38 mitogen-activated protein kinase (MAPK) pathway [24].

This bipolar function of mTNF, which not only can act as a ligand but also mediates reverse signaling into cells expressing this molecule, is a unique hallmark of several members of the TNF superfamily [25].

Regarding biological activities, it was shown that as a ligand, mTNF is able to exert cytotoxic activities, is involved in host defense against intracellular bacteria like *Mycobacterium tuberculosis*, mediates activation of endothelial cells as well as cytokine production by monocytes and also induces resistance to apoptosis in CD4+ T cells [25, 26]. As a receptor, mTNF exerts its biological functions in immune responses by modulation of T-cell, natural killer cell or macrophage function, cytokine suppression, NF-κB activation or apoptosis of the mTNF-bearing cell [25, 26].

Immunopathogenic Role of Transmembrane TNF in Inflammatory Bowel Disease

The pivotal importance of mTNF in IBD pathogenesis was shown in animal models, in which intestinal inflammation was induced upon transfer of naïve T cells into mTNF RAG2–/– mice, which had a mutated TNF that could not be cleaved into sTNF [27]. These data demonstrate that the systemic effects of TNF are not required for induction and perpetuation of chronic mucosal inflammation in the intestine. In concordance with these results, recent data also indicated that specific neutralization of mTNF, but not sTNF, was able to induce remission in T-cell-mediated colitis [28]. These data imply that not only the development but also the maintenance of intestinal inflammation is mTNF dependent and that sTNF does not seem to play a critical role in this process.

While existing data show only low mTNF expression on normal macrophages and T cells [29], recent experiments demonstrated that mTNF expression was more frequently found on intestinal antigen-presenting cells (APCs) compared to T cells in IBD patients [17]. Immunohistochemical staining of intestinal cryosections revealed a significant upregulation of mTNF in CD14+ macrophages compared to CD4+ lymphocytes (fig. 1). It could be observed that intestinal mTNF-expressing CD14+ macrophages were able to activate TNFR2-expressing CD4+ T cells, resulting in increased resistance to apoptosis among CD4+ T cells, which perpetuate and aggravate the mucosal inflammatory reaction in IBD [17].

These data suggest that mTNF regulation in APCs, rather than in T cells, is involved in the immunopathogenesis of IBD. This notion is also supported by observations regarding the colitogenic potential of mTNF on APCs, rather than on T cells, in an experimental transfer colitis model [27]. The interplay between mTNF and its corresponding receptor TNFR2 has also been implicated in the development of granulomas, which is one specific characteristic of Crohn's disease [26].

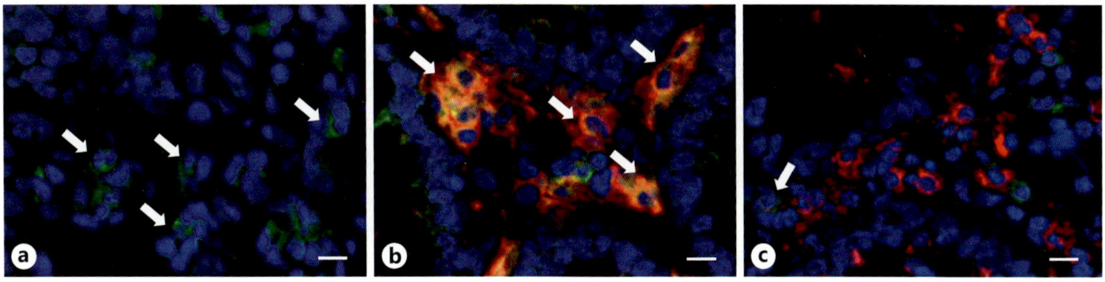

Fig. 1. Ex vivo immunofluorescence staining for transmembrane TNF (mTNF) with a fluorescent anti-TNF antibody in gut cryosections from patients with Crohn's disease. **a** Representative immunofluorescence staining for mTNF (arrows) with a fluorescent anti-TNF antibody (green) and antibodies against (**b**) CD14 or (**c**) CD4 (all red). Nuclei were counterstained with DAPI (blue). Double-positive cells are shown in yellow (arrows). The scale bars represent 10 μm. A higher percentage of mTNF+ cells was observed among intestinal CD14+ macrophages compared to CD4+ T cells in patients with Crohn's disease.

Overexpression of TNFR2, the corresponding receptor for mTNF signaling, in T cells has been shown to aggravate experimental colitis [30], and the absence of TNFR2 attenuated spontaneous development of colitis in T-cell receptor-α–/– mice [31]. A positive correlation was observed between the serum concentration of the soluble forms of TNFR2 and TNFR1 and disease activity in IBD patients [32], and overexpression of TNFR2 could also be found in the mucosal CD4+ T cells of IBD patients [17, 30]. Additionally, a functional polymorphism of TNFR2 is supposed to be associated with an increased risk of ulcerative colitis [33].

It has further been shown that mTNF expression in intestinal epithelial cells may also be involved in IBD pathogenesis, as mTNF leads to accelerated apoptosis induction in epithelial cells, thereby disrupting the barrier function in conjunction with IFN-γ [34].

Nevertheless, it also has to be taken into account that TNF signaling via TNFR2 can additionally induce apoptosis in CD4+ T cells and limits inflammation in an experimental T-cell transfer model [35]. These data indicate that TNFR2 has a pivotal function in mediating the resolution or perpetuation of mucosal inflammation in IBD, warranting further research.

Altogether, these data clearly indicate that mTNF plays a pivotal role in the inflammatory process in IBD and therefore represents an attractive target for therapeutic approaches, with monoclonal antibodies directed against it.

Binding of Anti-TNF Antibodies to Transmembrane TNF in Inflammatory Bowel Disease

The ligand-binding properties of anti-TNF antibody binding to sTNF and mTNF have been intensively studied to gain further insights into the molecular mechanism of action of anti-TNF antibodies. It was shown that all anti-TNF antibodies bind to sTNF with high affinity [36–39]. Nevertheless, differences between infliximab/adalimumab and etanercept were found in regard to their kinetic parameters of binding and the stability of complexes formed between the antibodies and sTNF trimers [40, 41].

Based on the pro-inflammatory capacity of mTNF, much attention has been paid to the binding of TNF antagonists to mTNF. Apart from pharmacokinetics, tissue penetration and serum half-life, the differential effects of the anti-TNF antibodies in regard to mTNF binding may explain the discrepant clinical efficacies of infliximab, adalimumab, certolizumab and etanercept, the last of which is ineffective in Crohn's disease treatment [42].

In this regard, it was also shown that etanercept is generally ineffective in the treatment of granulomatous diseases, which mainly develop from the interplay between mTNF and its corresponding receptor, TNFR2 [26]. Therefore, it is likely that sufficient neutralization of mTNF is a prerequisite to suppress granuloma formation, which etanercept does not seem to achieve.

The investigation of the binding characteristics of anti-TNF antibodies to mTNF has mostly been performed with cell lines transfected with native TNF or mutated mTNF that is resistant to TACE. However, when analyzing the results, it has to be taken into account that alternate proteases are also able to cleave mTNF at alternative intramembrane sites [43].

In several studies, it was shown that all anti-TNF antibodies are able to bind to different cell lines expressing transfected mTNF [36, 38, 41, 44]. The binding affinities were altogether a little lower than the ones toward sTNF [38]. It has to be noted that binding of etanercept to mTNF has been mostly described in experiments where noncleavable mTNF was stably overexpressed. In untransfected and activated primary lymphocytes, there have been divergent results. In a study on peripheral blood monocytes, the antibodies infliximab, adalimumab and etanercept exhibited similar binding capacities [45]. In blood T cells stimulated with PMA/ionomycin, similar binding of adalimumab, infliximab and etanercept was recorded [42]. In contrast, one study presented binding of infliximab to blood T lymphocytes stimulated with CD3/CD28, while this effect was absent with etanercept [46].

The variation between the anti-TNF agents in regard to mTNF cross-linking, rather than affinity, may explain the differences in the functional properties of the antibodies. It was shown that up to three molecules of infliximab are able to bind to mTNF, whereas etanercept is only able to form complexes at a 1:1 ratio, as both receptor arms bind to a single mTNF trimer [40, 41]. It was proposed that cross-linking of anti-TNF antibodies is required for therapeutic efficacy. The anti-TNF antibody infliximab, with therapeutical efficacy in IBD, is able to form more stable immune complexes, with greater avidity in binding to mTNF, than the clinically inefficient etanercept. As the rate of dissociation between etanercept and TNF is higher compared to that between infliximab and TNF, bioavailable mTNF-bearing cells are released more quickly to convey their pathological signals. The higher avidity of infliximab and other anti-TNF antibodies for mTNF is regarded as the reason for their clinical effectiveness in IBD when compared to etanercept [36, 41].

Functional Outcome of the Interaction between Anti-TNF Antibodies and Transmembrane TNF in Inflammatory Bowel Disease

The efficacy of anti-TNF antibodies in IBD has been attributed to several effects, such as regulation of intestinal cell adhesion molecule expression [47]; induction of intestinal fibroblast motility [48]; induction of regulatory T cells [49]; or, most recently, induction of regulatory macrophages in an Fc region-dependent manner [50].

Nevertheless, most existing data are related to the effects mediated by binding of anti-TNF antibodies to mTNF-bearing mucosal cells [51], which elicits downregulation of cytokine production or growth arrest, intracellular signaling cascades, cytotoxic effects or induction of apoptosis (fig. 2).

It was shown that the process of infliximab-induced reverse signaling led to downregulated production of the pro-inflammatory cytokines TNF-α, IL-1β, IL-6 and IL-8 in peripheral blood monocytes [52] and of IFN-γ in the mucosal T cells of Crohn's disease patients after infliximab treatment [53]. Moreover, infliximab treatment of Jurkat T cells transfected with mTNF led to upregulation of IL-10 and E-selectin and also resulted in the arrest of these cells in the G0/G1 phase of the cell cycle [36].

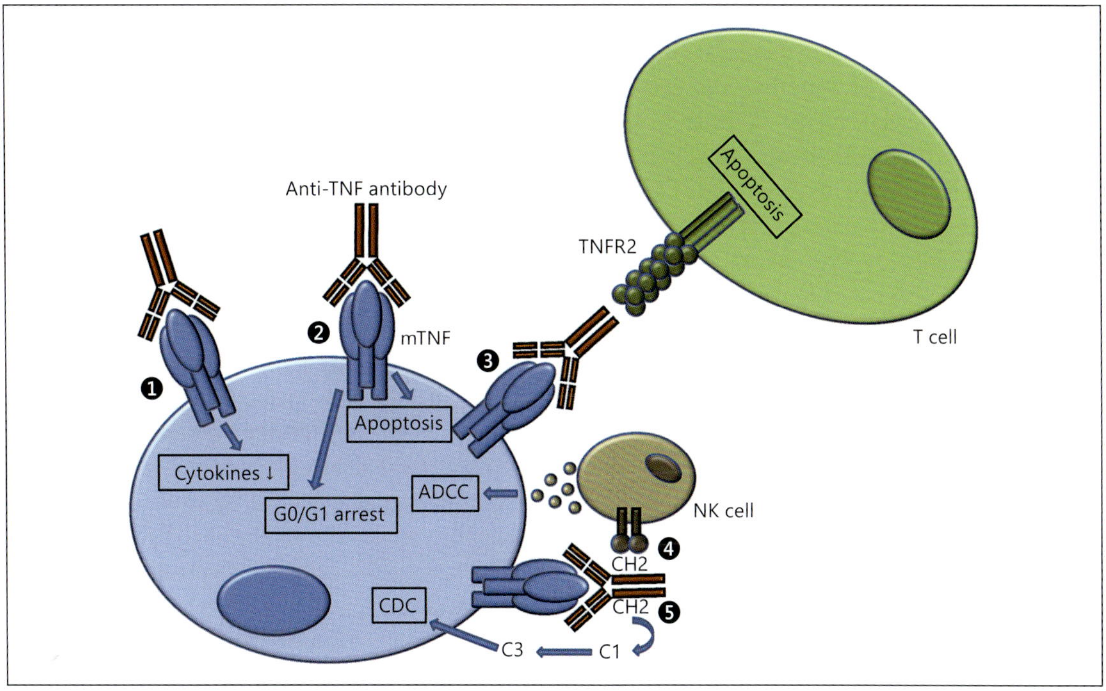

Fig. 2. Effects mediated by binding of anti-TNF antibodies to mTNF-bearing mucosal cells. (1) Suppression of pro-inflammatory cytokine production. (2) Arrest of the cell in the G0/G1 phase of the cell cycle. Direct induction of apoptosis via reverse signaling. (3) Indirect induction of apoptosis in TNFR2+CD4+ T-cells. (4) Antibody-dependent cell-mediated cytotoxicity. (5) Complement-dependent cytotoxicity.

Additional studies demonstrated that infliximab is able to act on several cellular targets. It transiently activates the p38 MAPK and p44/42 extracellular signal-regulated kinase in monocytic cells [54]. Differential phosphorylation of p38 MAPK was observed in Crohn's disease patients who did or did not respond to infliximab therapy [55]. A subsequent study demonstrated that infliximab and certolizumab pegol mediated reverse signaling via mTNF, leading to MAPK activation and TGF-β secretion, in turn leading to downregulation of the pro-inflammatory growth and differentiation factor 1 and IL-6 [56].

Further studies showed that elimination and clearance of active inflammatory cells from inflamed tissue was also achieved by cytotoxic effects. In complement-dependent cytotoxicity (CDC), an Fc-containing anti-TNF agent binds to the mTNF of the target cell, which is followed by activation of the complement cascade. In different cell lines (Jurkat T cells, CHO cells, melanoma cells), it was shown that infliximab and adalimumab were markedly more effective than etanercept in inducing CDC [37, 38, 57], while this effect was completely absent with certolizumab pegol [39]. This was explained by the missing Fc portion of IgG1 in certolizumab pegol [26, 39] and the lack of a specific CH1 domain in IgG1 for complement C3 activation by etanercept [26, 58]. Additionally, CDC induction in peripheral blood mononuclear cells could not be reproduced by infliximab, adalimumab or etanercept [38]. Therefore, it is still unclear if CDC is an important mechanism for anti-TNF agents' effects in IBD.

When analyzing antibody-dependent cell-mediated cytotoxicity (ADCC), there was similar potency for infliximab, adalimumab and etanercept in mTNF-transfected Jurkat T cells [57] and stronger potency for infliximab and adalimumab compared to etanercept in NS0 [39] or CHO [37] cells. In contrast, certolizumab pegol did not show any ADCC activity [39, 59]. This may be explained by the fact that compared to certolizumab pegol, the other agents carry the CH2 and CH3 domains of the Fc domain of IgG1 [26], which mediate binding to Fc receptors and granzyme B/perforin release from natural killer cells, leading to the lysis of the mTNF-expressing target cell.

There are few data regarding the most recently approved anti-TNF antibody golimumab, but a recent paper showed that it was able to bind to mTNF on Jurkat T cells. Golimumab also induced ADCC and CDC, which was comparable to infliximab and adalimumab [59].

Besides the described mechanisms, the central focus has been on accumulating data regarding regulation of apoptosis as the main mechanism of action of mTNF-bound anti-TNF agents [60, 61].

Augmented lamina propria T-cell activation and resistance to apoptosis have been identified as key factors in IBD pathogenesis, as these factors impair mucosal homeostasis and lead to unrestrained accumulation of activated lymphocytes that perpetuate the inflammatory response [62–64]. An elegant in vivo imaging study in Crohn's disease patients demonstrated that T-cell apoptosis occurred within the first few days after the initiation of anti-TNF therapy and correlated with the clinical response to treatment [65].

It was first believed that there is only direct induction of apoptosis due to reverse signaling through mTNF in mucosal T cells, elicited by mTNF-bound anti-TNF antibodies [16, 44]. It was described that infliximab-induced reverse signaling led to directly induced cell death via induction of the caspase 8-mitochondrial permeability pathway, in which induction of the pro-apoptotic proteins bak and bax lead to apoptotic effects [16, 44, 46, 66]. Adalimumab appeared to have a similar mechanism, inducing caspase 3-dependent apoptosis [67]. Differences in the propensity of infliximab and etanercept to induce apoptosis were observed in peripheral blood and mucosal lymphocytes from Crohn's disease patients. Infliximab, but not etanercept, induced T-cell apoptosis in a mixed lymphocyte reaction with monocyte-derived dendritic cells [46]. However, other data could not verify direct induction of apoptosis in vitro in anti-TNF antibody-treated blood lymphocytes from Crohn's disease patients [39, 52].

Subsequent data indicated that there is indirect induction of apoptosis by anti-TNF antibodies in IBD. It was shown the anti-TNF antibodies infliximab, adalimumab, and certolizumab pegol, but not etanercept, bind to mTNF and thereby block the interaction between mTNF on CD14+ macrophages and TNFR2 on lamina propria T cells and suppress TNFR2-mediated signaling, resulting in the induction of T-cell apoptosis. The finding that anti-TNF antibodies only induced apoptosis indirectly by blocking the mTNF/TNFR2 pathway further characterized the pivotal role of mTNF in the molecular mechanism of action of anti-TNF antibodies in IBD [17]. Furthermore, a recently published study demonstrated that mTNF expression on mucosal target cells is predictive of the clinical efficacy of anti-TNF antibodies. In an in vivo molecular imaging study in 25 Crohn's disease patients, mTNF expression on intestinal immune cells was visualized by topical administration of a fluorescent anti-TNF antibody (adalimumab), followed by confocal laser endomicroscopy for mTNF imaging (fig. 3). It was demonstrated that Crohn's disease patients with high numbers of mTNF+ intestinal cells showed a significantly higher rate of response to subsequently initiated anti-TNF therapy than patients with low numbers of mTNF+ cells did [68]. These results indicate that it might be of interest to specifically target the mTNF/TNFR2 interaction in the future, rather than total TNF. These

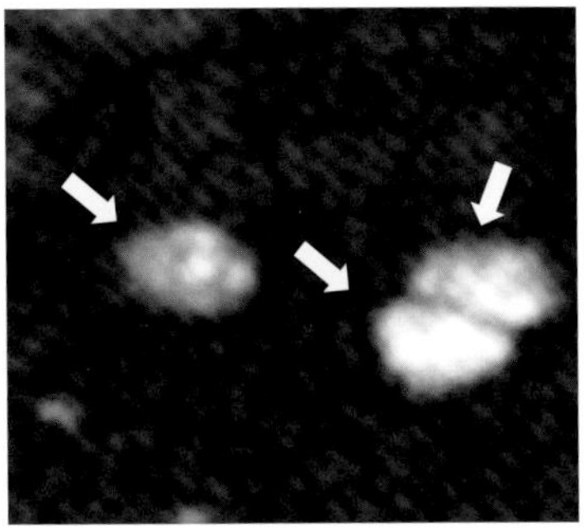

Fig. 3. In vivo molecular imaging of intestinal mTNF+ immune cells in a Crohn's disease patient. In vivo topical administration of a Good Manufacturing Practices-conforming fluorescent anti-TNF antibody to the inflamed mucosa of a Crohn's disease patient yielded specific signals for mTNF+ mucosal cells (arrows).

study results indicate that in vivo imaging of molecular targets may be useful for the development of individualized therapy and for the optimization of biological therapeutic approaches.

Conclusion

A growing understanding of the immunopathogenic role of TNF in IBD is essential for appreciation of its role as the molecular target of anti-TNF antibody treatment. Recent studies clearly indicate that mTNF-expressing effector cells, rather than sTNF, are critically involved in the induction and perpetuation of chronic mucosal inflammation in IBD. The high-avidity binding of clinically effective anti-TNF antibodies to mTNF and subsequent cross-linking and multimer formation are regarded as decisive factors in exertion of their therapeutic functions. It was shown that binding of anti-TNF agents to mTNF-bearing cells leads to downregulation of cytokine production, along with growth arrest, modulation of intracellular signaling cascades, cytotoxic effects and direct or indirect induction of apoptosis. The majority of these data have been obtained using in vitro systems, and their relevance to the in vivo situation has to be carefully analyzed.

As approximately 40% of IBD patients do not clinically benefit from anti-TNF treatment, there is a dire clinical need to establish predictive biomarkers for the therapeutic response in order to avoid the exposure of nonresponders to anti-TNF therapy, thus enhancing safety and cost-effective use of this treatment. The in vivo assessment of mucosal mTNF expression via a molecular imaging procedure with a fluorescent anti-TNF antibody to predict the therapeutic response opens new avenues for personalized medicine in IBD.

Another intriguing question is the secondary loss of response of IBD patients to anti-TNF therapy. Although pharmacokinetic analyses regarding through levels and anti-drug antibodies may explain this phenomenon in some patients, the mechanistic background for these treatment failures needs to be elucidated.

Further understanding of the mechanism of action of anti-TNF antibodies and their interaction with mTNF-expressing intestinal cells will elucidate the involved signaling pathways, present novel targets for treatment, enable rational prediction of the response based on the molecular mechanism of action and contribute to fully realizing the whole potential of this substance class.

References

1 Podolsky DK: Inflammatory bowel disease. N Engl J Med 2002;347:417–429.

2 Strober W, Fuss I, Mannon P: The fundamental basis of inflammatory bowel disease. J Clin Invest 2007;117:514–521.

3 MacDonald TT, Hutchings P, Choy MY, Murch S, Cooke A: Tumour necrosis factor-alpha and interferon-gamma production measured at the single cell level in normal and inflamed human intestine. Clin Exp Immunol 1990;81:301–305.

4 Reimund JM, Wittersheim C, Dumont S, Muller CD, Baumann R, Poindron P, Duclos B: Mucosal inflammatory cytokine production by intestinal biopsies in patients with ulcerative colitis and Crohn's disease. J Clin Immunol 1996;16:144–150.

5 Breese EJ, Michie CA, Nicholls SW, Murch SH, Williams CB, Domizio P, Walker-Smith JA, MacDonald TT: Tumor necrosis factor alpha-producing cells in the intestinal mucosa of children with inflammatory bowel disease. Gastroenterology 1994;106:1455–1466.
6 Plevy SE, Landers CJ, Prehn J, Carramanzana NM, Deem RL, Shealy D, Targan SR: A role for TNF-alpha and mucosal T helper-1 cytokines in the pathogenesis of Crohn's disease. J Immunol 1997;159:6276–6282.
7 Van Deventer SJ: Tumour necrosis factor and Crohn's disease. Gut 1997;40: 443–448.
8 Neurath MF, Finotto S, Fuss I, Boirivant M, Galle PR, Strober W: Regulation of T-cell apoptosis in inflammatory bowel disease: to die or not to die, that is the mucosal question. Trends Immunol 2001;22:21–26.
9 Targan SR, Hanauer SB, van Deventer SJ, Mayer L, Present DH, Braakman T, DeWoody KL, Schaible TF, Rutgeerts PJ: A short-term study of chimeric monoclonal antibody cA2 to tumor necrosis factor alpha for Crohn's disease. Crohn's Disease cA2 Study Group. N Engl J Med 1997;337:1029–1035.
10 Hanauer SB, Sandborn WJ, Rutgeerts P, Fedorak RN, Lukas M, MacIntosh D, Panaccione R, Wolf D, Pollack P: Human anti-tumor necrosis factor monoclonal antibody (adalimumab) in Crohn's disease: the CLASSIC-I trial. Gastroenterology 2006;130:323–333.
11 Sandborn WJ, Feagan BG, Stoinov S, Honiball PJ, Rutgeerts P, Mason D, Bloomfield R, Schreiber S; PRECISE 1 Study Investigators: Certolizumab pegol for the treatment of Crohn's disease. N Engl J Med 2007;357:228–238.
12 Rutgeerts P, Sandborn WJ, Feagan BG, Reinisch W, Olson A, Johanns J, Traver S, Rachmilewitz D, Hanauer SB, Lichtenstein GR, de Villiers WJ, Present D, Sands BE, Colombel JF: Infliximab for induction and maintenance therapy for ulcerative colitis. N Engl J Med 2005; 353:2462–2476.
13 Sandborn WJ, van Assche G, Reinisch W, Colombel JF, D'Haens G, Wolf DC, Kron M, Tighe MB, Lazar A, Thakkar RB: Adalimumab induces and maintains clinical remission in patients with moderate-to-severe ulcerative colitis. Gastroenterology 2012;142:257–265.
14 Sandborn WJ, Feagan BG, Marano C, Zhang H, Strauss R, Johanns J, Adedokun OJ, Guzzo C, Colombel JF, Reinisch W, Gibson PR, Collins J, Järnerot G, Hibi T, Rutgeerts P; PURSUIT-SC Study Group: Subcutaneous golimumab induces clinical response and remission in patients with moderate-to-severe ulcerative colitis. Gastroenterology 2014;146: 85–95.
15 Sandborn WJ, Hanauer SB, Katz S, Safdi M, Wolf DG, Baerg RD, Tremaine WJ, Johnson T, Diehl NN, Zinsmeister AR: Etanercept for active Crohn's disease: a randomized, double-blind, placebo-controlled trial. Gastroenterology 2001;121: 1088–1094.
16 Van Deventer SJ: Transmembrane TNF-alpha, induction of apoptosis, and the efficacy of TNF-targeting therapies in Crohn's disease. Gastroenterology 2001; 121:1242–1246.
17 Atreya R, Zimmer M, Bartsch B, Waldner MJ, Atreya I, Neumann H, Hildner K, Hoffman A, Kiesslich R, Rink AD, Rau TT, Rose-John S, Kessler H, Schmidt J, Neurath MF: Antibodies against tumor necrosis factor (TNF) induce T-cell apoptosis in patients with inflammatory bowel diseases via TNF receptor 2 and intestinal CD14+ macrophages. Gastroenterology 2011;141: 2026–2038.
18 Wajant H, Pfizenmaier K, Scheurich P: Tumor necrosis factor signaling. Cell Death Differ 2003;10:45–65.
19 Grell M, Douni E, Wajant H, Löhden M, Clauss M, Maxeiner B, Georgopoulos S, Lesslauer W, Kollias G, Pfizenmaier K, Scheurich P: The transmembrane form of tumor necrosis factor is the prime activating ligand of the 80 kDa tumor necrosis factor receptor. Cell 1995;83: 793–802.
20 Black RA, Rauch CT, Kozlosky CJ, Peschon JJ, Slack JL, Wolfson MF, Castner BJ, Stocking KL, Reddy P, Srinivasan S, Nelson N, Boiani N, Schooley KA, Gerhart M, Davis R, Fitzner JN, Johnson RS, Paxton RJ, March CJ, Cerretti DP: A metalloproteinase disintegrin that releases tumour-necrosis factor-alpha from cells. Nature 1997;385:729–733.
21 Brynskov J, Foegh P, Pedersen G, Ellervik C, Kirkegaard T, Bingham A, Saermark T: Tumour necrosis factor alpha converting enzyme (TACE) activity in the colonic mucosa of patients with inflammatory bowel disease. Gut 2002;51: 37–43.
22 Bazzoni F, Beutler B: The tumor necrosis factor ligand and receptor families. N Engl J Med 1996;334:1717–1725.
23 Grell M, Wajant H, Zimmermann G, Scheurich P: The type 1 receptor (CD120a) is the high-affinity receptor for soluble tumor necrosis factor. Proc Natl Acad Sci U S A 1998;95:570–575.
24 Waetzig GH, Seegert D, Rosenstiel P, Nikolaus S, Schreiber S: p38 mitogen-activated protein kinase is activated and linked to TNF-alpha signaling in inflammatory bowel disease. J Immunol 2002; 168:5342–5351.
25 Eissner G, Kolch W, Scheurich P: Ligands working as receptors: reverse signaling by members of the TNF superfamily enhance the plasticity of the immune system. Cytokine Growth Factor Rev 2004;15:353–366.
26 Horiuchi T, Mitoma H, Harashima S, Tsukamoto H, Shimoda T: Transmembrane TNF-alpha: structure, function and interaction with anti-TNF agents. Rheumatology (Oxford) 2010;49:1215–1228.
27 Corazza N, Brunner T, Buri C, Rihs S, Imboden MA, Seibold I, Mueller C: Transmembrane tumor necrosis factor is a potent inducer of colitis even in the absence of its secreted form. Gastroenterology 2004;127:816–825.
28 Perrier C, de Hertogh G, Cremer J, Vermeire S, Rutgeerts P, Van Assche G, Szymkowski DE, Ceuppens JL: Neutralization of membrane TNF, but not soluble TNF, is crucial for the treatment of experimental colitis. Inflamm Bowel Dis 2013;19:246–253.
29 Ware CF, Crowe PD, Grayson MH, Androlewicz MJ, Browning JL: Expression of surface lymphotoxin and tumor necrosis factor on activated T, B, and natural killer cells. J Immunol 1992;149: 3881–3888.
30 Holtmann MH, Douni E, Schütz M, Zeller G, Mudter J, Lehr HA, Gerspach J, Scheurich P, Galle PR, Kollias G, Neurath MF: Tumor necrosis factor-receptor 2 is up-regulated on lamina propria T cells in Crohn's disease and promotes experimental colitis in vivo. Eur J Immunol 2002;32:3142–3151.

31 Mizoguchi E, Mizoguchi A, Takedatsu H, Cario E, de Jong YP, Ooi CJ, Xavier RJ, Terhorst C, Podolsky DK, Bhan AK: Role of tumor necrosis factor receptor 2 (TNFR2) in colonic epithelial hyperplasia and chronic intestinal inflammation in mice. Gastroenterology 2002;122: 134–144.
32 Owczarek D, Cibor D, Głowacki MK, Cieśla A, Mach P: TNF-α and soluble forms of TNF receptors 1 and 2 in the serum of patients with Crohn's disease and ulcerative colitis. Pol Arch Med Wewn 2012;122:616–623.
33 Pierik M, Vermeire S, Steen KV, Joossens S, Claessens G, Vlietinck R, Rutgeerts P: Tumour necrosis factor-alpha receptor 1 and 2 polymorphisms in inflammatory bowel disease and their association with response to infliximab. Aliment Pharmacol Ther 2004;20:303–310.
34 Bruewer M, Luegering A, Kucharzik T, Parkos CA, Madara JL, Hopkins AM, Nusrat A: Proinflammatory cytokines disrupt epithelial barrier function by apoptosis-independent mechanisms. J Immunol 2003;171:6164–6172.
35 Dayer Schneider J, Seibold I, Saxer-Sekulic N, Paredes BE, Saurer L, Mueller C: Lack of TNFR2 expression by CD4(+) T cells exacerbates experimental colitis. Eur J Immunol 2009;39:1743–1753.
36 Mitoma H, Horiuchi T, Tsukamoto H: Binding activities of infliximab and etanercept to transmembrane tumor necrosis factor-alpha. Gastroenterology 2004;126:934–935.
37 Arora T, Padaki R, Liu L, Hamburger AE, Ellison AR, Stevens SR, Louie JS, Kohno T: Differences in binding and effector functions between classes of TNF antagonists. Cytokine 2009;45: 124–131.
38 Kaymakcalan Z, Sakorafas P, Bose S, Scesney S, Xiong L, Hanzatian DK, Salfeld J, Sasso EH: Comparisons of affinities, avidities, and complement activation of adalimumab, infliximab, and etanercept in binding to soluble and membrane tumor necrosis factor. Clin Immunol 2009;131:308–316.
39 Nesbitt A, Fossati G, Bergin M, Stephens P, Stephens S, Foulkes R, Brown D, Robinson M, Bourne T: Mechanism of action of certolizumab pegol (CDP870): in vitro comparison with other anti-tumor necrosis factor alpha agents. Inflamm Bowel Dis 2007;13:1323–1332.
40 Santora LC, Kaymakcalan Z, Sakorafas P, Krull IS, Grant K: Characterization of noncovalent complexes of recombinant human monoclonal antibody and antigen using cation exchange, size exclusion chromatography, and BIAcore. Anal Biochem 2001;299:119–129.
41 Scallon B, Cai A, Solowski N, Rosenberg A, Song XY, Shealy D, Wagner C: Binding and functional comparisons of two types of tumor necrosis factor antagonists. J Pharmacol Exp Ther 2002;301: 418–426.
42 Tracey D, Klareskog L, Sasso EH, Salfeld JG, Tak PP: Tumor necrosis factor antagonist mechanisms of action: a comprehensive review. Pharmacol Ther 2008;117:244–279.
43 Friedmann E, Hauben E, Maylandt K, Schleeger S, Vreugde S, Lichtenthaler SF, Kuhn PH, Stauffer D, Rovelli G, Martoglio B: SPPL2a and SPPL2b promote intramembrane proteolysis of TNFalpha in activated dendritic cells to trigger IL-12 production. Nat Cell Biol 2006;8:843–848.
44 Mitoma H, Horiuchi T, Hatta N, Tsukamoto H, Harashima S, Kikuchi Y, Otsuka J, Okamura S, Fujita S, Harada M: Infliximab induces potent anti-inflammatory responses by outside-to-inside signals through transmembrane TNF-alpha. Gastroenterology 2005;128:376–392.
45 Shen C, Assche GV, Colpaert S, Maerten P, Geboes K, Rutgeerts P, Ceuppens JL: Adalimumab induces apoptosis of human monocytes: a comparative study with infliximab and etanercept. Aliment Pharmacol Ther 2005;21:251–258.
46 Van den Brande JM, Braat H, van den Brink GR, Versteeg HH, Bauer CA, Hoedemaeker I, van Montfrans C, Hommes DW, Peppelenbosch MP, van Deventer SJ: Infliximab but not etanercept induces apoptosis in lamina propria T-lymphocytes from patients with Crohn's disease. Gastroenterology 2003;124: 1774–1785.
47 Danese S, Sans M, Scaldaferri F, Sgambato A, Rutella S, Cittadini A, Piqué JM, Panes J, Katz JA, Gasbarrini A, Fiocchi C: TNF-alpha blockade down-regulates the CD40/CD40L pathway in the mucosal microcirculation: a novel anti-inflammatory mechanism of infliximab in Crohn's disease. J Immunol 2006;176: 2617–2624.
48 Di Sabatino A, Pender SL, Jackson CL, Prothero JD, Gordon JN, Picariello L, Rovedatti L, Docena G, Monteleone G, Rampton DS, Tonelli F, Corazza GR, MacDonald TT: Functional modulation of Crohn's disease myofibroblasts by anti-tumor necrosis factor antibodies. Gastroenterology 2007;133:137–149.
49 Ricciardelli I, Lindley KJ, Londei M, Quaratino S: Anti tumour necrosis-alpha therapy increases the number of FOXP3 regulatory T cells in children affected by Crohn's disease. Immunology 2008;125:178–183.
50 Vos AC, Wildenberg ME, Duijvestein M, Verhaar AP, van den Brink GR, Hommes DW: Anti-tumor necrosis factor-α antibodies induce regulatory macrophages in an Fc region-dependent manner. Gastroenterology 2011;140:221–230.
51 Wong M, Ziring D, Korin Y, Desai S, Kim S, Lin J, Gjertson D, Braun J, Reed E, Singh RR: TNFalpha blockade in human diseases: mechanisms and future directions. Clin Immunol 2008;126: 121–136.
52 Ringheanu M, Daum F, Markowitz J, Levine J, Katz S, Lin X, Silver J: Effects of infliximab on apoptosis and reverse signaling of monocytes from healthy individuals and patients with Crohn's disease. Inflamm Bowel Dis 2004;10: 801–810.
53 Agnholt J, Kaltoft K: Infliximab down-regulates interferon-gamma production in activated gut T-lymphocytes from patients with Crohn's disease. Cytokine 2001;15:212–222.
54 Waetzig GH, Seegert D, Rosenstiel P, Nikolaus S, Schreiber S: p38 mitogen-activated protein kinase is activated and linked to TNF-alpha signaling in inflammatory bowel disease. J Immunol 2002; 168:5342–5351.
55 Waetzig GH, Rosenstiel P, Nikolaus S, Seegert D, Schreiber S: Differential p38 mitogen-activated protein kinase target phosphorylation in responders and non-responders to infliximab. Gastroenterology 2003;125:633–634.
56 Derer S, Till A, Haesler R, Sina C, Grabe N, Jung S, Nikolaus S, Kuehbacher T, Groetzinger J, Rose-John S, Rosenstiel PC, Schreiber S: mTNF reverse signaling induced by TNFα antagonists involves a GDF-1 dependent pathway: implications for Crohn's disease. Gut 2013;62:376–386.

57 Mitoma H, Horiuchi T, Tsukamoto H, Tamimoto Y, Kimoto Y, Uchino A, To K, Harashima S, Hatta N, Harada M: Mechanisms for cytotoxic effects of anti-tumor necrosis factor agents on transmembrane tumor necrosis factor alpha-expressing cells: comparison among infliximab, etanercept, and adalimumab. Arthritis Rheum 2008;58:1248–1257.

58 Shohet JM, Pemberton P, Carroll MC: Identification of a major binding site for complement C3 on the IgG1 heavy chain. J Biol Chem 1993;268:5866–5871.

59 Ueda N, Tsukamoto H, Mitoma H, Ayano M, Tanaka A, Ohta S, Inoue Y, Arinobu Y, Niiro H, Akashi K, Horiuchi T: The cytotoxic effects of certolizumab pegol and golimumab mediated by transmembrane tumor necrosis factor α. Inflamm Bowel Dis 2013;19:1224–1231.

60 Atreya R, Neurath MF: New therapeutic strategies for treatment of inflammatory bowel disease. Mucosal Immunol 2008; 1:175–182.

61 Neurath MF: Cytokines in inflammatory bowel disease. Nat Rev Immunol 2014; 14:329–342.

62 Boirivant M, Marini M, Di Felice G, Pronio AM, Montesani C, Tersigni R, Strober W: Lamina propria T cells in Crohn's disease and other gastrointestinal inflammation show defective CD2 pathway-induced apoptosis. Gastroenterology 1999;116:557–565.

63 Ina K, Itoh J, Fukushima K, Kusugami K, Yamaguchi T, Kyokane K, Imada A, Binion DG, Musso A, West GA, Dobrea GM, McCormick TS, Lapetina EG, Levine AD, Ottaway CA, Fiocchi C: Resistance of Crohn's disease T cells to multiple apoptotic signals is associated with a Bcl-2/Bax mucosal imbalance. J Immunol 1999;163:1081–1090.

64 Atreya R, Mudter J, Finotto S, Müllberg J, Jostock T, Wirtz S, Schütz M, Bartsch B, Holtmann M, Becker C, Strand D, Czaja J, Schlaak JF, Lehr HA, Autschbach F, Schürmann G, Nishimoto N, Yoshizaki K, Ito H, Kishimoto T, Galle PR, Rose-John S, Neurath MF: Blockade of interleukin 6 trans signaling suppresses T-cell resistance against apoptosis in chronic intestinal inflammation: evidence in Crohn disease and experimental colitis in vivo. Nat Med 2000;6: 583–588.

65 Van den Brande JM, Koehler TC, Zelinkova Z, Bennink RJ, te Velde AA, ten Cate FJ, van Deventer SJ, Peppelenbosch MP, Hommes DW: Prediction of antitumour necrosis factor clinical efficacy by real-time visualisation of apoptosis in patients with Crohn's disease. Gut 2007; 56:509–517.

66 Lügering A, Schmidt M, Lügering N, Pauels HG, Domschke W, Kucharzik T: Infliximab induces apoptosis in monocytes from patients with chronic active Crohn's disease by using a caspase-dependent pathway. Gastroenterology 2001;121:1145–1157.

67 Shen C, Van Assche G, Rutgeerts P, Ceuppens JL: Caspase activation and apoptosis induction by adalimumab: demonstration in vitro and in vivo in a chimeric mouse model. Inflamm Bowel Dis 2006;12:22–28.

68 Atreya R, Neumann H, Neufert C, Waldner MJ, Billmeier U, Zopf Y, Willma M, App C, Münster T, Kessler H, Maas S, Gebhardt B, Heimke-Brinck R, Reuter E, Dörje F, Rau TT, Uter W, Wang TD, Kiesslich R, Vieth M, Hannappel E, Neurath MF: In vivo imaging using fluorescent antibodies to tumor necrosis factor predicts therapeutic response in Crohn's disease. Nat Med 2014;20:313–318.

Raja Atreya
Medical Clinic 1, Friedrich-Alexander University Erlangen-Nürnberg
Ulmenweg 18
DE–91054 Erlangen (Germany)
E-Mail raja.atreya@uk-erlangen.de

Rogler G, Herfarth H, Hibi T, Nielsen OH (eds): Anti-Tumor Necrosis Factor Therapy in Inflammatory Bowel Disease.
Front Gastrointest Res. Basel, Karger, 2015, vol 34, pp 73–82 (DOI: 10.1159/000381445)

Apoptosis of T Cells and Monocytes

Torsten Kucharzik

Department of General Medicine and Gastroenterology, Lüneburg Hospital, University of Hamburg, Hamburg, Germany

Abstract

Defective apoptosis of mucosal cell populations seems to be a relevant pathogenetic mechanism in inflammatory bowel disease (IBD). Consequently, it has been suggested that induction of apoptosis in various effector cells may be a relevant therapeutic mechanism in IBD. Indeed, it was shown that different drugs used for treatment of IBD have the capacity to induce apoptosis in T cells or monocytes in vitro and in vivo. The clinical relevance of these findings has remained questionable so far. TNF-α is one of the most relevant proinflammatory mediators in IBD, and anti-TNF treatment has been shown to be of particular benefit for patients with IBD. During the last couple of years, it was shown that various anti-TNF agents can induce apoptosis in activated monocytes and lymphocytes in vitro and in vivo. This mechanism requires reverse signaling via transmembranous TNF, thereby eliciting a signal transduction cascade that results in programmed cell death. Although other mechanisms might also contribute to the clinical effect of anti-TNF, current data suggest that apoptosis induction in mononuclear cells is associated with clinical efficacy of anti-TNF agents. As apoptosis induction in activated monocytes or T cells may be regarded as an important therapeutic mechanism for anti-TNF agents in IBD and other chronic inflammatory disorders, identification of mechanisms that target apoptotic pathways might result in future therapeutic strategies for IBD.

Introduction

Inflammatory bowel disease (IBD) is characterized by a dense infiltrate of mucosal cells that mainly consist of activated T cells and macrophages.

Extensive studies over the last few decades have shown that activated T cells [1, 2] as well as monocytes and macrophages [3, 4] play an intriguing role in the pathogenesis of IBD. Increased proliferation or insufficient apoptosis might contribute to increased numbers of inflammatory cells in IBD mucosa. Apoptosis is involved in the regulation and function of the immune system and also in the removal of potentially harmful cells. Dysfunction or dysregulation of the apoptotic program has been implicated in multiple immune disorders, including rheumatoid arthritis (RA). In addition, there is more and more evidence that intrinsic defects in

Table 1. Induction of apoptosis by different therapeutics used in IBD

Therapeutic agent in IBD	Targeted cell population	Reference(s)
Steroids	monocytes, lymphocytes	Schmidt et al. [11], Schmidt et al. [12]
Sulfasalazine	lymphocytes	Doering et al. [10]
Infliximab	monocytes, lymphocytes	Lugering et al. [14], Van den Brande et al. [41], Di Sabatino et al. [45], Van den Brande et al. [47]
Adalimumab	monocytes, lymphocytes	Shen et al. [40], Atreya et al. [49]
Golimumab	monocytes, lymphocytes	Ueda et al. [50]
Methotrexate	lymphocytes	Genestier et al. [16], Cutolo et al. [17], Nielsen et al. [69]
Azathioprine	lymphocytes	Tiede et al. [15]
Cyclosporine	lymphocytes	Naujokat et al. [18], Steiner et al. [70]
Tacrolimus	lymphocytes	Migita et al. [19]
Thalidomide	monocytes	Gockel et al. [20], Panousis et al. [71]

the control of programmed cell death in the mucosal compartment are implicated in the pathogenesis of IBD [5–9]. The properties of apoptosis induction in the lamina propria T cells of patients with Crohn's disease (CD) or ulcerative colitis have been determined, and it was shown that mucosal T cells are highly resistant to apoptosis [8, 10]. As apoptosis of activated T cells is an important mechanism of peripheral immune tolerance, these findings may explain the chronicity and perpetuation of inflammatory reactions in IBD mucosa. Recent observations suggest that the apoptosis defect in mucosal T cells in CD occurs at the level of the mitochondria, in the intrinsic pathway of apoptosis [9]. As defective apoptosis of mucosal cell populations appears to be an important pathogenetic mechanism for mucosal inflammation in IBD, it has been speculated that removal of potentially harmful cells by induction of apoptosis might be a therapeutic tool in IBD.

Over the last few years, various therapeutic agents have therefore been examined regarding their capacity to induce apoptosis in effector cell populations in IBD. It was shown that most agents used for IBD treatment, such as steroids [11, 12], sulfasalazine [10], infliximab [13, 14], azathioprine [15], methotrexate [16, 17], cyclosporine [18], tacrolimus [19] and thalidomide [20], have the capacity to induce apoptosis in monocytes or lymphocytes (table 1). Different molecular apoptotic pathways seem to be utilized by different drugs, which might explain the differential therapeutic effects of these agents.

Although a variety of in vitro studies have shown that apoptosis can be induced in lymphocytes and monocytes by various drugs used in IBD, it remains unclear whether apoptosis also occurs in vivo and, more importantly, if induction of apoptosis is indeed the integral effect of these drugs.

TNF-α is one of the predominant proinflammatory mediators of inflammation in IBD, and induction of apoptosis has been intensively investigated for different anti-TNF agents during the last couple of years. This chapter will focus on the role of anti-TNF agents and their capacity to induce apoptosis in lymphocytes and monocytes as well as the importance of anti-TNF-induced apoptosis as a relevant mechanism of action in IBD.

Anti-TNF Agents in the Treatment of Inflammatory Bowel Disease

Multiple studies over the last few decades provided evidence that TNF is a crucial proinflammatory cytokine in various inflammatory disorders, and it has therefore been targeted therapeutically [21–23]. The initial form of TNF is a 26 kDa transmembrane protein (transmembrane TNF, or mTNF). After cleavage from the cell surface by a metalloproteinase called TNF-α-converting enzyme, TNF is released as a 17 kDa protein (soluble TNF, or sTNF). After trimerization, it binds to two different receptors: TNF receptor (TNF-R) I (p55), the primary receptor for sTNF, which is constitutively expressed by most cell types, and TNF-RII (p75), the main receptor for mTNF, which is expressed in a highly regulated manner [24]. TNF is predominantly expressed by tissue macrophages and T cells and stimulates inflammation by activating gene transcription through IKK/NF-kB and JNK/AP-1 signaling, thereby inducing cytokine and chemokine expression, among other effects.

In CD, the lamina propria of the gut contains abundant TNF-producing cells, and increased concentrations of TNF have also been found in the stool of children with CD [25, 26]. The in vivo action of TNF-α seems pleiotropic and may also be relevant to the pathogenesis of IBD [27, 28]. Different therapeutic strategies, such as the use of steroids, pentoxifylline, and thalidomide, have been shown to reduce TNF expression in various models [29–32]. As an example of a small molecule with TNF-inhibiting functions, thalidomide has proven effective in the therapy of refractory CD but is seldom used because of its severe side effects [33–35].

For the past 20 years, various anti-TNF agents have been established for the treatment of IBD. The first was infliximab, a chimeric antibody specific for human TNF that was generated by grafting a mouse Fab region into a 75% human IgG1 constant region. This was followed by other anti-TNF agents, such as adalimumab, certolizumab and golimumab, which all appear to have more or less clinical efficacy in IBD.

Other anti-TNF agents, such as onercept, CDP571 and the TNF-R fusion protein etanercept, never played a significant role in IBD treatment because of a lack of data on clinical efficacy.

Although the current clinical data do not allow a final comparison regarding the efficacy of the different anti-TNF reagents, it can be concluded that (I.) anti-TNF antibodies are efficient in the therapy of CD and ulcerative colitis and that (II.) in contrast to RA, receptor-binding approaches are inefficient in these conditions, even though the receptor fusion-protein constructs are capable of binding sTNF as well as membrane-bound TNF. These observations suggest that mere neutralization of TNF is not the only therapeutic effect and that different mechanisms might be involved in IBD and RA.

Induction of Apoptosis by Anti-TNF Action in vitro and in vivo

Much data, such as data on the clinical inefficacy of receptor-fusion constructs as well as on long-lasting therapeutic effects, suggest that anti-TNF therapy is based on more than mere neutralization of sTNF and also exerts its function through different mechanisms. Indeed, multiple studies showed that anti-TNF antibodies are likely to directly interact with different cellular subsets of the immune system, such as monocytes, lymphocytes and epithelial cells, and various molecular mechanisms have been described recently.

Multiple observations over the last few decades have indicated that programmed cell death plays a central role during the development of organisms [36]. Apoptosis is a relevant mechanism in the function of the immune system, and various data have shown that dysregulation of apoptotic cell death may be a relevant mechanism in inflammatory disorders such as RA [37]. Similarly, several reports suggested that mucosal T cells found in the inflamed mucosa of CD patients are resistant to apoptotic stimuli [5, 6, 9]. Therefore, proapoptotic stimulation seems to be an intriguing therapeutic mechanism. Indeed, early studies analyzing the lamina propria cellular infiltrate after infliximab challenge showed a significant loss

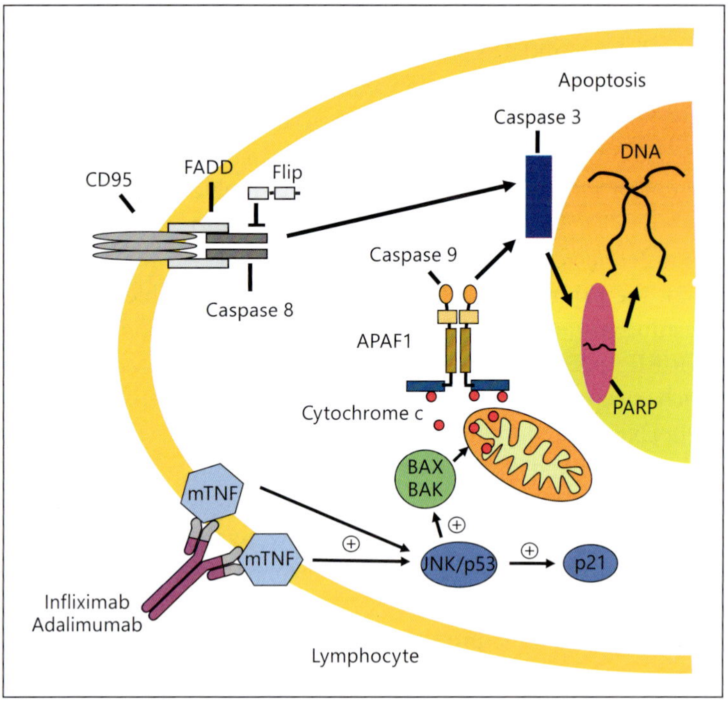

Fig. 1. Apoptosis induction by reverse signaling. Apoptosis induced by anti-TNF agents in lymphocytes and monocytes is linked to reverse signaling of transmembrane TNF, thereby inducing JNK/p53 activation, resulting in the mitochondrial pathway of apoptosis. Fas ligation is not involved in this apoptotic process.

of CD68+ monocytes as well as CD4+ and CD8+ T lymphocytes [38]. A later report by our group showed that infliximab induces apoptosis in freshly isolated monocytes [14]. Corresponding observations were found by Waetzig et al. [39]. The induction of apoptosis does not seem to require the Fas/FasL signal transduction pathway, but rather involves upregulation of Bax/Bak, followed by mitochondrial release of cytochrome c (fig. 1). Shen et al. recently extended these observations by showing that the humanized anti-TNF antibody adalimumab is also capable of inducing monocyte apoptosis, whereas the recombinant fusion protein etanercept is not [40]. Additionally, there is convincing in vitro evidence that the anti-TNF antibody infliximab induces monocyte apoptosis. Similarly, in vitro induction of T cell apoptosis by infliximab in peripheral blood lymphocytes as well as in lamina propria lymphocytes was shown by ten Hove et al. [13] and confirmed by others [41–43]. Induction of apoptosis mainly occurs in the inflamed tissue of IBD patients, rather than in uninflamed tissue, suggesting that upregulation or increased expression of TNF on inflamed cells is required for the apoptotic process [44]. As apoptosis is supposed to rapidly occur in vivo, this mechanism would explain the fast therapeutic effect of anti-TNF agents seen in CD and also the observation that in some patients, therapeutic effects extend far beyond the circulating half-life of the antibody. However, the nature of the process also makes it difficult to analyze the process more carefully in vivo and to correlate it with therapeutic effects. Corresponding to the observations found in monocytes, the effect was absent when cells were incubated with etanercept, suggesting that the lack of efficacy of this reagent in the treatment of CD might be related to the induction of apoptosis. Further confirming these observations, one report showed that the reduced rate of apoptotic T cells found in the lamina propria of patients suffering from active CD is reverted after infliximab treatment [45], although the results not only potentially reflect direct apoptotic effects but also might include other immunomodulatory effects 10 weeks after drug administration. In vivo induction of apoptosis could be demonstrated for adalimumab in a chimeric mouse model [46]. A successful approach to detect in vivo apoptosis after anti-TNF treatment in humans was demonstrated by van den Brande et al., who employed scintigraphic annexin V labeling [47]. An observation that does not fit within this view is that the soluble Fab fragment certolizumab, which has been shown to exert anti-inflammatory effects in patients with CD, does not appear to induce apoptosis in mononuclear cells in vitro [48]. However, data from other groups could not confirm these observations [49]. In addition, in our own hands, Fab fragments from infliximab exert even stronger proapoptotic effects on monocytes, suggesting that the Fc part of the antibody is not required for apoptosis induction [14].

Mechanisms of Anti-TNF-Induced Apoptosis

There is ample evidence that the immunosuppressive efficacy of anti-TNF agents (infliximab, adalimumab and golimumab) not only is mediated by binding of sTNF but also involves direct interference with intracellular signaling events, a process described as 'reverse signaling' [43, 50, 51]. Initially, the conservation of the cytoplasmatic part of mTNF across various species suggested that the transmembrane ligand might transduce bidirectional signals [52], and further observations demonstrated that a dimeric form of the type I sTNF receptor is indeed able to dephosphorylate mTNF. Binding of the sTNF receptor to mTNF induced an increase in intracellular calcium levels [53], further substantiating the presence of an associated signaling pathway, in a macrophage cell line. More recent data showed that reverse signaling might serve as a silencing signal, as monocytes were found to be resistant to lipopolysaccharide (LPS) stimulation after incubation with TNF-binding agents [54, 55]. Mitoma et al. showed that stably transfected Jurkat T cells constitutively expressing mutant forms of mTNF undergo apoptosis after incubation with infliximab, suggesting that this effector mechanism, described in earlier reports, is linked to reverse signaling [43]. The induction of apoptosis was associated with induced interleukin-10 production and G0/G1 cycle arrest, and all events were inhibited by substitution of the intracytoplasmatic serine residues of mTNF. A detailed analysis of intracellular signaling pathways showed upregulation of Bax, Bak and $p21^{WAF/CIP1}$ and phosphorylation of c-JUN kinase. In contrast, etanercept was not capable of inducing similar events, whereas two TNF-binding reagents induced E-selectin expression, indicating that at least two different signal transduction pathways are involved. The data also confirm previous results obtained from peripheral and lamina propria T cells regarding induction of apoptosis [41] and further extend these observations, as effects mediated by TNF-RI and TNF-RII can be excluded.

The finding of apoptosis induction in lymphocytes by anti-TNF and exploration of the underlying mechanisms was recently extended by the observation that different clinically effective anti-TNF antibodies are able to induce T cell apoptosis in IBD only when mucosal TNF-R2(+) T cells are cocultured with mTNF-expressing CD14(+) macrophages [49]. The finding that anti-TNF antibodies induce apoptosis indirectly by targeting the mTNF/TNF-R2 pathway may have important implications for the development of new therapeutic strategies in IBD.

In a different setting, Kirchner et al. demonstrated that anti-TNF reagents also potentially exert their effects on monocytes through two different mechanisms [54]: whereas the secretion of 'death factor x' by monocytes after LPS stimulation was dependent on protein kinase C, the secretion of LPS-induced cytokines was not. Interestingly, the latter was not observed after incubation with etanercept, whereas the anti-TNF antibodies 195F and infliximab as well as etanercept suppressed the release of endothelial apoptotic factors.

Mitoma et al. recently demonstrated that JNK activation might be crucial for cellular responses to infliximab. In their publication, MAPK activation was shown in transfected Jurkat T cells, and induction of apoptosis after infliximab challenge correlated with JNK phosphorylation, whereas both phenomena were absent after incubation with etanercept [43]. Our group recently showed that another anti-TNF agent, thalidomide, which is also capable of inducing monocyte apoptosis, is associated with activation of Act1, while JNK1/2, p38 and ERK1/2 remain unaffected [20]. It therefore appears likely that different proapoptotic anti-TNF agents use different signaling pathways that all result in programmed cell death.

Among the various possible routes, one probable pathway for the proapoptotic action of TNF-α antagonists in IBD could be related to inhibited expression of the FLIP and NF-kB proteins, which are abundant in IBD and other chronic inflammatory disorders, such as RA, and which are fundamental to the process of inflammation. Upregulation of the FLIP and NF-kB proteins confers the ability to induce apoptosis in various cell populations and has been identified in IBD as well as in RA patients [56–59].

Are Apoptosis-Related Mechanisms Relevant to the Clinical Efficacy of Anti-TNF Agents?

Several groups have convincingly shown that anti-TNF agents such as infliximab, adalimumab and golimumab can induce apoptosis in monocytes and lymphocytes in vitro and in vivo. However, the relevant question is whether the apoptosis-related mechanisms associated with these agents are important for the clinical efficacy of these drugs. This question is difficult to answer, as there is no simple method to quantify apoptosis in vivo, given that dying cells are usually rapidly removed by macrophages.

Hlavaty et al. developed an apoptotic pharmacogenetic index as a clinical predictor of a response to infliximab treatment. The apoptotic index was based on well-characterized polymorphisms in Fas, Fas ligand and caspase 9, which are known to be associated with low apoptotic activity. With this technique, the authors were able to demonstrate that the response to treatment positively correlates with apoptosis, while nonresponse is associated with a low apoptotic index [60]. These data suggest that apoptosis is indeed linked to the clinical response to anti-TNF agents. The view that induction of apoptosis of mTNF-expressing cells has clinical implications has recently been further confirmed by the observation that the number of mTNF-expressing cells, as determined by confocal laser endomicroscopy, correlates with clinical responses to anti-TNF treatment [61].

Considering these observations, there seems to be a simple link between the capacity for induction of apoptosis in lymphocytes or monocytes and clinical efficacy in IBD: anti-TNF agents, such as infliximab and adalimumab, that have clinical efficacy in IBD exert strong proapoptotic effects. In contrast, etanercept, which has been reported not to induce apoptosis in monocytes and lymphocytes, has no clinical efficacy in IBD (table 2). However, the situation is more complex. Other authors showed that the TNF-R fusion protein sTNF receptor I, also exerts proapoptotic effects in monocytes via reverse signaling [62]. These data raise the question of why receptor fusion proteins are not efficacious in CD, even though they have proapoptotic properties. In addition, recent data have shown that certolizumab, which exhibits clinical efficacy in CD, does not induce apoptosis in immune cells, even though it had even higher TNF-binding capacities compared to infliximab in these studies [63]. These data suggest that apoptosis is not required for clinical efficacy.

Table 2. Correlation of the clinical efficacy of various anti-TNF agents in IBD with the capacity to induce apoptosis

Anti-TNF agent	Binds to sTNF-α	Binds to mTNF-α	Monocyte apoptosis	Lymphocyte apoptosis	Clinical response in CD	Clinical response in UC	Reference(s)
Infliximab	+++	+++	+++	+++	+++	+++	Lugering et al. [14], Van den Brande et al. [41], Atreya et al. [49], ten Hove et al. [13], Mitoma et al. [43], Di Sabatino et al. [45], Van den Brande et al. [47]
Adalimumab	+++	+++	+++	+++	+++	+++	Atreya et al. [49], Mitoma et al. [43], Shen et al. [46]
Etanercept	+++	+	+/–	+/–	–	n.d.	Van den Brande et al. [41], Mitoma et al. [43]
Onercept	+++	+++	yes	n.d.	–	n.d.	Waetzig et al. [62]
Certolizumab	+++	+++	no	no	++	n.d.	Nesbitt et al. [48], Atreya et al. [49], Ueda et al. [50]
Golimumab	+++	+++	+/–	+/–	n.d.	+++	Ueda et al. [50]
Thalidomide	+	+	yes	n.d.	+	n.d.	Gockel et al. [20]

n.d. = Not determined; UC = ulcerative colitis.

Other preliminary data have shown that immune cell apoptosis after infliximab treatment can be detected in responders as well as nonresponders, while phosphorylation of the p38 downstream effectors ATF-2 and Hsp27 differs between the two groups [64]. These results support the view that differential signaling via the p38 MAPK pathway, but not necessarily induction of apoptosis, might contribute to the diversity of responses to infliximab treatment.

Even more confusing and in contrast to data described earlier are reports suggesting that etanercept and infliximab induce apoptosis in macrophages, but not lymphocytes, in RA joints [65]. These data raise the question of whether macrophages and lymphocytes in RA behave differently compared to those in CD. In contrast, more recent data detected induction of lymphocyte apoptosis in RA patients, although there was high interindividual variation [66, 67].

In sum, even though there are more and more data suggesting that induction of apoptosis by anti-TNF drugs is at least in part linked to clinical efficacy in IBD, there are still many open questions, and it is conceivable that other mechanisms might also contribute to the clinical efficacy of anti-TNF agents.

As more and more biosimilars for anti-TNF drugs will be on the market over the next couple of years, implementation of standardized tests for evaluating the capacity to induce apoptosis in monocyte and lymphocyte populations has already been proposed, suggesting the importance of these mechanisms in drug efficacy [68].

Summary

Defects in the apoptosis of mucosal cell populations are an important factor in the pathogenesis of IBD. A variety of therapeutic agents that are used for the treatment of IBD have the capacity to induce apoptosis in immune cells, such as monocytes/macrophages and lymphocytes, in vitro. It has been shown that reverse signaling by transmembranous TNF is required for inducing a signaling cascade that results in apoptotic cell death. TNF fusion proteins such as etanercept do not induce reverse signaling, which may explain the clinical inefficacy of these drugs. It therefore appears likely that apoptosis is a relevant mechanism in anti-TNF treatment and also potentially in other drug treatments that are currently used in IBD. However, induction of apoptosis cannot explain every clinical feature of anti-TNF antibody treatment. In addition, results for different anti-TNF drugs regarding their capacity to induce apoptosis in different immune cells are partially inconclusive. It therefore appears likely that other mechanisms might also play an important mechanistic role. It is also conceivable that different anti-TNF agents act via different pathways.

The molecular apoptotic pathways that are affected by different drugs used in the treatment of IBD are likely to be different, which might explain the drugs' additional or even synergistic therapeutic effects.

Identification of underlying apoptotic pathways in the future might help to identify targets that may be used as therapeutic tools in IBD. This might also help to further identify predictors of response. As both monocytes/macrophages and T lymphocytes contribute substantially to the pathogenesis of mucosal inflammation in IBD, therapeutic induction of apoptosis may affect both of these cell populations. Further insight into the apoptotic pathways may also help to identify mechanisms that might explain primary anti-TNF-refractory IBD as a basis for new strategies for the treatment of patients with IBD.

References

1 Neurath MF, Finotto S, Glimcher LH: The role of Th1/Th2 polarization in mucosal immunity. Nat Med 2002;8:567–573.

2 Strober W, Fuss IJ, Blumberg RS: The immunology of mucosal models of inflammation. Annu Rev Immunol 2002; 20:495–549.

3 Rugtveit J, Nilsen EM, Bakka A, et al: Cytokine profiles differ in newly recruited and resident subsets of mucosal macrophages from inflammatory bowel disease. Gastroenterology 1997;112: 1493–1505.

4 Rogler G: Update in inflammatory bowel disease pathogenesis. Curr Opin Gastroenterol 2004;20:311–317.

5 Boirivant M, Marini M, Di Felice G, et al: Lamina propria T cells in Crohn's disease and other gastrointestinal inflammation show defective CD2 pathway-induced apoptosis. Gastroenterology 1999;116:557–565.

6 Ina K, Itoh J, Fukushima K, et al: Resistance of Crohn's disease T cells to multiple apoptotic signals is associated with a Bcl-2/Bax mucosal imbalance. J Immunol 1999;163:1081–1090.

7 Atreya R, Mudter J, Finotto S, et al: Blockade of interleukin 6 trans signaling suppresses T-cell resistance against apoptosis in chronic intestinal inflammation: evidence in crohn disease and experimental colitis in vivo. Nat Med 2000;6:583–588.

8 Itoh J, de La Motte C, Strong SA, et al: Decreased Bax expression by mucosal T cells favours resistance to apoptosis in Crohn's disease. Gut 2001;49:35–41.

9 Sturm A, Leite AZ, Danese S, et al: Divergent cell cycle kinetics underlie the distinct functional capacity of mucosal T cells in Crohn's disease and ulcerative colitis. Gut 2004;53:1624–1631.

10 Doering J, Begue B, Lentze MJ, et al: Induction of T lymphocyte apoptosis by sulphasalazine in patients with Crohn's disease. Gut 2004;53:1632–1638.

11 Schmidt M, Pauels HG, Lugering N, et al: Glucocorticoids induce apoptosis in human monocytes: potential role of IL-1 beta. J Immunol 1999;163:3484–3490.

12 Schmidt M, Lugering N, Lugering A, et al: Role of the CD95/CD95 ligand system in glucocorticoid-induced monocyte apoptosis. J Immunol 2001;166:1344–1351.

13 ten Hove T, van Montfrans C, Peppelenbosch MP, et al: Infliximab treatment induces apoptosis of lamina propria T lymphocytes in Crohn's disease. Gut 2002;50:206–211.

14 Lugering A, Schmidt M, Lugering N, et al: Infliximab induces apoptosis in monocytes from patients with chronic active Crohn's disease by using a caspase-dependent pathway. Gastroenterology 2001;121:1145–1157.

15 Tiede I, Fritz G, Strand S, et al: CD28-dependent Rac1 activation is the molecular target of azathioprine in primary human CD4+ T lymphocytes. J Clin Invest 2003;111:1133–1145.

16 Genestier L, Paillot R, Fournel S, et al: Immunosuppressive properties of methotrexate: apoptosis and clonal deletion of activated peripheral T cells. J Clin Invest 1998;102:322–328.

17 Cutolo M, Bisso A, Sulli A, et al: Antiproliferative and antiinflammatory effects of methotrexate on cultured differentiating myeloid monocytic cells (THP-1) but not on synovial macrophages from patients with rheumatoid arthritis. J Rheumatol 2000;27:2551–2557.

18 Naujokat C, Daniel V, Bauer TM, et al: Cell cycle- and activation-dependent regulation of cyclosporin A-induced T cell apoptosis. Biochem Biophys Res Commun 2003;310:347–354.
19 Migita K, Eguchi K: FK 506-mediated T-cell apoptosis induction. Transplant Proc 2001;33:2292–2293.
20 Gockel HR, Lugering A, Heidemann J, et al: Thalidomide induces apoptosis in human monocytes by using a cytochrome c-dependent pathway. J Immunol 2004;172:5103–5109.
21 Feldmann M, Maini RN: Anti-TNF alpha therapy of rheumatoid arthritis: what have we learned? Annu Rev Immunol 2001;19:163–196.
22 Rutgeerts P, Van Assche G, Vermeire S: Optimizing anti-TNF treatment in inflammatory bowel disease. Gastroenterology 2004;126:1593–1610.
23 Derkx B, Taminiau J, Radema S, et al: Tumour-necrosis-factor antibody treatment in Crohn's disease. Lancet 1993; 342:173–174.
24 Locksley RM, Killeen N, Lenardo MJ: The TNF and TNF receptor superfamilies: integrating mammalian biology. Cell 2001;104:487–501.
25 Breese EJ, Michie CA, Nicholls SW, et al: Tumor necrosis factor alpha-producing cells in the intestinal mucosa of children with inflammatory bowel disease. Gastroenterology 1994;106:1455–1466.
26 Nicholls S, Stephens S, Braegger CP, et al: Cytokines in stools of children with inflammatory bowel disease or infective diarrhoea. J Clin Pathol 1993;46:757–760.
27 Carlos TM, Harlan JM: Leukocyte-endothelial adhesion molecules. Blood 1994; 84:2068–2101.
28 Levi M, ten Cate H, van der Poll T, et al: Pathogenesis of disseminated intravascular coagulation in sepsis. JAMA 1993; 270:975–979.
29 Barnes PJ: Anti-inflammatory actions of glucocorticoids: molecular mechanisms. Clin Sci (Lond) 1998;94:557–572.
30 Diab-Assef M, Reimund JM, Ezenfis J, et al: The phosphodiesterase inhibitor, pentoxifylline, alters rat intestinal epithelial cell proliferation via changes in the expression of transforming growth factors. Scand J Gastroenterol 2002;37:206–214.
31 Reimund JM, Dumont S, Muller CD, et al: In vitro effects of oxpentifylline on inflammatory cytokine release in patients with inflammatory bowel disease. Gut 1997;40:475–480.
32 Bauditz J, Wedel S, Lochs H: Thalidomide reduces tumour necrosis factor alpha and interleukin 12 production in patients with chronic active Crohn's disease. Gut 2002;50:196–200.
33 Gordon JN, Goggin PM: Thalidomide and its derivatives: emerging from the wilderness. Postgrad Med J 2003;79: 127–132.
34 Ehrenpreis ED, Kane SV, Cohen LB, et al: Thalidomide therapy for patients with refractory Crohn's disease: an open-label trial. Gastroenterology 1999; 117:1271–1277.
35 Vasiliauskas EA, Kam LY, Abreu-Martin MT, et al: An open-label pilot study of low-dose thalidomide in chronically active, steroid-dependent Crohn's disease. Gastroenterology 1999;117:1278–1287.
36 Danial NN, Korsmeyer SJ: Cell death: critical control points. Cell 2004;116: 205–219.
37 Pope RM: Apoptosis as a therapeutic tool in rheumatoid arthritis. Nat Rev Immunol 2002;2:527–535.
38 Baert FJ, D'Haens GR, Peeters M, et al: Tumor necrosis factor alpha antibody (infliximab) therapy profoundly downregulates the inflammation in Crohn's ileocolitis. Gastroenterology 1999;116: 22–28.
39 Waetzig GH, Seegert D, Rosenstiel P, et al: p38 mitogen-activated protein kinase is activated and linked to TNF-alpha signaling in inflammatory bowel disease. J Immunol 2002;168:5342–5351.
40 Shen C, Assche GV, Colpaert S, et al: Adalimumab induces apoptosis of human monocytes: a comparative study with infliximab and etanercept. Aliment Pharmacol Ther 2005;21:251–258.
41 Van den Brande JM, Braat H, van den Brink GR, et al: Infliximab but not etanercept induces apoptosis in lamina propria T-lymphocytes from patients with Crohn's disease. Gastroenterology 2003; 124:1774–1785.
42 Di Sabatino A, Ciccocioppo R, Cinque B, et al: Defective mucosal T cell death is sustainably reverted by infliximab in a caspase dependent pathway in Crohn's disease. Gut 2004;53:70–77.
43 Mitoma H, Horiuchi T, Hatta N, et al: Infliximab induces potent anti-inflammatory responses by outside-to-inside signals through transmembrane TNF-alpha. Gastroenterology 2005;128:376–392.
44 Eder P, Lykowska-Szuber L, Krela-Kazmierczak I, et al: Anti-TNF antibodies do not induce the apoptosis of lamina propria mononuclear cells in uninflamed intestinal tissue in patients with Crohn's disease. Folia Histochem Cytobiol 2013;51:239–243.
45 Di Sabatino A, Ciccocioppo R, Benazzato L, et al: Infliximab downregulates basic fibroblast growth factor and vascular endothelial growth factor in Crohn's disease patients. Aliment Pharmacol Ther 2004;19:1019–1024.
46 Shen C, Van Assche G, Rutgeerts P, et al: Caspase activation and apoptosis induction by adalimumab: demonstration in vitro and in vivo in a chimeric mouse model. Inflamm Bowel Dis 2006;12:22–28.
47 Van den Brande JM, Koehler TC, Zelinkova Z, et al: Prediction of antitumour necrosis factor clinical efficacy by real-time visualisation of apoptosis in patients with Crohn's disease. Gut 2007; 56:509–517.
48 Nesbitt A, Fossati G, Bergin M, et al: Mechanism of action of certolizumab pegol (CDP870): in vitro comparison with other anti-tumor necrosis factor alpha agents. Inflamm Bowel Dis 2007; 13:1323–1332.
49 Atreya R, Zimmer M, Bartsch B, et al: Antibodies against tumor necrosis factor (TNF) induce T-cell apoptosis in patients with inflammatory bowel diseases via TNF receptor 2 and intestinal CD14(+) macrophages. Gastroenterology 2011;141:2026–2038.
50 Ueda N, Tsukamoto H, Mitoma H, et al: The cytotoxic effects of certolizumab pegol and golimumab mediated by transmembrane tumor necrosis factor alpha. Inflamm Bowel Dis 2013;19: 1224–1231.
51 Mitoma H, Horiuchi T, Tsukamoto H, et al: Mechanisms for cytotoxic effects of anti-tumor necrosis factor agents on transmembrane tumor necrosis factor alpha-expressing cells: comparison among infliximab, etanercept, and adalimumab. Arthritis Rheum 2008;58: 1248–1257.
52 Smith CA, Farrah T, Goodwin RG: The TNF receptor superfamily of cellular and viral proteins: activation, costimulation, and death. Cell 1994;76:959–962.

53 Watts AD, Hunt NH, Wanigasekara Y, et al: A casein kinase I motif present in the cytoplasmic domain of members of the tumour necrosis factor ligand family is implicated in 'reverse signalling'. EMBO J 1999;18:2119–2126.
54 Kirchner S, Holler E, Haffner S, et al: Effect of different tumor necrosis factor (TNF) reactive agents on reverse signaling of membrane integrated TNF in monocytes. Cytokine 2004;28:67–74.
55 Kirchner S, Boldt S, Kolch W, et al: LPS resistance in monocytic cells caused by reverse signaling through transmembrane TNF (mTNF) is mediated by the MAPK/ERK pathway. J Leukoc Biol 2004;75:324–331.
56 Monteleone I, Monteleone G, Fina D, et al: A functional role of flip in conferring resistance of Crohn's disease lamina propria lymphocytes to FAS-mediated apoptosis. Gastroenterology 2006;130: 389–397.
57 Caprioli F, Stolfi C, Caruso R, et al: Transcriptional and post-translational regulation of Flip, an inhibitor of Fas-mediated apoptosis, in human gut inflammation. Gut 2008;57:1674–1680.
58 Palao G, Santiago B, Galindo M, et al: Down-regulation of FLIP sensitizes rheumatoid synovial fibroblasts to Fas-mediated apoptosis. Arthritis Rheum 2004;50:2803–2810.
59 Schedel J, Gay RE, Kuenzler P, et al: FLICE-inhibitory protein expression in synovial fibroblasts and at sites of cartilage and bone erosion in rheumatoid arthritis. Arthritis Rheum 2002;46: 1512–1518.
60 Hlavaty T PM, Joossens S, Claessens G, Van Schuerbeek N, Rutgeerts P, Vermeire S: Prediction of response to infliximab in luminal and fistulizing Crohn's disease based on a decision making model using an apoptotic pharmacogenetic index and clinical predictors. Gastroenterology 2005;128:A309.
61 Atreya R, Neumann H, Neufert C, et al: In vivo imaging using fluorescent antibodies to tumor necrosis factor predicts therapeutic response in Crohn's disease. Nat Med 2014;20:313–318.
62 Waetzig GH, Rosenstiel P, Arlt A, et al: Soluble tumor necrosis factor (TNF) receptor-1 induces apoptosis via reverse TNF signaling and autocrine transforming growth factor-beta1. FASEB J 2005; 19:91–93.
63 Fossati G, Nebitt AM: Effect of the anti-TNF agents adalimumab, infliximab and certolizumab pegol on the induction of apoptosis in activated peripheral blood lymphocytes. Gastroenterology 2004; 128:A512.
64 Waetzig GH, Rosenstiel P, Nikolaus S, et al: Differential p38 mitogen-activated protein kinase target phosphorylation in responders and nonresponders to infliximab. Gastroenterology 2003;125:633–634; author reply 635–636.
65 Catrina AI, Trollmo C, af Klint E, et al: Evidence that anti-tumor necrosis factor therapy with both etanercept and infliximab induces apoptosis in macrophages, but not lymphocytes, in rheumatoid arthritis joints: extended report. Arthritis Rheum 2005;52:61–72.
66 Coury F, Ferraro-Peyret C, Le Cam S, et al: Peripheral blood lymphocytes from patients with rheumatoid arthritis are differentially sensitive to apoptosis induced by anti-tumour necrosis factor-alpha therapy. Clin Exp Rheumatol 2008;26:234–239.
67 Makrygiannakis D, Catrina AI: Apoptosis as a mechanism of action of tumor necrosis factor antagonists in rheumatoid arthritis. J Rheumatol 2012;39:679–685.
68 Urbano PC, Soccol VT, Azevedo VF: Apoptosis and the FLIP and NF-kappa B proteins as pharmacodynamic criteria for biosimilar TNF-alpha antagonists. Biologics 2014;8:211–220.
69 Nielsen CH, Albertsen L, Bendtzen K, et al: Methotrexate induces poly(ADP-ribose) polymerase-dependent, caspase 3-independent apoptosis in subsets of proliferating CD4+ T cells. Clin Exp Immunol 2007;148:288–295.
70 Steiner S, Daniel C, Fischer A, et al: Cyclosporine A regulates pro-inflammatory cytokine production in ulcerative colitis. Arch Immunol Ther Exp (Warsz) 2015;63:53–63.
71 Panousis K, Nikolaou VS, Tsaganos T, et al: Thalidomide prolongs survival after experimental musculoskeletal injury, through an effect on mononuclear apoptosis. J Surg Res 2014;188:198–205.

Torsten Kucharzik, MD, PhD
Department of General Medicine and Gastroenterology
Lüneburg Hospital, University of Hamburg, Bögelstrasse 1
DE–21339 Lueneburg (Germany)
E-Mail Torsten.Kucharzik@klinikum-lueneburg.de

Rogler G, Herfarth H, Hibi T, Nielsen OH (eds): Anti-Tumor Necrosis Factor Therapy in Inflammatory Bowel Disease.
Front Gastrointest Res. Basel, Karger, 2015, vol 34, pp 83–89 (DOI: 10.1159/000381446)

Neutralisation of Soluble Tumor Necrosis Factor

Erwin Dreesen · Ann Gils

Laboratory for Therapeutic and Diagnostic Antibodies, Department of Pharmaceutical and Pharmacological Sciences, KU Leuven, Leuven, Belgium

Abstract

The pleiotropic cytokine tumor necrosis factor-alpha (TNF) plays a pivotal role in the pathogenesis of inflammatory bowel disease (IBD). At physiological concentrations, TNF is beneficial in protecting the host against infections. At high concentrations, TNF increases inflammation, ultimately resulting in tissue damage. Increased TNF levels have been reported in the intestinal mucosa, serum and stool of patients with active IBD. Active soluble TNF exists as a homotrimer and preferentially binds to TNF receptor 1, thereby inducing the expression of a multitude of pro-inflammatory and cell survival genes. Neutralizing soluble TNF is an important therapeutic strategy. Currently, four anti-TNF biological agents are approved for the treatment of IBD. Infliximab (Remicade® and its two biosimilars, Inflectra™ and Remsima inflammatory burden), adalimumab (Humira®) and golimumab (Simponi®) are bivalent monoclonal antibodies. Certolizumab pegol (Cimzia®) is a PEGylated monovalent Fab antibody fragment. All four molecules have been shown to be effective for inducing and maintaining remission in IBD. The pharmacokinetic profile of biological agents is influenced by many patient-, disease- and drug-specific factors, such as body weight, concomitant immunosuppressive medication and immunogenicity. These inter- and intra-individual differences contribute to the problem of inadequate response and loss of response. Further insights into the pathophysiology of IBD and the pharmacokinetics of anti-TNF biological agents will contribute to therapeutic advances, such as the development of novel therapeutic strategies and the monitoring of pharmacological parameters (i.e. therapeutic drug monitoring).

Introduction

Inflammatory bowel disease (IBD) includes a spectrum of chronic inflammatory disorders of the gastrointestinal tract. Crohn's disease (CD) and ulcerative colitis (UC) are considered as the two extremes [1]. The etiology of IBD remains unclear. Genetic susceptibility and environmental factors lead to the development of an inflamed gastrointestinal tract, producing pro-inflammatory cytokines that further activate immune cells [2]. The pleiotropic cytokine tumor necrosis factor-alpha (TNF) plays a pivotal role in the pathogenesis of IBD. At physiological concentrations, the effect of TNF is beneficial since it augments host defense against infections. High concentrations, however, lead to excessive inflammation and consequent tissue damage [3]. Elevated TNF levels are found in the intestinal mucosa, serum and stool of patients with active IBD [4–9]. TNF drives the adaptive immune response, modulates immune cell function, triggers epithelial apoptosis, induces endothelial expression of adhesion molecules and regulates matrix metalloproteinase expression, ultimately leading to tissue degradation and damage [3, 10]. Neutralizing TNF has been proven to be very effective in the treatment of immune-mediated inflammatory disorders, including CD and UC [11].

Production of Soluble Tumor Necrosis Factor-Alpha

TNF is produced by a wide variety of cell types, including immune cells (e.g. lymphocytes, monocytes and macrophages) and nonimmune cells (e.g. endothelial cells, fibroblasts and smooth muscle cells). Initially, TNF is expressed on the cell surface as a transmembrane type II protein (tmTNF) composed of 233 amino acids (26 kDa) [12]. The extracellular domain can be released through enzymatic cleavage by TNF-converting enzyme (TACE), a disintegrin and metalloproteinase, hydrolyzing the Ala^{76}-Val^{77} bond [13]. The action of TACE results in shedding of the 157 amino-acid (17 kDa) soluble TNF monomer (sTNF) [14]. Both tmTNF and sTNF coexist as mono-, di- and trimers, but only the trimeric forms are biologically active [15].

Lymphotoxin-alpha (LTα) is a close homolog of trimeric sTNF. It is also a homotrimer, composed of 17 kDa monomers. Unlike TNF, LTα is not produced as a membrane-bound protein, but rather only exists in a secreted, soluble form.

Mechanism of Action

tmTNF and sTNF exert their biological activity by binding to two structurally distinct type I transmembrane TNF receptors (TNFRs) on target cells: the 55 kDa TNFR1 and the 75 kDa TNFR2. Virtually every cell type in the human body expresses TNFR1, whereas expression of TNFR2 is typically restricted to cells of the immune system [16]. TNFR1 is constitutively expressed, whereas expression of TNFR2 is subject to downstream regulation [16]. The receptors share an extracellular TNF-binding domain structure, although their affinities differ. sTNF exhibits 20 times higher affinity for TNFR1, whereas binding of sTNF to TNFR2 has rapid on and off kinetics [16, 17]. Therefore, TNFR2 might act as a 'ligand passer' for TNFR1, increasing the concentration of TNF at the cell surface [18]. tmTNF preferentially binds to TNFR2. Both receptors activate different intracellular signaling pathways to induce gene transcription. The cytoplasmic portion of TNFR1, but not TNFR2, contains a death domain [19, 20]. Binding of sTNF to TNFR1 activates the cytoplasmic-associated death domain protein [20], leading to the activation of nuclear factor kappaB (NFκB). NFκB is a transcription factor that drives expression of a multitude of pro-inflammatory and cell survival genes. Interleukin (IL)-1 and IL-6 are upregulated, and leukocyte migration is enhanced by induced expression of adhesion molecules. Activation of NFκB prevents macrophage and lymphocyte apoptosis at sites of inflammation [21]. While TNFR1 is responsible for the pro-inflammatory properties of TNF, TNFR2 mediates the immunoregulatory action of TNF.

TACE can also release the extracellular portion of TNFR1 and TNFR2, resulting in formation of the soluble TNFRs (sTNFRs) sTNFR1 and sTNFR2. sTNFR1 and sTNFR2 can bind TNF, acting as natural inhibitors that compete with the membrane-bound receptors.

LTα exerts similar biological activities as TNF. It also engages TNFR1 and TNFR2, but unlike for TNF, TNFR2 does not operate as a 'ligand passer' for LTα [22].

Neutralisation of Soluble Tumor Necrosis Factor-Alpha

Since TNF plays a pivotal role in the pathogenesis of chronic inflammatory diseases, neutralizing its actions is an important therapeutic strategy. The developed therapies are biological agents that block TNF activity. Five biological agents have been shown to be effective in the treatment of patients with IBD as well as other chronic inflammatory disorders (e.g. rheumatoid arthritis and psoriasis). Currently, four out of five are approved for the treatment of IBD. Infliximab, adalimumab and golimumab are full-length bivalent IgG1 monoclonal antibodies (mAbs). Infliximab (Remicade®) is a chimeric mAb comprising human and murine variable regions [23] that is administered via the intravenous (IV) route at 5 mg/kg every 8 weeks in both UC and CD patients [24]. The US Food and Drug Administration (FDA) and the European Medicines Agency (EMA) approved Remicade® as the first anti-TNF biological agent for the treatment of CD in 1998 and 1999, respectively. Recently, two biosimilars of infliximab (Inflectra™ and Remsima™) were approved. Adalimumab (Humira®) is a human IgG1 mAb derived from phage display [25] and is administered via the subcutaneous (SC) route at 40 mg once every 2 weeks in both UC and CD [26]. Golimumab (Simponi®), which was recently approved by the FDA and the EMA, is a mAb derived from transgenic mice engineered to express human IgG [27] and is administered via the SC route at 50 mg or 100 mg once every 4 weeks in UC [28, 29]. Certolizumab pegol (Cimzia®), approved by the FDA and Switzerland for the treatment of CD, is a monovalent Fab antibody fragment covalently linked to two cross-linked chains of a 20 kDa polyethylene glycol moiety to increase its half-life in vivo and to enhance solubility. Cimzia® is administered via the SC route at 400 mg once every 4 weeks in CD (for a review, see [30]). Etanercept (Enbrel®), a genetically engineered fusion protein comprising two identical chains of recombinant human TNFR2 fused to the Fc portion of human IgG1, has been shown to be safe but not effective in the treatment of CD [31]. Etanercept is the only anti-TNF agent that also binds to LTα [3].

Binding, Affinity and in vitro Potency

Bivalent mAbs can bind to both the monomeric and the trimeric forms of sTNF. The formation of multimeric complexes was shown to be dynamic in nature. Size exclusion chromatography revealed that the most stable complex consists of three molecules of mAb and three molecules of TNF, generating a complex of approximately 600 kDa. This complex is cleared very rapidly from the body, thereby allowing very efficient removal of excess TNF [32]. In contrast, etanercept can only bind to a single sTNF trimer, resulting in small, unstable 1:1 complexes, leading to dissociation of TNF [33].

Golimumab, adalimumab, infliximab and etanercept bind with approximately 20- to 1,400-fold lower affinity to tmTNF compared with sTNF. The reduced affinity for tmTNF might reflect steric or charge hindrance [27]. The dissociation equilibrium constant for the binding of sTNF to immobilized anti-TNF agents, measured by surface plasmon resonance, was 18 pM for golimumab, 11 pM for etanercept, 44 pM for infliximab and 127 pM for adalimumab [27]. Neutralisation of the cytotoxic effect of sTNF on a human rhabdomyosarcoma cell line was inhibited by all anti-TNF agents, revealing half-maximal inhibitory concentration values of 6.5 ng/ml for golimumab, 0.8 ng/ml for etanercept, 24.2 ng/ml for infliximab and 36.4 ng/ml for adalimumab [27].

These in vitro measurements suggest that a lower serum concentration of golimumab compared with infliximab or adalimumab would provide a similar pharmacological effect in patients. In addition to the increased affinity and the low half-maximal inhibitory concentration, the same study also demonstrated high conformational stability for golimumab, allowing a liquid formulation at 100 mg/ml.

Pharmacokinetics of Anti-Tumor Necrosis Factor-Alpha Agents

A drug can only exert its pharmacological effect when a sufficiently high concentration is attained in the circulation and subsequently at the site of action, which is the bowel in the case of IBD. The blood concentration of the anti-TNF biologics is the result of the absorption, the distribution and the elimination.

The *absorption* of an anti-TNF biologic is influenced by the route of administration. Out of the four anti-TNF biologics available to treat CD and UC, only infliximab is administered via the IV route. IV administration allows large volumes to be administered and results in a rapid central distribution, with low variability in bioavailability and high peak concentrations. Peak concentrations are reached immediately post-infusion and are reported to be ~100 μg/ml [34]. The disadvantage of IV administration is the need for administration at a specialized center, which makes it inconvenient for the patient and increases costs. In addition, rapid infusion may precipitate adverse events. Adalimumab, certolizumab pegol and golimumab are administered via the SC route. Systemic absorption occurs most likely via the lymphatic system, which slowly drains into the vascular compartment. It was shown that the absorption of adalimumab from the site of administration into the vascular compartment takes 131 ± 56 hours [35]. The extent of absorption is influenced by the presence of pre-systemic antibody degradation by proteolytic enzymes. It is hypothesized that this degradation is saturable, leading to an increase in bioavailability with increasing doses of antibody. For adalimumab, the mean bioavailability is estimated to be 62%. The disadvantages of SC administration are the inability to administer large volumes due to the pain associated with the injection of large volumes, the inability to administer high doses due to limited solubility at approximately 100 mg/ml, the inter-individual differences in bioavailability and the increased risk of immunogenicity [36].

Antibody *distribution* depends on the rate and extent of antibody extravasation and distribution within tissue and elimination from tissue. Due to their large size and hydrophilicity, antibodies distribute mainly within the central compartment. The volume of distribution for infliximab was reported to range between 4.5 and 6 l [34, 37, 38], which is similar to the distribution volume reported for adalimumab (5.1–8 l) [35].

Owing to their large size, IgGs are not filtered by the kidney, and therefore, renal excretion does not contribute to the *elimination* of anti-TNF antibodies. This is also true for certolizumab pegol, which, due to PEGylation of the antibody fragment, is above the glomerular filtration limit. Elimination of antibodies and conjugated antibody derivatives occurs via lysosomal proteolytic catabolism after receptor-mediated endocytosis. However, salvage and recirculation routes prevent rapid elimination [39]. The neonatal Fc receptor (FcRn), mainly expressed on endothelial cells, protects biologics from catabolism, thereby prolonging their half-lives [40]. IgG is taken up into the endosomes of catabolic cells by fluid-phase pinocytosis. IgGs have low affinity at physiological pH but bind to the FcRn at low pH via the Fc receptor of the IgG molecule. The FcRn-IgG complex is returned to the central compartment, whereas unbound IgG is degraded in the lysosomes [41]. Since this system is saturable, the elimination kinetics are nonlinear at high doses.

Immunogenicity, concomitant immunosuppressive medication and drug loss through a 'leaky gut' also influence the clearance of anti-TNF biologics. The half-life of anti-TNF biologics is in the range of 8–20 days [3].

Future Perspectives

The introduction of anti-TNF biopharmaceuticals has revolutionized the treatment of IBD. Despite their widespread use in everyday clinical practice, the precise mechanism of action remains unclear. It is clear that simple neutralisation of sTNF is not the full story. In recent years, novel therapeutic strategies have been applied, mainly targeting leukocyte trafficking and pro-inflammatory cytokines, such as IL-6, IL-12 and IL-23 [42]. Vedolizumab (Entyvio®) is a humanized mAb directed against the $\alpha_4\beta_7$ integrin, an adhesion molecule on lymphocytes. Vedolizumab selectively inhibits migration and trafficking of lymphocytes in the inflamed gut. Ustekinumab (Stelara®) is a fully human mAb that blocks the activity of IL-12 and IL-23, two pro-inflammatory cytokines that play an important role in IBD. Tofacitinib (Xeljanz®) is a novel, orally administered small molecule that inhibits Janus-activated kinase, thereby inhibiting the intracellular signaling cascade of pro-inflammatory cytokines. Small molecules that inhibit other intracellular signalers, e.g. NFκB, are currently under development. Although many therapeutic targets are currently under investigation, optimizing neutralisation of (soluble) TNF remains subject of further investigation. Several alternative strategies are in the therapeutic pipeline. To overcome the inconvenience of parenteral dosing, oral therapies have been developed. Vandenbroucke *et al.* engineered an *L. lactis* strain to secrete mono- and bivalent murine TNF-neutralizing nanobodies and provided proof of concept for the oral administration of this strain to achieve *in situ* secretion of anti-TNF nanobodies [43]. This approach could overcome not only patient discomfort but also the adverse effects of traditional anti-TNF therapy since systemic nanobody levels were undetectable. One other strategy is oral use of thioketal nanoparticles containing anti-TNF small interfering RNA to inhibit TNF gene expression specifically at sites of inflammation [44]. Along with these innovative drug delivery strategies, the therapeutic spectrum for IBD will soon expand with the market introduction of infliximab biosimilars. Though they might lower the pressure on national healthcare budgets, many concerns about interchangeability, immunogenicity profiles and extrapolation across indications remain. More refined implementation of the currently available anti-TNF drugs through therapeutic drug monitoring and stratified medicine is another way to overcome (cost) efficacy and safety obstacles.

References

1 Vermeire S, Van Assche G, Rutgeerts P: Classification of inflammatory bowel disease: the old and the new. Curr Opin Gastroenterol 2012;28:321–326.
2 Basso PJ, Fonseca MT, Bonfá G, Alves VB, Sales-Campos H, Nardini V, Cardoso CR: Association among genetic predisposition, gut microbiota, and host immune response in the etiopathogenesis of inflammatory bowel disease. Braz J Med Biol Res 2014;47:727–737.
3 Tracey D, Klareskog L, Sasso EH, Salfeld JG, Tak PP: Tumor necrosis factor antagonist mechanisms of action: a comprehensive review. Pharmacol Ther 2008;117:244–279.
4 Murch SH, Lamkin VA, Savage MO, Walker-Smith JA, MacDonald TT: Serum concentrations of tumour necrosis factor alpha in childhood chronic inflammatory bowel disease. Gut 1991;32: 913–917.
5 Braegger CP, Nicholls S, Murch SH, Stephens S, MacDonald TT: Tumour necrosis factor alpha in stool as a marker of intestinal inflammation. Lancet 1992; 339:89–91.
6 Murch SH, Braegger CP, Walker-Smith JA, MacDonald TT: Location of tumour necrosis factor alpha by immunohistochemistry in chronic inflammatory bowel disease. Gut 1993;34: 1705–1709.

7 Komatsu M, Kobayashi D, Saito K, Furuya D, Yagihashi A, Araake H, Tsuji N, Sakamaki S, Niitsu Y, Watanabe N: Tumor necrosis factor-alpha in serum of patients with inflammatory bowel disease as measured by a highly sensitive immuno-PCR. Clin Chem 2001;47:1297–1301.

8 Breese EJ, Michie CA, Nicholls SW, Murch SH, Williams CB, Domizio P, Walker-Smith JA, MacDonald TT: Tumor necrosis factor alpha-producing cells in the intestinal mucosa of children with inflammatory bowel disease. Gastroenterology 1994;106:1455–1466.

9 Nicholls S, Stephens S, Braegger CP, Walker-Smith JA, MacDonald TT: Cytokines in stools of children with inflammatory bowel disease or infective diarrhoea. J Clin Pathol 1993;46:757–760.

10 Apostolaki M, Armaka M, Victoratos P, Kollias G: Cellular mechanisms of TNF function in models of inflammation and autoimmunity. Curr Dir Autoimmun 2010;11:1–26.

11 Billiet T, Rutgeerts P, Ferrante M, Van Assche G, Vermeire S: Targeting TNF-α for the treatment of inflammatory bowel disease. Expert Opin Biol Ther 2014;14:75–101.

12 Kriegler M, Perez C, DeFay K, Albert I, Lu SD: A novel form of TNF/cachectin is a cell surface cytotoxic transmembrane protein: ramifications for the complex physiology of TNF. Cell 1988;53:45–53.

13 Wolfsberg TG, White JM: ADAMs in fertilization and development. Dev Biol 1996;180:389–401.

14 Black RA, Rauch CT, Kozlosky CJ, Peschon JJ, Slack JL, Wolfson MF, Castner BJ, Stocking KL, Reddy P, Srinivasan S, Nelson N, Boiani N, Schooley KA, Gerhart M, Davis R, Fitzner JN, Johnson RS, Paxton RJ, March CJ, Cerretti DP: A metalloproteinase disintegrin that releases tumour-necrosis factor-alpha from cells. Nature 1997;385:729–733.

15 Smith RA, Baglioni C: The active form of tumor necrosis factor is a trimer. J Biol Chem 1987;262:6951–6954.

16 Grell M, Douni E, Wajant H, Löhden M, Clauss M, Maxeiner B, Georgopoulos S, Lesslauer W, Kollias G, Pfizenmaier K, Scheurich P: The transmembrane form of tumor necrosis factor is the prime activating ligand of the 80 kDa tumor necrosis factor receptor. Cell 1995;83:793–802.

17 Grell M, Wajant H, Zimmermann G, Scheurich P: The type 1 receptor (CD120a) is the high-affinity receptor for soluble tumor necrosis factor. Proc Natl Acad Sci U S A 1998;95:570–575.

18 Tartaglia LA, Pennica D, Goeddel DV: Ligand passing: the 75-kDa tumor necrosis factor (TNF) receptor recruits TNF for signaling by the 55-kDa TNF receptor. J Biol Chem 1993;268:18542–18548.

19 Tartaglia LA, Ayres TM, Wong GH, Goeddel DV: A novel domain within the 55 kd TNF receptor signals cell death. Cell 1993;74:845–853.

20 Hsu H, Xiong J, Goeddel DV: The TNF receptor 1-associated protein TRADD signals cell death and NF-kappa B activation. Cell 1995;81:495–504.

21 Baud V, Karin M: Signal transduction by tumor necrosis factor and its relatives. Trends Cell Biol 2001;11:372–377.

22 Medvedev AE, Espevik T, Ranges G, Sundan A: Distinct roles of the two tumor necrosis factor (TNF) receptors in modulating TNF and lymphotoxin alpha effects. J Biol Chem 1996;271:9778–9784.

23 Knight DM, Trinh H, Le J, Siegel S, Shealy D, McDonough M, Scallon B, Moore MA, Vilcek J, Daddona P: Construction and initial characterization of a mouse-human chimeric anti-TNF antibody. Mol Immunol 1993;30:1443–1453.

24 Mouser JF, Hyams JS: Infliximab: a novel chimeric monoclonal antibody for the treatment of Crohn's disease. Clin Ther 1999;21:932–942.

25 Jespers LS, Roberts A, Mahler SM, Winter G, Hoogenboom HR: Guiding the selection of human antibodies from phage display repertoires to a single epitope of an antigen. Biotechnology (N Y) 1994;12:899–903.

26 Stack WA, Mann SD, Roy AJ, Heath P, Sopwith M, Freeman J, Holmes G, Long R, Forbes A, Kamm MA: Randomised controlled trial of CDP571 antibody to tumour necrosis factor-alpha in Crohn's disease. Lancet 1997;349:521–524.

27 Shealy DJ, Cai A, Staquet K, Baker A, Lacy ER, Johns L, Vafa O, Gunn G, Tam S, Sague S, Wang D, Brigham-Burke M, Dalmonte P, Emmell E, Pikounis B, Bugelski PJ, Zhou H, Scallon BJ, Giles-Komar JM: Characterization of golimumab, a human monoclonal antibody specific for human tumor necrosis factor α. MAbs 2010;2:428–439.

28 Sandborn WJ, Feagan BG, Marano C, Zhang H, Strauss R, Johanns J, Adedokun OJ, Guzzo C, Colombel JF, Reinisch W, Gibson PR, Collins J, Järnerot G, Hibi T, Rutgeerts P, PURSUIT-SC Study Group: Subcutaneous golimumab induces clinical response and remission in patients with moderate-to-severe ulcerative colitis. Gastroenterology 2014;146:85–95.

29 Sandborn WJ, Feagan BG, Marano C, Zhang H, Strauss R, Johanns J, Adedokun OJ, Guzzo C, Colombel JF, Reinisch W, Gibson PR, Collins J, Järnerot G, Rutgeerts P, Group P-MS: Subcutaneous golimumab maintains clinical response in patients with moderate-to-severe ulcerative colitis. Gastroenterology 2014;146:96–109.

30 Goel N, Stephens S: Certolizumab pegol. MAbs 2010;2:137–147.

31 Sandborn WJ, Hanauer SB, Katz S, Safdi M, Wolf DG, Baerg RD, Tremaine WJ, Johnson T, Diehl NN, Zinsmeister AR: Etanercept for active Crohn's disease: a randomized, double-blind, placebo-controlled trial. Gastroenterology 2001;121:1088–1094.

32 Santora LC, Kaymakcalan Z, Sakorafas P, Krull IS, Grant K: Characterization of noncovalent complexes of recombinant human monoclonal antibody and antigen using cation exchange, size exclusion chromatography, and BIAcore. Anal Biochem 2001;299:119–129.

33 Scallon B, Cai A, Solowski N, Rosenberg A, Song XY, Shealy D, Wagner C: Binding and functional comparisons of two types of tumor necrosis factor antagonists. J Pharmacol Exp Ther 2002;301:418–426.

34 Klotz U, Teml A, Schwab M: Clinical pharmacokinetics and use of infliximab. Clin Pharmacokinet 2007;46:645–660.

35 Weisman MH, Moreland LW, Furst DE, Weinblatt ME, Keystone EC, Paulus HE, Teoh LS, Velagapudi RB, Noertersheuser PA, Granneman GR, Fischkoff SA, Chartash EK: Efficacy, pharmacokinetic, and safety assessment of adalimumab, a fully human anti-tumor necrosis factor-alpha monoclonal antibody, in adults with rheumatoid arthritis receiving concomitant methotrexate: a pilot study. Clin Ther 2003;25:1700–1721.

36 Lobo ED, Hansen RJ, Balthasar JP: Antibody pharmacokinetics and pharmacodynamics. J Pharm Sci 2004;93:2645–2668.

37 Fasanmade AA, Adedokun OJ, Ford J, Hernandez D, Johanns J, Hu C, Davis HM, Zhou H: Population pharmacokinetic analysis of infliximab in patients with ulcerative colitis. Eur J Clin Pharmacol 2009;65:1211–1228.
38 Fasanmade AA, Adedokun OJ, Blank M, Zhou H, Davis HM: Pharmacokinetic properties of infliximab in children and adults with Crohn's disease: a retrospective analysis of data from 2 phase III clinical trials. Clin Ther 2011;33:946–964.
39 Brambell FW, Hemmings WA, Morris IG: A theoretical model of gamma-globulin catabolism. Nature 1964;203:1352–1354.
40 Kuo TT, Baker K, Yoshida M, Qiao SW, Aveson VG, Lencer WI, Blumberg RS: Neonatal Fc receptor: from immunity to therapeutics. J Clin Immunol 2010;30:777–789.
41 Wang W, Wang EQ, Balthasar JP: Monoclonal antibody pharmacokinetics and pharmacodynamics. Clin Pharmacol Ther 2008;84:548–558.
42 Löwenberg M, D'Haens G: Novel targets for inflammatory bowel disease therapeutics. Curr Gastroenterol Rep 2013;15:311.
43 Vandenbroucke K, de Haard H, Beirnaert E, Dreier T, Lauwereys M, Huyck L, Van Huysse J, Demetter P, Steidler L, Remaut E, Cuvelier C, Rottiers P: Orally administered L. lactis secreting an anti-TNF Nanobody demonstrate efficacy in chronic colitis. Mucosal Immunol 2010;3:49–56.
44 Wilson DS, Dalmasso G, Wang L, Sitaraman SV, Merlin D, Murthy N: Orally delivered thioketal nanoparticles loaded with TNF-α-siRNA target inflammation and inhibit gene expression in the intestines. Nat Mater 2010;9:923–928.

Ann Gils
Laboratory for Therapeutic and Diagnostic Antibodies
Department of Pharmaceutical and Pharmacological Sciences, Katholieke Universiteit Leuven
Campus Gasthuisberg, O&N2, PB 820, Herestraat 49
BE–3000 Leuven (Belgium)
E-Mail ann.gils@pharm.kuleuven.be

Rogler G, Herfarth H, Hibi T, Nielsen OH (eds): Anti-Tumor Necrosis Factor Therapy in Inflammatory Bowel Disease.
Front Gastrointest Res. Basel, Karger, 2015, vol 34, pp 90–94 (DOI: 10.1159/000381447)

Recommended Screening Procedures before Treatment with Anti-TNF Agents

Christian Maaser

University Teaching Hospital Lüneburg, Department of Gastroenterology Outpatients' Center, Lueneburg, Germany

Abstract

As the current treatment algorithms for patients with chronic inflammatory bowel disease have become more aggressive, often involving anti-TNF therapy, with the aim of reaching deep remission rather than just clinical improvement, the risk of relevant complications has increased. The aim of this review is to point out various potential areas of increased risk and to list necessary precautions to be taken before introducing anti-TNF therapy to keep the risk of complications as low as possible. The main focus is therefore on potential infectious complications, as these are the most frequent complications and as there are effective primary and secondary preventive strategies. Primary strategies include checking and, if necessary, updating the immunization record as well as providing specific advice on lifestyle. Secondary preventive strategies include the detection and treatment of acute or chronic infections, e.g. latent tuberculosis. In addition, special aspects to be considered in elderly patients with inflammatory bowel disease before treatment initiation are mentioned. By following these precautions, we are hopefully more effective in treating our patients, with an acceptable level of risk.

Introduction

Anti-TNF therapy has become one of the major pillars for the treatment of Crohn's disease as well as ulcerative colitis. While the benefit of various anti-TNF agents has clearly been shown in multiple clinical trials, reflected by induction of a long-term response and remission, several potential risk and side effects have to be taken into account. Two major areas of side effects are an increased risk of infectious complications as well as an increased risk of developing specific neoplasias. In order to decrease the risk, certain screening procedures are recommended before the initiation of anti-TNF treatment.

Main Points

Rule Out Acute Intestinal Infections

Before the initiation of anti-TNF therapy, acute infections should be ruled out as the cause of the underlying symptoms instead of the suspected flare of the chronic disease. As most patients with inflammatory bowel disease who are considered for anti-

TNF treatment are already receiving immunosuppressive therapy, e.g. prednisolone or azathioprine, they are at an increased risk for two specific infections: cytomegalovirus (CMV) and *Clostridium difficile* infections. The risk of a *Clostridium* infection, for example, has been shown to increase three times in patients receiving glucocorticosteroids [1]. As both of these infections can present with bloody diarrhea, a differential diagnosis of an acute flare of the underlying chronic disease cannot be made based on clinical symptoms alone. Therefore, testing a stool sample for *Clostridium difficile* toxin and antigen as well as performing PCR for CMV in EDTA blood and/or immunohistochemistry for CMV in tissue from colonic biopsies should be considered [2, 3]. In addition, depending on the local specific infectious risk, testing for further infectious organisms should be considered. For example, *Yersinia, Salmonella* and *Campylobacter* can all cause clinical symptoms mimicking an acute flare.

Rule Out Abscess Formation

Due to the transmural inflammatory pathology of the disease, Crohn's disease patients are at an increased risk of developing an abscess. Patients should therefore be carefully asked about symptoms and examined for potential abscesses. In addition to analyzing clinical signs and inflammatory blood parameters, such as elevated C-reactive protein and elevated leukocytes, analysis might include cross-sectional imaging, e.g. by transabdominal ultrasound and/or MRI and by perianal ultrasound/pelvic MRI in cases in which perianal fistulas are present [4]. In addition, in the case of perianal fistulas, seton placement before the start of medical treatment should be discussed with a surgeon experienced in the treatment of perianal fistulas.

Rule Out Acute Nonintestinal Infections

Due to the immunosuppressive effect of anti-TNF medication, keeping its long half-life in mind, any additional acute nonintestinal infection should be ruled out by carefully asking about potential clinical signs of infection, including fever, cough, and urinary tract infection. In the case of symptoms suggestive of an acute infection, further diagnostic work-up and treatment of the infection should be started before anti-TNF therapy starts to avoid serious infectious complications. In addition, careful attention should be given to patients who live in or have traveled to areas endemic for mycoses, such as histoplasmosis.

Rule Out Chronic Infections

Serious courses of a chronic hepatitis B infection after initiation of immunosuppressive therapy have been reported. Therefore, testing for antibodies against hepatitis B surface antigen and hepatitis B core antigen is recommended before treatment start. In seronegative patients, vaccination is recommended. As the vaccine is a non-live vaccine, vaccination can be started after initiation of anti-TNF therapy; however, the effectiveness should be controlled and might sometimes lead to the recommendation of an extra booster vaccination. In hepatitis B surface antigen-positive patients, who are at risk for severe reactivation, preventive therapy with a nucleoside/nucleotide analog is indicated [5].

Screening for hepatitis C, however, is not required, as experience has shown that anti-TNF therapy does not lead to progression of chronic hepatitis C infection [6].

As immunosuppressive therapy can potentially have a negative influence on the human immunodeficiency virus load, it is recommended that patients at risk for this type of infection be screened [7].

Rule Out (Latent) Tuberculosis

As the risk of granulomatous infections, e.g. tuberculosis (TB) and listeriosis, is increased in anti-TNF-treated patients, certain safety precautions have to be taken.

Screening for (Latent) Tuberculosis [7]

Before the introduction of screening procedures, one of the most prominent opportunistic infections was TB (144/100,000 with infliximab versus

27/100,000 in the general population) [8]. The risk varies depending on several factors, e.g. the country, infections of family members, socio-economic status and the travel history of the patient. Therefore, a careful history is one very important aspect of screening. Has the patient ever had contact with a person with open TB? Is the patient from a country with a high prevalence of TB or has he/she traveled to such countries? Furthermore, in most countries, a chest x-ray as well as one further testing method is required. For a long time, PPD skin testing was one of the most common methods to test for (latent) TB. However, immunosuppression can lead to false-negative results on the one hand, and prior vaccination can lead to false-positive results on the other hand. Furthermore, the test can become positive due to infection with nontuberculous mycobacteria containing similar antigens. This would lead to unnecessary prophylactic therapy, e.g. isoniazid treatment, with a risk of severe side effects and drug interactions. In addition, the patient has to return for reading of the test 48–72 hours after application. Due to these disadvantages, guidelines in many countries have been changed, and an interferon-gamma release assay is now the required/alternative testing method. This assay is based on the detection of interferon-gamma released by antigen-stimulated lymphocytes and is not influenced by prior TB vaccination. Currently, there are two tests available: the QuantiFERON-TB Gold test and the T-SPOT. TB test. These tests are not affected by prior BCG vaccination, but the blood must be processed within 12 hours.

In the case of a positive test without further signs of active TB, most guidelines recommend careful reevaluation of the anti-TNF treatment. In the case of no further treatment options, prophylactic treatment with isoniazid, e.g. for 4 weeks before the introduction of anti-TNF, is required and needs to be continued for several months in combination with the anti-TNF therapy.

Check and Update Immunization Record

While the risk of some infections can be reduced by maintaining good food hygiene and avoiding certain 'high-risk' food products, other infections can be prevented by adequate vaccination [9]. Taking a careful history of the vaccination record should be part of the routine work-up before the start of anti-TNF therapy. Ideally, in the case of missing recommended vaccinations, those missing should be applied before initiation of treatment. In general, one has to keep in mind that live vaccines, e.g. against rubella and chicken pox, are contraindicated in patients under immunosuppression and therefore cannot be performed once anti-TNF has been started. In contrast, non-live vaccines, e.g. against influenza, pneumococcus, and hepatitis B, can be applied even during anti-TNF therapy. However, the success/effect of the vaccination can be reduced under immunosuppression.

Provide Lifestyle Advice

The pretreatment patient visit should also include general health maintenance advice [10]. For example, some infectious agents can be transmitted by contaminated food. One granulomatous infection that patients treated with anti-TNF are at an increased risk of developing is listeriosis. Patients should therefore be advised to avoid unpasteurized milk, soft cheese and raw meat, especially if on double immunosuppression [11, 12]. However, there have been various outbreaks reported, with *Listeria* transmitted by a great variety of different infected foods, so even when the above-mentioned food recommendations are carefully considered, complete safety cannot be guaranteed.

Furthermore, the risk of infectious complications in patients receiving anti-TNF therapy when travelling to areas endemic for TB or mycoses should be discussed. Patients should be aware of this increased risk so that they are able to make informed decisions regarding their travel plans.

Table 1. Screening procedures before anti-TNF treatment

Screen for (latent) TB	Chest x-ray, IGRA, (PPD skin test)
Screen for acute intestinal infection	CMV PCR from EDTA blood, *Clostridium difficile* antigen/toxin from stool
Screen for acute nonintestinal infection	Clinical signs, e.g. fever, cough or urinary tract infection?
Screen for chronic infections	Anti-HBsAg and anti-HBc antibodies; anti-HIV testing optional
Screen for abscess	Clinical signs? Cross-sectional imaging, e.g. MRI, transabdominal ultrasound and/or endorectal ultrasound, optional
Check and update immunization record	See country-specific recommendations
Check for cardiac insufficiency	Clinical signs? Cardiac ultrasound optional
Provide general health advice	Food hygiene, travel, sun protection

IGRA = Interferon-gamma release assay; HBsAg = hepatitis B surface antigen; HBc = hepatitis B core antigen; HIV = human immunodeficiency virus.

In addition to good food hygiene, patients should be informed about an increased risk of developing melanoma while under anti-TNF therapy [13] and should therefore be advised to use sun protection as well as to seek periodic professional skin cancer screenings. Some guidelines suggest yearly screening [14].

Furthermore, patients should be informed about a slightly increased risk of developing lymphoma [13]. Though there is no preventive measure, patients should be asked to report potentially swollen lymph nodes in the future.

As the role of anti-TNF in the development of malignancies is not clearly known, a careful history of past malignancies should be taken, and the risk/benefit ratio should be carefully considered in those with a positive history [15].

Rule Out Severe Cardiac Insufficiency

In a randomized study evaluating infliximab in patients with moderate to severe heart failure (New York Heart Association Functional Class III/IV), infliximab at a dose of 10 mg/kg was associated with an increased incidence of death and hospitalization due to worsening of heart failure [16]. Due to this potential increased risk, anti-TNF therapy, e.g. infliximab at doses >5 mg/kg, is contraindicated in patients with moderate to severe heart failure. In patients with a cardiac history, cardiac function should be evaluated before treatment start.

Special Note Regarding the Elderly Patient with Inflammatory Bowel Disease

As the potential side effects and risk of serious infections as well as cancer development are highest in the older patient population (age 65 and higher), the potential benefit of anti-TNF therapy in the elderly should be carefully weighed against the potential risks [17].

Conclusions

To ensure safe immunosuppressive therapy with an anti-TNF agent, specific pretherapeutic examinations (see table 1) are mandatory for every patient. However, one has to keep in mind that in addition, an individual risk/benefit evaluation should be performed and that alternative options, e.g. surgical options, should be taken into consideration.

References

1 Schneeweiss S, Setoguchi S, Weinblatt ME, Katz JN, Avorn J, Sax PE, Levin R, Solomon DH: Anti-tumor necrosis factor alpha therapy and the risk of serious bacterial infections in elderly patients with rheumatoid arthritis. Arthritis Rheum 2007;56:1754–1764.

2 Goodman AL, Murray CD, Watkins J, Griffiths PD, Webster DP: CMV in the gut: a critical review of CMV detection in the immunocompetent host with colitis. Eur J Clin Microbiol Infect Dis 2015; 34:13–18.

3 Landsman MJ, Sultan M, Stevens M, Charabaty A, Mattar MC: Diagnosis and management of common gastrointestinal tract infectious diseases in ulcerative colitis and Crohn's disease patients. Inflamm Bowel Dis 2014;20:2503–2510.

4 Panes J, Bouhnik Y, Reinisch W, Stoker J, Taylor SA, Baumgart DC, Danese S, Halligan S, Marincek B, Matos C, Peyrin-Biroulet L, Rimola J, Rogler G, van Assche G, Ardizzone S, Ba-Ssalamah A, Bali MA, Bellini D, Biancone L, Castiglione F, Ehehalt R, Grassi R, Kucharzik T, Maccioni F, Maconi G, Magro F, Martín-Comín J, Morana G, Pendsé D, Sebastian S, Signore A, Tolan D, Tielbeek JA, Weishaupt D, Wiarda B, Laghi AJ: Imaging techniques for assessment of inflammatory bowel disease: joint ECCO and ESGAR evidence-based consensus guidelines. Crohns Colitis 2013;7:556–585.

5 Seetharam A, Perrillo R, Gish R: Immunosuppression in patients with chronic hepatitis B. Curr Hepatol Rep 2014;13: 235–244.

6 Campbell S, Ghosh S: Infliximab therapy for Crohn's disease in the presence of chronic hepatitis C infection. Eur J Gastroenterol Hepatol 2001;13:191–192.

7 Rahier JF, Magro F, Abreu C, Armuzzi A, Ben-Horin S, Chowers Y, Cottone M, de Ridder L, Doherty G, Ehehalt R, Esteve M, Katsanos K, Lees CW, Macmahon E, Moreels T, Reinisch W, Tilg H, Tremblay L, Veereman-Wauters G, Viget N, Yazdanpanah Y, Eliakim R, Colombel JF; European Crohn's and Colitis Organisation (ECCO): Second European evidence-based consensus on the prevention, diagnosis and management of opportunistic infections in inflammatory bowel disease. J Crohns Colitis 2014;8:443–468.

8 Wallis RS, Broder MS, Wong JY, Hanson ME, Beenhouwer DO: Granulomatous infectious diseases associated with tumor necrosis factor antagonists. Clin Infect Dis 2004;38:1261–1265.

9 Lodhia N: The appropriate use of vaccines in patients with inflammatory bowel disease. J Clin Gastroenterol 2014; 48:395–401.

10 Moscandrew M, Mahadevan U, Kane S: General health maintenance in IBD. Inflamm Bowel Dis 2009;15:1399–1409.

11 Slifman NR, Gershon SK, Lee JH, Edwards ET, Braun MM: Listeria monocytogenes infection as a complication of treatment with tumor necrosis factor alpha-neutralizing agents. Arthritis Rheum 2003;48:319–324.

12 Wing EJ, Gregory SH: Listeria monocytogenes: clinical and experimental update. J Infect Dis 2002;185(suppl 1):S18–S24.

13 Biancone L, Onali S, Petruzziello C, Calabrese E, Pallone F: Cancer and immunomodulators in inflammatory bowel diseases. Inflamm Bowel Dis 2015;21: 674–698.

14 Preiß JC, Bokemeyer B, Buhr HJ, Dignaß A, Häuser W, Hartmann F, Herrlinger KR, Kaltz B, Kienle P, Kruis W, Kucharzik T, Langhorst J, Schreiber S, Siegmund B, Stallmach A, Stange EF, Stein J, Hoffmann JC: Updated German clinical practice guideline on 'Diagnosis and treatment of Crohn's disease' 2014. Z Gastroenterol 2014;52:1431–1484.

15 Beaugerie L: Management of inflammatory bowel disease patients with a cancer history. Curr Drug Targets 2014;15: 1042–1048.

16 Chung ES, Packer M, Lo KH, Fasanmade AA, Willerson JT; Anti-TNF Therapy Against Congestive Heart Failure Investigators: Randomized, double-blind, placebo-controlled, pilot trial of infliximab, a chimeric monoclonal antibody to tumor necrosis factor-alpha, in patients with moderate-to-severe heart failure: results of the anti-TNF Therapy Against Congestive Heart Failure (ATTACH) trial. Circulation 2003;107: 3133–3140.

17 Stallmach A, Hagel S, Gharbi A, Settmacher U, Hartmann M, Schmidt C, Bruns T: Medical and surgical therapy of inflammatory bowel disease in the elderly – prospects and complications. J Crohns Colitis 2011;5:177–188.

Christian Maaser, MD
Klinikum Lüneburg, Ambulanzzentrum Gastroenterologie
Boegelstrasse 1
DE–21339 Lueneburg (Germany)
E-Mail Christian.maaser@klinikum-lüneburg.de

Rogler G, Herfarth H, Hibi T, Nielsen OH (eds): Anti-Tumor Necrosis Factor Therapy in Inflammatory Bowel Disease.
Front Gastrointest Res. Basel, Karger, 2015, vol 34, pp 95–99 (DOI: 10.1159/000381448)

The Risk of Formation of Neutralizing Antibodies

Joshua Clark • Atsushi Sakuraba

Section of Gastroenterology, Hepatology and Nutrition, University of Chicago Medicine, Chicago, Ill., USA

Abstract

Tumor necrosis factor (TNF)-α is a key cytokine that drives the dysregulated immune response in inflammatory bowel diseases. Anti-TNF-α agents are the most widely used biologics that have been manufactured to specifically target either or both circulating and membrane-bound TNF-α, thus preventing its pro-inflammatory actions during disease progression. Despite its undoubted efficacy, one-third of inflammatory bowel disease patients receiving anti-TNF-α agents are primary nonresponders, and about half of the patients who initially respond lose their response over time (secondary loss of response). The majority of these cases can be explained by immunogenicity, which is when the property of a foreign biologic produces an immune response within the human body and can lead to lower drug levels in association with a reduced response and serious adverse effects that cause patients to withdraw from treatment. Combination therapy with immunomodulators is the major strategy to suppress immunogenicity and to achieve a durable response.

Introduction

The immunopathogeneses of inflammatory bowel diseases (IBDs), including Crohn's disease (CD) and ulcerative colitis (UC), are characterized by elevated levels of circulatory and mucosal pro-inflammatory cytokines [1–4]. Tumor necrosis factor (TNF)-α, which is produced by T cells and macrophages, is a key cytokine that drives the dysregulated immune response in IBDs [1, 5]. These cells are found in elevated numbers in the intestinal mucosa of IBD patients [6, 7]. The resulting increased TNF-α level contributes to the acute and chronic inflammation that characterizes these diseases [8]. Conventional medications, including 5-aminosalicylates, corticosteroids, and immunomodulators, such as azathioprine and mercaptopurine, have been used for many years for the treatment of CD and UC [9]. More recently, studies have shown that biologic agents are successful in inducing and maintaining remission of CD and UC and are favored in patients with moderate to severe disease [9]. Anti-TNF-α agents are the most widely used biologics that have been manufactured to specifically target either or both circulating and membrane-bound TNF-α, thus preventing its pro-inflammatory actions during disease progression. Approximately one-third of IBD patients receiving anti-TNF-α agents are primary nonresponders, and about half of the patients who initially respond lose their responses over time (secondary loss of response) [10, 11]. Possible explanations for the failure/loss of response are immunogenicity against the biologic, enhanced clearance of the biologic, an alternate mechanism of inflammation (a nonTNF pathway), and noninflammatory conditions (strictures or irritable bowel). In the present chapter, we will focus on immunogenicity, which is the capacity of the foreign biologic to produce an immune response within the human body.

Formation of Neutralizing Antibodies

Biologics are nonnative proteins manufactured from exogenous sources that are targeted against a specific cell type or component. Anti-TNF-α agents are among the most widely used biologics [10–12]. Some of these agents are partial murine-human chimeric monoclonal antibodies, while others are fully humanized antibodies [13]. Infliximab, which was the first anti-TNF-α biologic to be introduced into clinical practice, is one example of a chimeric monoclonal antibody with a 25% murine component located at the antigen-binding variable domain [10, 14]. This murine component is recognized by the body as a foreign antigen and can provoke a response by the immune system (immunogenicity) [13, 15, 16]. Fully humanized antibodies, such as adalimumab, golimumab and certolizumab pegol, have been developed but have not yet been proven to be successful in completely preventing immunogenicity [17–19]. When a biologic is introduced into the body, the immune system uses lymphocytes to create antibodies that specifically target the foreign agent. An antibody created in response to a biologic specifically binds to distinct sites on the molecule and can be neutralizing [15]. As neutralizing antibodies created by the immune system attack a biologic agent, the drug level lowers, and most often, a loss of response occurs due to the inability to suppress TNF-α. Furthermore, once anti-drug antibodies have formed, any subsequent doses of the biologic agent that are of the same dosage will continue to be neutralized, likely rendering it ineffective. This effect remains true for patients switching to a different anti-TNF-α agent [20–23]. Patients who have developed antibodies against the first agent are at a higher risk of developing antibodies against a subsequent agent [24].

Anti-TNF-α agents are effective in treating the symptoms and mucosal inflammation of IBDs. However, a single dose is not sufficient to cause disease remission, and once an agent is discontinued, patients often relapse, and the signs and symptoms of inflammation return. Based on the findings of clinical trials, patients who have received only one dose or episodic treatment of infliximab have higher rates of anti-drug antibody (human anti-chimeric antibody or antibody to infliximab (ATI)) formation, leading to a less successful long-term outcome, while those who have received scheduled maintenance infusions are much less likely to produce these antibodies and have better clinical outcomes [15, 25]. For this reason, anti-TNF-α agents are administered in a series of treatments to patients with CD and UC to provide a durable response.

With scheduled treatments, however, immunogenicity cannot be fully eliminated. Although anti-TNF-α agents have shown success in achieving short- and long-term remission, this effectiveness, especially when they are used alone, can begin to decrease over time. The development of anti-drug antibodies appears to be the cause of loss of response in a majority of the cases [13, 26]. Concurrent treatment with immunosuppressives, such as azathioprine/6-mercaptopurine or methotrexate, can reduce this incidence.

The following four anti-TNF-α agents are currently approved for IBD treatment in the United States: infliximab, adalimumab, certolizumab pegol and golimumab. As previously mentioned, infliximab is a partial murine-human chimeric antibody, while adalimumab, certolizumab pegol and golimumab are fully humanized. Studies have shown slight variances in the incidence of anti-drug antibody formation for each agent. Depending on the study, it has been reported that 30–61%

of patients who have been treated with infliximab without immunosuppressives develop antibodies [16]. In addition, 44% of patients who have been treated with adalimumab without immunosuppressives have developed anti-drug antibodies (antibody to adalimumab) [27], and 8.3% of patients who have been treated with certolizumab pegol without immunosuppressives have developed antibodies [28]. In patients who have been treated with golimumab without concurrent immunosuppressives, 13.5% have been found to develop antibodies [18]. Although these numbers most likely do not represent the exact percentages of the entire population of IBD patients due to the limited number of participants in each study, they represent the overall trends of antibody formation against biologic drugs. Based on these results, infliximab seems to trigger an immune response more often than the fully humanized biologics.

In nearly all cases, neutralizing antibodies are not present before the initial doses of the biologic are administered, yet they can be found shortly after the initial administration. Neutralizing antibody formation is highest during the induction phase of a treatment. During this time, the patient is given an initial 'loading dose', which consists of infusions at week 0, week 2, and week 6 in the case of infliximab. For the 6 months following the loading dose, patients are at a higher risk of developing ATI. During these two time periods, patients are the most susceptible to neutralizing antibody formation. In very rare cases, however, patients have been found to carry pre-existing antibodies that neutralize the biologic agent [29]. In these instances, patients who have never been subjected to biologic treatments show the presence of neutralizing antibodies in the blood. Although information is limited on pre-existing antibodies, they are believed to be components of the natural antibody population or of the adaptive immune response to environmental antigens [30]. While it has been determined that neutralizing antibodies are formed in response to biologics, there has been no evidence in support of a correlation between sex, disease location, smoking, or the use of mesalamine or corticosteroids and the formation of neutralizing antibodies at the time of infusion or injection [16, 31]. In psoriasis, younger age has been associated with an increased risk of neutralizing antibody formation [31]. Immunological activity in young patients may affect the development of antibodies; however, the clear etiology remains unknown [8].

Another disadvantage of the development of neutralizing antibodies to biologics is increased risks of acute and delayed infusion reactions and delayed hypersensitivity reactions, especially in the case of infliximab [15]. These reactions are most typically characterized by dizziness, headache, diaphoresis, and nausea, but more severe reactions can present with fever, dyspnea and/or stridor, palpitations, or hypotension. Patients with positive neutralizing antibodies are at a higher risk of infusion reactions compared to those who have not developed them [15]. Additionally, CD patients with infusion reactions are less likely to be in remission at 1 and 5 years and are more likely to require surgery [10].

Prevention and Suppression of Neutralizing Antibodies

Although neutralizing antibodies have negative impacts on biologics, there are several effective strategies for preventing their formation, including scheduled maintenance infusions, as described above, the use of hydrocortisone premedication, and the use of combination therapy with immunomodulators [11].

In a randomized controlled trial, Farrell et al. have demonstrated that patients premedicated with hydrocortisone show a reduced level of ATI compared to those given placebo [32]. This group found that the rate of developing ATI was numerically, but not significantly, reduced (26% vs. 42%). They also demonstrated that administering a second infusion within 8 weeks of the first or concurrent immunosuppressive therapy significantly reduced the incidence of ATI formation (odds ratios of 0.13 and 0.19, respectively). Hydrocortisone premedication is now widely prescribed to patients receiving infliximab infusions.

The concomitant use of immunomodulators is another common method for preventing the formation of neutralizing antibodies. Immunomodulators suppress the immune system and possibly prevent a response to foreign agents, i.e. biologics, from occurring. When used in conjunction with biologics, immunomodulators suppress the formation of neutralizing antibodies and help to maintain remission. When used in low doses, methotrexate, a common immunosuppressant, protects against the formation of antibodies, as shown by the increased responses of patients to biologic drugs. In the Study of Biologic and Immunomodulator Naïve Patients in Crohn's Disease (SONIC), ATIs were detected in 1 of 116 patients (0.9%) receiving combination therapy and 15 of 103 patients (14.6%) receiving infliximab monotherapy [33]. Concomitant immunosuppression reduces antibody formation and has been found to be associated with increased infliximab trough levels [16, 34]. Together, these methods of suppressing neutralizing antibody formation yield a more successful treatment outcome. Few studies have investigated the optimal dose of immunomodulator to reduce immunogenicity, and results are still inconclusive [35, 36]. The addition of an immunomodulator, however, can be associated with increased risks of lymphoma, skin cancer and infections, and the benefit needs to be carefully evaluated for each individual patient [37].

Conclusion

Biologics are new agents used for the treatment of CD and UC that have yielded high success rates in reducing symptoms and achieving remission. However, immunogenicity can trigger the formation of anti-drug antibodies, leading to lower drug levels in association with a reduced response and serious adverse effects that cause patients to withdraw from treatment. Combination therapy with immunomodulators is the major strategy to increase the success of suppressing anti-drug antibody formation. However, the benefits of combination therapy must be weighed against the risks for each individual patient.

References

1 Sakuraba A, Sato T, Kamada N, et al: Th1/Th17 immune response is induced by mesenteric lymph node dendritic cells in Crohn's disease. Gastroenterology 2009;137:1736–1745.

2 Ebert EC: Infliximab and the TNF-alpha system. Am J Physiol Gastrointest Liver Physiol 2009;296:G612–G620.

3 Podolsky DK: Inflammatory bowel disease. N Engl J Med 2002;347:417–429.

4 Sato T, Nakai T, Tamura N, et al: Osteopontin/Eta-1 upregulated in Crohn's disease regulates the Th1 immune response. Gut 2005;54:1254–1262.

5 Plevy SE, Landers CJ, Prehn J, et al: A role for TNF-alpha and mucosal T helper-1 cytokines in the pathogenesis of Crohn's disease. J Immunol 1997;159:6276–6282.

6 Ebert EC, Das KM, Mehta V, et al: Non-response to infliximab may be due to innate neutralizing anti-tumour necrosis factor-alpha antibodies. Clin Exp Immunol 2008;154:325–331.

7 Breese EJ, Michie CA, Nicholls SW, et al: Tumor necrosis factor alpha-producing cells in the intestinal mucosa of children with inflammatory bowel disease. Gastroenterology 1994;106:1455–1466.

8 Braegger CP, Nicholls S, Murch SH, et al: Tumour necrosis factor alpha in stool as a marker of intestinal inflammation. Lancet 1992;339:89–91.

9 Hanauer SB: Medical therapy for ulcerative colitis 2004. Gastroenterology 2004;126:1582–1592.

10 Hanauer SB, Feagan BG, Lichtenstein GR, et al: Maintenance infliximab for Crohn's disease: the ACCENT I randomised trial. Lancet 2002;359:1541–1549.

11 Hanauer SB, Sandborn WJ, Rutgeerts P, et al: Human anti-tumor necrosis factor monoclonal antibody (adalimumab) in Crohn's disease: the CLASSIC-I trial. Gastroenterology 2006;130:323–333; quiz 591.

12 Schreiber S, Khaliq-Kareemi M, Lawrance IC, et al: Maintenance therapy with certolizumab pegol for Crohn's disease. N Engl J Med 2007;357:239–250.

13 Cassinotti A, Travis S: Incidence and clinical significance of immunogenicity to infliximab in Crohn's disease: a critical systematic review. Inflamm Bowel Dis 2009;15:1264–1275.

14 Rutgeerts P, D'Haens G, Targan S, et al: Efficacy and safety of retreatment with anti-tumor necrosis factor antibody (infliximab) to maintain remission in Crohn's disease. Gastroenterology 1999; 117:761–769.
15 Kozuch PL, Hanauer SB: General principles and pharmacology of biologics in inflammatory bowel disease. Gastroenterol Clin North Am 2006;35: 757–773.
16 Baert F, Noman M, Vermeire S, et al: Influence of immunogenicity on the long-term efficacy of infliximab in Crohn's disease. N Engl J Med 2003;348: 601–608.
17 Sandborn WJ, Rutgeerts P, Enns R, et al: Adalimumab induction therapy for Crohn disease previously treated with infliximab: a randomized trial. Ann Intern Med 2007;146:829–838.
18 Emery P, Fleischmann RM, Moreland LW, et al: Golimumab, a human anti-tumor necrosis factor alpha monoclonal antibody, injected subcutaneously every four weeks in methotrexate-naive patients with active rheumatoid arthritis: twenty-four-week results of a phase III, multicenter, randomized, double-blind, placebo-controlled study of golimumab before methotrexate as first-line therapy for early-onset rheumatoid arthritis. Arthritis Rheum 2009;60: 2272–2283.
19 van Schouwenburg PA, Rispens T, Wolbink GJ: Immunogenicity of anti-TNF biologic therapies for rheumatoid arthritis. Nat Rev Rheumatol 2013;9: 164–172.
20 Hyrich KL, Lunt M, Watson KD, et al: Outcomes after switching from one anti-tumor necrosis factor alpha agent to a second anti-tumor necrosis factor alpha agent in patients with rheumatoid arthritis: results from a large UK national cohort study. Arthritis Rheum 2007;56: 13–20.
21 Plasencia C, Pascual-Salcedo D, García-Carazo S, et al: The immunogenicity to the first anti-TNF therapy determines the outcome of switching to a second anti-TNF therapy in spondyloarthritis patients. Arthritis Res Ther 2013;15:R79.
22 Gisbert JP, Marín AC, McNicholl AG, et al: Systematic review with meta-analysis: the efficacy of a second anti-TNF in patients with inflammatory bowel disease whose previous anti-TNF treatment has failed. Aliment Pharmacol Ther 2015;2:613–623.
23 Yanai H, Lichtenstein L, Assa A, et al: Levels of drug and antidrug antibodies are associated with outcome of interventions after loss of response to infliximab or adalimumab. Clin Gastroenterol Hepatol 2015;13:522–530.e2.
24 Bartelds GM, Wijbrandts CA, Nurmohamed MT, et al: Anti-infliximab and anti-adalimumab antibodies in relation to response to adalimumab in infliximab switchers and anti-tumour necrosis factor naive patients: a cohort study. Ann Rheum Dis 2010;69:817–821.
25 Hanauer SB, Wagner CL, Bala M, et al: Incidence and importance of antibody responses to infliximab after maintenance or episodic treatment in Crohn's disease. Clin Gastroenterol Hepatol 2004;2:542–553.
26 Reinisch W, Sandborn WJ, Rutgeerts P, et al: Long-term infliximab maintenance therapy for ulcerative colitis: the ACT-1 and -2 extension studies. Inflamm Bowel Dis 2012;18:201–211.
27 Wang SL, Hauenstein S, Ohrmund L, et al: Monitoring of adalimumab and antibodies-to-adalimumab levels in patient serum by the homogeneous mobility shift assay. J Pharm Biomed Anal 2013; 78–79:39–44.
28 Lichtenstein GR, Thomsen OØ, Schreiber S, et al: Continuous therapy with certolizumab pegol maintains remission of patients with Crohn's disease for up to 18 months. Clin Gastroenterol Hepatol 2010;8:600–609.
29 Steenholdt C, Palarasah Y, Bendtzen K, et al: Pre-existing IgG antibodies cross-reacting with the Fab region of infliximab predict efficacy and safety of infliximab therapy in inflammatory bowel disease. Aliment Pharmacol Ther 2013; 37:1172–1183.
30 Xue L, Rup B: Evaluation of pre-existing antibody presence as a risk factor for posttreatment anti-drug antibody induction: analysis of human clinical study data for multiple biotherapeutics. AAPS J 2013;15:893–896.
31 Bito T, Nishikawa R, Hatakeyama M, et al: Influence of neutralizing antibodies to adalimumab and infliximab on the treatment of psoriasis. Br J Dermatol 2014;170:922–929.
32 Farrell RJ, Alsahli M, Jeen YT, et al: Intravenous hydrocortisone premedication reduces antibodies to infliximab in Crohn's disease: a randomized controlled trial. Gastroenterology 2003;124: 917–924.
33 Colombel JF, Sandborn WJ, Reinisch W, et al: Infliximab, azathioprine, or combination therapy for Crohn's disease. N Engl J Med 2010;362:1383–1395.
34 Ben-Horin S, Waterman M, Kopylov U, et al: Addition of an immunomodulator to infliximab therapy eliminates anti-drug antibodies in serum and restores clinical response of patients with inflammatory bowel disease. Clin Gastroenterol Hepatol 2013;11:444–447.
35 Hayes MJ, Stein AC, Sakuraba A: Comparison of efficacy, pharmacokinetics, and immunogenicity between infliximab mono- versus combination therapy in ulcerative colitis. J Gastroenterol Hepatol 2014;29:1177–1185.
36 Yarur AJ, Kubiliun MJ, Czul F, et al: Concentrations of 6-thioguanine nucleotide correlate with trough levels of infliximab in patients with inflammatory bowel disease on combination therapy. Clin Gastroenterol Hepatol 2015, in press, DOI: 10.1016/j.cgh.2014.12.026.
37 Molnar T, Farkas K, Nagy F, et al: Lymphomas in two IBD patients treated with anti-TNF-alpha mono or combination therapy: is hepatosplenic lymphoma really the 'old maid'? Inflamm Bowel Dis 2011;17:2025–2026.

Atsushi Sakuraba, MD, PhD
Section of Gastroenterology, Hepatology and Nutrition
Department of Medicine, The University of Chicago
5841 S. Maryland Ave. MC 4076, Chicago, IL 60637 (USA)
E-Mail asakurab@medicine.bsd.uchicago.edu

Rogler G, Herfarth H, Hibi T, Nielsen OH (eds): Anti-Tumor Necrosis Factor Therapy in Inflammatory Bowel Disease.
Front Gastrointest Res. Basel, Karger, 2015, vol 34, pp 100–103 (DOI: 10.1159/000381578)

TNF Antagonist Trough Concentrations and Treatment Efficacy in Inflammatory Bowel Disease

Niels Vande Casteele

University of Leuven, Therapeutic and Diagnostic Antibodies, Leuven, Belgium and University of California San Diego, Division of Gastroenterology, IBD Center, La Jolla, Ca., USA

Abstract

Inter-individual differences in responses and remission rates have been observed in patients with inflammatory bowel diseases treated with TNF antagonists. These differences, together with the risk of loss of response in patients initially responding to treatment, have led researchers to investigate the exposure-response relationships for these biopharmaceutical agents. Different retrospective studies have found a correlation between TNF antagonist trough concentration and patient response, remission and mucosal healing. Moreover, recent cohort and post hoc studies have found clinically significant cut-off concentrations that are correlated with short- and long-term outcomes. Current evidence indicates that the therapeutic drug monitoring of TNF antagonists with individualized dosing has the potential to change and optimize empiric dosing regimens.

Introduction

Substantial inter-individual variability in the pharmacokinetics (PK) of TNF antagonists has been observed in inflammatory bowel disease (IBD) patients [1]. The PK profile of a monoclonal antibody describes the absorption, distribution, metabolization and elimination of a drug and is dependent on drug, patient and disease characteristics [2]. The description of the time course of a drug inside of the body represents the exposure of a patient to the drug. In clinical practice, the drug trough concentration – the lowest serum concentration just before the next administration – is often used as a measurement of drug exposure. Because drug PK and pharmacodynamics are intertwined, investigators have focused on exploring the exposure-response relationships that could explain some of the observed variability in patient response. From the literature, it is known that 70–90% of IBD patients respond to TNF antagonists and that remission is achieved in only 20–50% of patients with standard dosing regimens [3]. Retrospective cohort studies and phase III clinical trial post hoc analyses have investigated the correlations between TNF antagonist trough concentration and response, remission and mucosal healing.

Main Points

Nearly a decade ago, Maser et al. showed in a cohort of 105 Crohn's disease patients treated with infliximab that the rate of clinical remission was higher (82 vs. 6%; p = 0.001), the C-reactive protein (CRP) concentration was lower (2.0 vs. 11.8 mg/l; p = 0.001) and the rate of endoscopic improvement was higher (88 vs. 33%; p = 0.001) in patients with detectable infliximab trough concentrations compared to those with undetectable concentrations [4]. Seow et al. showed in a cohort of 115 ulcerative colitis patients treated with infliximab that the rates of clinical remission and endoscopic improvement were higher (69 vs. 15%; p = 0.001 and 76 vs. 28%; p = 0.001, respectively) and the risk of colectomy was lower (55 vs. 7%, odds ratio 0.11; 95% confidence interval 0.03–0.34; p = 0.001) in patients with detectable infliximab trough concentrations compared to those with undetectable concentrations [5]. The exposure-response relationship for adalimumab was evaluated in 258 ulcerative colitis patients during induction therapy (160/80 mg at week 0/2 and 40 mg every other week) in the ULTRA2 trial, which showed by quartile analysis that higher adalimumab trough concentrations were associated with higher rates of remission [6]. Recently, in the PURSUIT trial evaluating golimumab for the treatment of ulcerative colitis, a similar positive exposure-response relationship was observed [7].

These findings have incentivized investigators to delineate a cut-off TNF antagonist trough concentration that is correlated with (a change in) the CRP level, the clinical scoring index and/or mucosal healing [8–11]. In patients who have lost response to a drug, the determination of the TNF antagonist trough concentration as a surrogate marker to guide treatment intervention or follow-up testing could potentially be cost-saving. In patients with an apparent loss of response (e.g., based on clinical symptoms), the TNF antagonist trough concentration should be measured. If it is found to be suboptimal, then the patient would likely benefit from dose escalation or a switch to another TNF antagonist (the latter in the case of detectable antidrug antibodies). However, if the concentration is found to be (supra)optimal, then endoscopy can be used to rule out other causes of IBD symptoms (which should be addressed if present) or to confirm active disease, in which case the patient should be switched to a drug class with another mechanism of action [12, 13]. A multicenter randomized clinical trial conducted in North America will compare a testing based approach to the conventional approach of dose escalation in ulcerative colitis and Crohn's disease patients losing response to infliximab or adalimumab (NCT01960426).

In conjunction, the TNF antagonist trough concentration was found to have a predictive value, both during the induction phase and the maintenance phase. In a post hoc analysis of the ACCENT I trial, Cornillie et al. found that Crohn's disease patients with a sustained response to infliximab throughout the first year of treatment had a significantly higher median infliximab trough concentration at week 6 during induction compared to patients who did not have a sustained response (12.9 and 8.8 μg/ml, respectively; p = 0.0135). Moreover, an infliximab trough concentration cut-off of ≥3.5 μg/ml at week 14 was predictive of a durable sustained response to the drug throughout the first year of treatment (positive predictive value = 56% and negative predictive value = 83%) [14]. Regarding infliximab maintenance therapy in Crohn's disease patients, Drobne et al. assessed a cohort of 81 patients with available serum samples at the time of antimetabolite withdrawal after 6 months of combination therapy, finding that patients with infliximab trough concentrations of ≥5 μg/ml had a lower risk for loss of response to the drug during follow-up (0% lost response) compared to patients with lower but detectable (≥0.3 μg/ml) (20% lost response) and undetectable (<0.3 μg/ml) (86% lost response) infliximab concentrations. The median follow-up after withdrawal of the antimetabolite was 29 months (interquartile range 15–45) [15]. In a post hoc analysis of the ACT-1 and ACT-2 trials, Adedokun et al. found a correlation between infliximab concentration and efficacy in ulcerative colitis patients. The investigators found that an infliximab concentration of ≥5.1 μg/ml at week 14 predicted the outcome of clinical response at week 30, with a positive predictive value of 74% and a negative predictive value of 54%. Interestingly, at weeks 8, 30 and 54, the proportions of patients achieving clinical remission did not increase above a certain infliximab concentration [16]. In a large cohort study including 285 ulcerative colitis patients treated with infliximab with a median follow-up of 5 years and of which 112 had available serum samples, an infliximab trough concentration of >2.5 μg/ml at week 14 of treatment was predictive of relapse-free survival ($p < 0.001$) and colectomy-free survival ($p = 0.034$) [17].

Based on this causal relationship between the TNF antagonist trough concentration and clinical outcome, the hypothesis of treating patients to reach a target trough concentration was evaluated in the randomized controlled TAXIT trial. In this trial, which included 263 IBD responder patients on maintenance infliximab, dose optimization based on individual trough concentration resulted in a more efficient use of the drug. Dose escalation in Crohn's disease patients with a suboptimal infliximab trough concentration to reach a concentration of ≥3 and ≤7 μg/ml resulted in a significant increase in the proportion of patients in clinical remission (65 before vs. 88% after; $p = 0.02$) and a concomitant decrease in the CRP concentration (4.3 before vs. 3.2 mg/l after; $p < 0.001$). Dose de-escalation in Crohn's disease and ulcerative colitis patients with a supraoptimal infliximab trough concentration to reach a concentration of ≤7 and ≥3 μg/ml did not have a significant effect on the proportion of patients in clinical remission or the CRP concentration, but it did result in significant drug cost savings of 28%. After the initial dose optimization phase, the randomized maintenance phase of the study did not show an additional effect of continuing concentration-based dosing over clinically based dosing [18].

Conclusions and Future Directions

Exposure-response relationships have become apparent for TNF antagonists based on the results of different retrospective cohort studies and phase III clinical trial post hoc analyses and has been confirmed prospectively for infliximab in the randomized TAXIT trial. The ongoing TAILORIX trial (NCT01442025) will investigate the value of early dose optimization (after induction) in Crohn's disease patients starting infliximab. Prospective studies evaluating a dose-to-target approach with other TNF antagonists (adalimumab and golimumab) are to be expected. Furthermore, population PK-pharmacodynamic modeling will identify the covariates responsible for some of the observed variability and will, together with a Bayesian approach, give a better estimate of the ideal individual dose to achieve target drug exposure. In summary, therapeutic drug monitoring with individualized dosing has the potential to change how patients are treated with TNF antagonists, if it is proven to be safe and more effective than the current empiric way of dosing, which is based on symptoms.

References

1 Ordas I, Mould DR, Feagan BG, et al: Anti-TNF monoclonal antibodies in inflammatory bowel disease: pharmacokinetics-based dosing paradigms. Clin Pharmacol Ther 2012;91:635–646.

2 Lobo ED, Hansen RJ, Balthasar JP: Antibody pharmacokinetics and pharmacodynamics. J Pharm Sci 2004;93:2645–2668.

3 Papamichael K, Gils A, Rutgeerts P, et al: Role for therapeutic drug monitoring during induction therapy with TNF antagonists in IBD: evolution in the definition and management of primary nonresponse. Inflamm Bowel Dis 2015;21:182–197.

4 Maser EA, Villela R, Silverberg MS, et al: Association of trough serum infliximab to clinical outcome after scheduled maintenance treatment for Crohn's disease. Clin Gastroenterol Hepatol 2006;4:1248–1254.

5 Seow CH, Newman A, Irwin SP, et al: Trough serum infliximab: a predictive factor of clinical outcome for infliximab treatment in acute ulcerative colitis. Gut 2010;59:49–54.

6 Mostafa NM, Eckert D, Pradhan RS, et al: P333 exposure-efficacy relationship (ER) for adalimumab during induction phase of treatment of adult patients with moderate to severe ulcerative colitis (UC). United European Gastroenterol J 2013;1:A221–A222.

7 Sandborn WJ, Feagan BG, Marano C, et al: Subcutaneous golimumab induces clinical response and remission in patients with moderate-to-severe ulcerative colitis. Gastroenterology 2014;146:85–95.

8 Vande Casteele N, Khanna R, Levesque BG, et al: The relationship between infliximab concentrations, antibodies to infliximab and disease activity in Crohn's disease. Gut 2014, DOI: 10.1136/gutjnl-2014-307883.

9 Levesque BG, Greenberg GR, Zou G, et al: A prospective cohort study to determine the relationship between serum infliximab concentration and efficacy in patients with luminal Crohn's disease. Aliment Pharmacol Ther 2014;39:1126–1135.

10 Imaeda H, Takahashi K, Fujimoto T, et al: Clinical utility of newly developed immunoassays for serum concentrations of adalimumab and anti-adalimumab antibodies in patients with Crohn's disease. J Gastroenterol 2014;49:100–109.

11 Roblin X, Marotte H, Rinaudo M, et al: Association between pharmacokinetics of adalimumab and mucosal healing in patients with inflammatory bowel diseases. Clin Gastroenterol Hepatol 2014;12:80–84.e2.

12 Feagan BG, Rutgeerts P, Sands BE, et al: Vedolizumab as induction and maintenance therapy for ulcerative colitis. N Engl J Med 2013;369:699–710.

13 Sandborn WJ, Feagan BG, Rutgeerts P, et al: Vedolizumab as induction and maintenance therapy for Crohn's disease. N Engl J Med 2013;369:711–721.

14 Cornillie F, Hanauer SB, Diamond RH, et al: Postinduction serum infliximab trough level and decrease of C-reactive protein level are associated with durable sustained response to infliximab: a retrospective analysis of the ACCENT I trial. Gut 2014;63:1721–1727.

15 Drobne D, Bossuyt P, Breynaert C, et al: Withdrawal of immunomodulators after co-treatment does not reduce trough level of infliximab in patients with Crohn's disease. Clin Gastroenterol Hepatol 2015;13:514–521.e4.

16 Adedokun OJ, Sandborn WJ, Feagan BG, et al. Association between serum concentration of infliximab and efficacy in adult patients with ulcerative colitis. Gastroenterology 2014;147:1296–1307.e5.

17 Loste MA, Vande Casteele N, Vermeire S, et al: A panel to predict long-term outcome of infliximab therapy for patients with ulcerative colitis. Clin Gastroenterol Hepatol 2015;13:531–538.

18 Vande Casteele N, Ferrante M, Van Assche G, et al: Trough Concentrations of Infliximab Guide Dosing for Patients With Inflammatory Bowel Disease. Gastroenterology 2015, DOI: 10.1053/j.gastro.2015.02.031.

Dr. Niels Vande Casteele
University of Leuven, Therapeutic and Diagnostic Antibodies
Herestraat 49, PO Box 820
BE–3000 Leuven (Belgium)
E-Mail niels.vandecasteele@kuleuven.be

Rogler G, Herfarth H, Hibi T, Nielsen OH (eds): Anti-Tumor Necrosis Factor Therapy in Inflammatory Bowel Disease.
Front Gastrointest Res. Basel, Karger, 2015, vol 34, pp 104–106 (DOI: 10.1159/000381579)

What Is a Biosimilar?

Dario Neri

Department of Chemistry and Applied Biosciences, Swiss Federal Institute of Technology (ETH Zurich), Zurich, Switzerland

Abstract

Biosimilars, also known as 'follow-on biologics', are biopharmaceutical products developed with the aim to mimic an innovator product as closely as possible, once the relevant patent protection has expired. Biosimilars and the corresponding innovator products are typically therapeutic proteins that may have the same amino acid sequence but for which complete identity is hard to achieve in practice due to the complex nature of protein structures. In most territories, the approval process for biosimilars requires the execution of clinical trials. Typically, the approval of a biosimilar product does not automatically imply interchangeability with the innovator product.

Introduction

Most biopharmaceuticals on the market are therapeutic proteins, which are produced using recombinant DNA technology [1]. Once the corresponding patents have expired, it may be attractive for competitor companies to develop 'biosimilars', which match the structure and properties of the innovator product as closely as possible. Typically, biosimilars are sold at a lower price compared to the innovator product, if only because the biosimilar product represents a 'copy' and does not require lengthy discovery activity.

Some biopharmaceuticals on the market, those which are produced in *Escherichia coli* or in yeast, are not glycosylated and are therefore easier to copy, yielding biosimilar products that display biochemical properties (e.g., very similar mass spectrometric, electrophoretic and chromatographic profiles, as well as biological activity and pharmacokinetic properties) closely matching those of the original product. Nonetheless, even in this more favorable situation, it is hard to formally demonstrate complete identity between an innovator product and the corresponding biosimilar since certain post-translational modifications (e.g., transamidation reactions) or different protein folding properties may be difficult to detect, even for polypeptides with an identical amino acid sequence and using sophisticated analytical methods. When considering glycosylated products produced in mammalian cells (e.g., monoclonal antibodies), the differences may become more substantial, as the distribution of various oligosaccharide structures on the protein

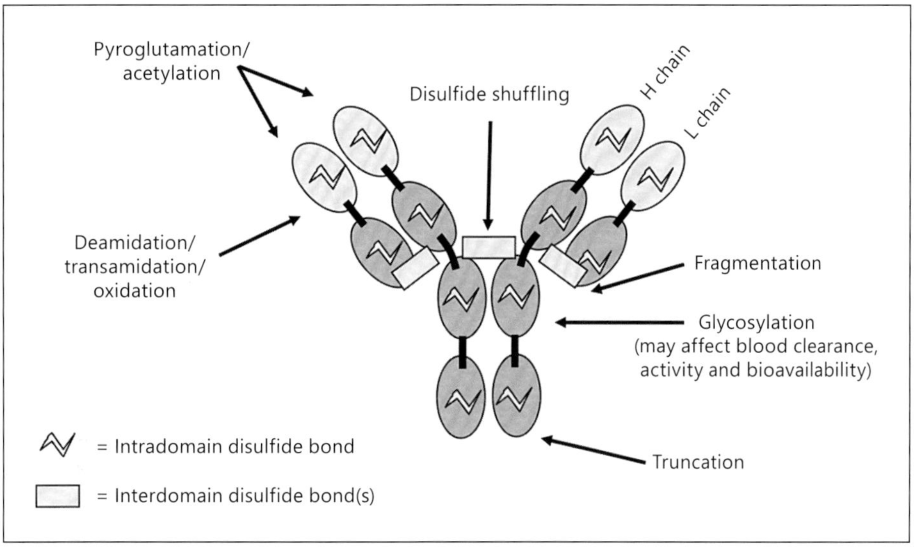

Fig. 1. Schematic representation of the domain structure of an antibody product in IgG format. The main structural features (e.g., immunoglobulin domains, disulfide bonds, and heavy and light chains) and some of the possible post-translational modifications that may lead to differences between closely related products are indicated.

depends on many parameters, including the host cell type and the fermentation conditions. Importantly, protein glycosylation has been shown to affect pharmacokinetics and, in the case of antibodies, the ability to recruit natural killer cells as a result of an alteration in affinity for Fcγ receptors [2, 3].

Main Points

In this Section, we focus on antibody biosimilars, as these molecules represent the main topic of the book. Biosimilar products aim to reproduce the properties of the innovator antibody by using a gene that codes for an identical amino acid sequence. However, since different companies use different plasmids and cell lines, copies of the original product can only be 'similar', not identical. Furthermore, variations in the methodologies used for cultured cell growth and downstream purification may lead to differences between an innovator product and the corresponding biosimilars.

Figure 1 schematically summarizes some of the main elements of chemical variability that can be found in clinical-grade preparations of antibody molecules. Antibodies produced in mammalian cells under different experimental conditions may exhibit modifications to the N-terminus and to the polypeptide chain (transamidase reactions, proteolytic degradation, or heterogeneity of the C-terminus). Furthermore, shuffling of disulfide bridges may occur. However, the most important source of chemical differences between antibody preparations is related to variations in N-linked glycoforms, which can be found on the conserved Asn297 residue. One has to remember that antibody glycosylation typically leads to several types of oligosaccharide structures that co-exist within the same product and that may vary to some extent from batch to bath [4].

In order to facilitate comparisons, companies involved in biosimilar product development may collect documentation about the batch-to-batch variability of the innovator product and use this information as a reference for their own biosimilar products [5].

Conclusions and Future Directions

Biosimilar products that have gained marketing authorization in some European countries include erythropoietins, G-CSF, FSH, hGH and a monoclonal antibody (a biosimilar of Infliximab) [1]. Broader distribution of biosimilars for Infliximab in Europe is expected after 2015, when the corresponding patents will expire.

On one hand, companies involved in the development of biosimilars may use information related to batch-to-batch variability of the innovator product as a benchmark to indicate that the specifications of their own product fall within previously accepted variations of the reference compound. On the other hand, some subtle variations in the manufacturing of biopharmaceuticals have previously been shown to have a substantial clinical impact. For example, changes in manufacturing conditions for a monoclonal antibody led to variations in pharmacokinetic properties and antibody potency in Phase III clinical trials (see [6]). Sometimes, seemingly minor experimental variations may have profound clinical consequences. One of the most prominent examples is related to changes in the formulation of recombinant erythropoietin preparations and the introduction of rubber stopping into the syringes used for this product. These changes were most likely responsible for a dramatic increase in the incidence of pure red-cell anemia following administration of the recombinant protein as a result of increased and persistent immunogenicity of the product [7]. Thus, small variations in manufacturing conditions may have big effects on therapeutic proteins. For these reasons, only the execution of comparative clinical trials and the broad distribution of a biosimilar product, along with suitable measures for product tracking and pharmacovigilance activities, can unambiguously indicate whether a substantial bioequivalence with the innovator product can be expected.

References

1 Walsh G: Biopharmaceutical benchmarks 2014. Nat Biotechnol 2014;32:992–1000.

2 Sinclair AM, Elliott S: Glycoengineering: the effect of glycosylation on the properties of therapeutic proteins. J Pharm Sci 2005;94:1626–1635.

3 Umaña P, Jean-Mairet J, Moudry R, Amstutz H, Bailey JE: Engineered glycoforms of an anti-neuroblastoma IgG1 with optimized antibody-dependent cellular cytotoxic activity. Nat Biotechnol 1999;17:176–180.

4 Nallet S, Fornelli L, Schmitt S, Parra J, Baldi L, Tsybin JO, Wurm FO: Glycan variability on a recombinant IgG antibody transiently produced in HEK-293E cells. N Biotech 2012;29:471–476.

5 Schiestl M, Stangler T, Torella C, Cepeljnik T, Toll H, Grau R: Acceptable changes in quality attributes of glycosylated biopharmaceuticals. Nat Biotechnol 2014;29:310–312.

6 Dove A: Betting on biogenerics. Nat Biotechnol 2001;19:117–120.

7 Woodcock J, Griffin J, Behrman R, Cherney B, Crescenzi T, Fraser B, Hixon D, Joneckis C, Kozlowski S, Rosenberg A, Schrager L, Shacter E, Temple R, Webber K, Winkle H: The FDA assessment of follow-on products: a historical perspective. Nat Rev Drug Discov 2007;6:437–442.

Dario Neri
Department of Chemistry and Applied Biosciences
Swiss Federal Institute of Technology (ETH Zurich), Vladimir Prelog Weg 4
CH–8093 Zurich (Switzerland)
E-Mail dario.neri@pharma.ethz.ch

Rogler G, Herfarth H, Hibi T, Nielsen OH (eds): Anti-Tumor Necrosis Factor Therapy in Inflammatory Bowel Disease.
Front Gastrointest Res. Basel, Karger, 2015, vol 34, pp 107–112 (DOI: 10.1159/000381580)

Is Extrapolation of Safety and Efficacy Data Possible?

Mark Ainsworth

Department of Medical Gastroenterology, Copenhagen University Hospital, Herlev, Denmark

Abstract

A biosimilar drug is a biologic medicinal product intended to be similar in structure and effect to an already marketed biologic medicinal product (the originator) for which safety and efficacy has already been established to a degree that would allow for the extrapolation of safety and efficacy data from the originator to the biosimilar, making it unnecessary to supply full documentation for the biosimilar. Due to the often extremely complicated structure of most biologics, biosimilarity can only be declared if careful physicochemical testing, in vitro and in vivo studies of biological activity, and limited clinical studies indicate no clinically relevant differences between an originator and the intended biosimilar (a so-called comparability exercise). Recently, a biosimilar to Remicade (infliximab) called Remsima has gained approval from European regulators. The scope of the comparability exercise leading to the approval of Remsima is reviewed. While the data supporting the biosimilarity of Remsima in general appears to be convincing and while the concept of the extrapolation of indications as such is not questioned, the extrapolation of indications in this specific case has by some been questioned due to the lack of knowledge of the exact modes of action of the drug and of the potential differences in the modes of action of the drug between indications. Considering the at least theoretical risk of the comparability exercise failing to detect differences in safety and efficacy that will be revealed at a later stage will, adequate post-marketing measures are needed in order to detect any signs of changes in safety and efficacy. Finally, the concepts of drift and evolution leading to divergence between an originator and a biosimilar must also be taken into account when using biosimilars in everyday clinical practice.

Introduction

A biosimilar is a biologic medicinal product (usually manufactured using recombinant gene technology) developed to be similar to an original biologic medicinal product for which safety and efficacy has already been convincingly demonstrated, thus allowing for the extrapolation of the safety and efficacy data for the original biologic [1, 2]. Thus, the concept of a biosimilar rests on a positive answer to the question posed in the title of this chapter. If extrapolation were considered unacceptable under any circumstances, even for biologics with a high degree of similarity, the concept of a biosimilar would be meaningless, as a full development program demonstrating safety and efficacy would always be necessary anyway. Regardless of this fundamental issue, the problem remains that describing the criteria for similarity between the biosimilar and the original needs to be fulfilled before it can be considered acceptable to extrapolate the safety and efficacy data for the original to the biosimilar.

Main Points

Biologics are usually large protein molecules with a complicated structure that are synthesized in a biological system. The structure is determined by not only the linear sequence of amino acids (primary structure) but also how segments of this sequence are folded (secondary structure) and how these segments are oriented three-dimensionally (tertiary structure). Furthermore, biologics may contain a number of protein subunits arranged in a three-dimensional structure (quaternary structure). Finally, many proteins are subject to glycosylation and post-translational modifications (such as acetylation, phosphorylation, methylation, sumoylation) [3]. Thus, merely demonstrating that an intended biosimilar has the same amino acid sequence as the originator product will not suffice. A thorough physicochemical characterization, usually in combination with limited pre-clinical and clinical studies (a comparability exercise), is necessary [1] to demonstrate that the intended biosimilar can be considered sufficiently similar (in terms of higher-order structure and function) to the original to allow for the extrapolation of safety and efficacy results.

The challenge of demonstrating comparability is dependent on the size and the complexity of the original biologic. In that respect, therapeutic monoclonal antibodies like infliximab and adalimumab pose a special challenge, as they are large complex molecules consisting of several subunits (two heavy chains and two light chains joined by disulfide bonds) of glycosylated polypeptides. The biological function of the antibody is dependent on the exact three-dimensional structure of several regions such as the Fab region (the antigen-binding domain) and the Fc region, which is responsible for complement activation and the interaction of the antibody with Fc receptors, mediating a number of different immune responses. Even small changes in the manufacturing process may have a profound effect on these regions and thus affect the biologic activity of the antibody [4]. In recent years, analytical techniques have improved, making it easier to demonstrate that an intended biosimilar has the same physicochemical characteristics as the original biologic [5]. Nevertheless, physicochemical investigations are currently not considered to be sufficient to rule out differences in higher-order structure (secondary, tertiary and quaternary structure), post-translational modifications and aggregation [6]. In general, animal studies (in vivo and in vitro studies) as well as limited human studies, primarily studies of pharmacodynamics (PD) and pharmacokinetics (PK) [7], will also have to be performed in order to rule out any clinically relevant differences between the intended biosimilar and the original product.

The biosimilar infliximab (sold under the trade names Remsima® and Inflectra®, as described in the subsequent section titled Remsima) has recently been approved by the European Medicines Agency (EMA) [8]. Its approval was based on an extensive comparability program following a stepwise approach as recommended by both the EMA [9] and the U.S. Food and Drug Administration [6]. Regarding all major physicochemical characteristics, Remsima was similar to Remicade [8]. Furthermore, the biologic activity of Remsima was similar to that of Remicade. However, the scientific committee of the EMA 'noted a small difference in the amount of a fucosylated infliximab, translating into a lower binding affinity towards specific Fc receptors and a lower *ex vivo* antibody-dependent cellular cytotoxicity activity in the most sensitive antibody-dependent cellular cytotoxicity assay' [8]. However, as this difference did not have any influence on the activity of Remsima in other experimental models, which were considered to be more relevant to the pathophysiologic conditions in humans, it was not considered of clinical importance [8]. In addition to these physicochemical analyses and animal (in vitro and in vivo) studies, a limited clinical program was also performed [10] consisting of a PK/PD study in patients with ankylosing spondylitis and a clinical phase III safety and efficacy study in patients with rheumatoid arthritis. The PK/PD study demonstrated that regarding the area under the curve at steady state and the maximal concentration following infusion, Remsima was equivalent to Remicade, as the 90% confidence interval of the ratio of the mean of the two agents was within the accepted range of 80–125% [11]. Furthermore, clinical efficacy, as judged by the Assessment in Ankylosing Spondylitis criteria, was similar between the two compounds. In a larger phase III clinical study in patients with rheumatoid arthritis treated with methotrexate, the safety and efficacy of Remsima was similar to that of Remicade [12]. Based on the totality of evidence, it was concluded that Remsima was sufficiently similar to Remicade to allow for the extrapolation of the safety and efficacy results obtained for Remicade, i.e. a biosimilar. The EMA extended this extrapolation to include all indications studied for Remicade, i.e. the indications for which no studies have been performed with Remsima [8]. The decision of the EMA, particularly the decision to allow the extrapolation of indications, has been criticized [13–18]. Most of the sceptics do not provide any concrete reasons for their position apart from the previously mentioned general problems associated with demonstrating similarity between complex biotechnology-derived molecules such as monoclonal antibodies [13–15, 17]. The general rejection of the possibility to demonstrate similarity between two biologics appears unsubstantiated. It has to be borne in mind that an original biologic sold today is not identical to the biologic that was originally demonstrated to be safe and efficacious. Thus, for almost all biologics manufactured by recombinant gene technology, there have been numerous subsequent changes in the manufacturing process that at least in theory could change the efficacy and safety of the drug [19]. For each of these changes, the manufacturer of the original biologic has to perform a comparability exercise similar in nature to the one previously described (albeit often of a smaller magnitude due to the in-depth knowledge of the previous manufacturing process) [20]. Thus, flatly rejecting the concept of a biosimilar based on the standpoint that demonstrating comparability is never possible would in essence also prevent manufacturers of the originator biologic from adjusting/changing/improving manufacturing processes, a practice that is widely accepted by regulators, albeit largely unknown by clinicians. However, others have raised more specific concerns about the extrapolation of indications for which no clinical data are available. Specifically, concerns have been raised about the appropriateness of the clinical and in vitro studies to demonstrate that Remsima is sufficiently similar to Remicade to allow for the extrapolation of the entire set of indications approved for Remicade [16, 18, 21]. A call for the performance of comparative clinical studies for each indication is of course always a cautionary approach. However, such a requirement will defeat the purpose of a biosimilar, as it essentially will mean that any new biologic, even the ones that are intended to be similar to an existing biologic, will have to provide a full package of documentation as if it were a new biologic. Apart from losing the predicted economic savings [22, 23] associated with the introduction of biosimilars, the question remains whether requesting clinical studies for each indication is truly necessary [24].

Furthermore, it is questionable whether clinical studies designed to provide confirmatory evidence of the safety and the efficacy of the original biosimilar are optimal in this setting. Thus, in terms of ruling out any differences in efficacy between a biosimilar and the original, the study design and endpoints should be chosen to provide optimal sensitivity to demonstrate differences between two biologics (optimal discriminatory ability), not necessarily to provide evidence for a clinical benefit [25].

Based on the available data [8, 10–12], it appears well documented that Remsima is similar to Remicade to an extent that would allow for the extrapolation of data obtained for Remicade. It is, however, still an open question whether this extrapolation can be extended to include all indications approved for Remicade but for which there are no data on Remsima [16, 21]. In particular, the incomplete knowledge of the exact mechanism of action of infliximab in different indications and the possibility that the mechanism of action differs between different diseases makes it difficult to identify a specific test that could reliably assess and rule out differences in the mode of action of Remicade versus Remsima.

However, when integrating biosimilars into clinical practice, there are a number of problems that need to be considered. As previously mentioned, even small differences in the manufacturing process may lead to differences in the higher-order structure of the biosimilar compared to the originator product. This, in turn, may change (increase or decrease) the immunogenicity of the biosimilar compared to the originator product. Although assessment of differences in antigenicity is a key element in any comparability exercise [2, 26, 27], the relatively short duration and small exposure of the clinical studies available at the time of approval makes it necessary to pay special attention to this problem after approval. This, combined with the need to be able to detect other signals indicating differences between an originator and a biosimilar in terms of safety and efficacy, makes it necessary to pay special attention to pharmacovigilance for biosimilars [28, 29]. Standard pharmacovigilance activities usually focus on the active substance instead of the brand name. However, in the situation in which one or more biosimilars are on the market, this strategy will not provide the information needed. A system needs to be in place for accurately determining which specific biosimilar(s) the patient has been treated with, e.g. infliximab (Remicade) or infliximab (Remsima) (traceability). Such a system has not been agreed upon.

Adding to this problem is the well known problem of drift, evolution and divergence of biological drugs [30]. As previously described, even minute alterations in the manufacturing process may lead to small (or large) changes in the structure and the function of a biotechnologically derived biologic. Thus, unnoticed and unplanned deviations (drift) as well as planned changes (evolution) may change the higher-order structure of the biologic, as well as its function, over time. Eventually, drift and evolution can result in the biosimilar (as well as the currently marketed original product) becoming different from the specific version of the originator product that was initially marketed and that was subsequently used in the comparability exercise (divergence). This problem also has to be addressed during the post-marketing surveillance of the biosimilar (and the originator). Furthermore, this inevitable problem also raises concerns about the appropriateness of changing between an original product and a biosimilar when treating an individual patient (interchangeability) [27]. Although experience with biosimilar erythropoiesis-stimulating agents does not indicate that switching back and forth constitutes a safety risk [27], this practice may preclude traceability and could theoretically lead to patients experiencing alterations in disease control due to the previously described divergence between the originator product and a biosimilar.

Conclusions and Future Directions

In conclusion, the extrapolation of safety and efficacy results of the original product to the biosimilar may be possible if an appropriate comparability exercise has been carried out. This appears to be the case for the recently approved infliximab biosimilar Remsima. However, caution should be exercised when extrapolating these safety and efficacy results in indications obtained for the original biologic but for which no studies have been performed with the biosimilar. When using biosimilars, robust post-marketing surveillance of efficacy and safety (including immunogenicity) is paramount. A prerequisite for meaningful pharmacovigilance is the establishment of a system that will provide a high degree of traceability. Finally, even for highly similar biologics, interchangeability may be problematic due to the inevitable drift and evolution of biologics, which could lead to divergence between the biosimilar and the original drug over time.

References

1 Committee for Medicinal Products for Human Use (CHMP): Guideline on similar biological medicinal products. CHMP/437/04. 2005. http://www.ema.europa.eu/docs/en_GB/document_library/Scientific_guideline/2009/09/WC500003517.pdf (accessed May 17, 2015).

2 World Health Organization, Expert Committee on Biological Sterilization: Guidelines on evaluation of similar biotherapeutic products (SBPs), 2009. http://www.who.int/biologicals/areas/biological_therapeutics/BIOTHERAPEUTICS_FOR_WEB_22APRIL2010.pdf (accessed May 17, 2015).

3 Tsiftsoglou AS, Ruiz S, Schneider CK: Development and regulation of biosimilars: current status and future challenges. BioDrugs 2013;27:203–211.

4 Committee for Medicinal Products for Human Use (CHMP): Guideline on similar biological medicinal products containing monoclonal antibodies – non-clinical and clinical issues. EMA/CHMP/BMWP/403543/2010. 2012. http://www.ema.europa.eu/docs/en_GB/document_library/Scientific_guideline/2012/06/WC500128686.pdf (accessed May 17, 2015).

5 Berkowitz SA, Engen JR, Mazzeo JR, Jones GB: Analytical tools for characterizing biopharmaceuticals and the implications for biosimilars. Nat Rev Drug Discov 2012;11:527–540.

6 U.S. Department of Health and Human Services, Food and Drug Administration, Center for Drug Evaluation and Research (CDER), Center for Biologics Evaluation and Research (CBER): Guidance for industry: scientific considerations in demonstrating biosimilarity to a reference product. Draft guidance, 2012. http://www.fda.gov/downloads/Drugs/GuidanceComplianceRegulatoryInformation/Guidances/UCM291128.pdf (accessed May 17, 2015).

7 Wang YM, Chow AT: Development of biosimilars – pharmacokinetic and pharmacodynamic considerations. J Biopharm Stat 2010;20:46–61.

8 Committee for Medicinal Products for Human Use (CHMP): Assessment report: Inflectra. International non-proprietary name: Infliximab. Procedure No. EMEA/H/C/002778/0000. EMA/CHMP/589422/2013. 2013. http://www.ema.europa.eu/docs/en_GB/document_library/EPAR_-_Public_assessment_report/human/002778/WC500151490.pdf (accessed May 17, 2015).

9 Committee for Medicinal Products for Human Use (CHMP). Guideline on similar biological medicinal products containing biotechnology-derived proteins as active substance: non-clinical and clinical issues. EMEA/CHMP/BMWP/42832/2005. 2006. http://www.ema.europa.eu/docs/en_GB/document_library/Scientific_guideline/2009/09/WC500003920.pdf (accessed May 17, 2015).

10 McKeage K: A review of CT-P13: an infliximab biosimilar. BioDrugs 2014;28:313–321.

11 Park W, Hrycaj P, Jeka S, Kovalenko V, Lysenko G, Miranda P, et al: A randomised, double-blind, multicentre, parallel-group, prospective study comparing the pharmacokinetics, safety, and efficacy of CT-P13 and innovator infliximab in patients with ankylosing spondylitis: the PLANETAS study. Ann Rheum Dis 2013;72:1605–1612.

12 Yoo DH, Hrycaj P, Miranda P, Ramiterre E, Piotrowski M, Shevchuk S, et al: A randomised, double-blind, parallel-group study to demonstrate equivalence in efficacy and safety of CT-P13 compared with innovator infliximab when coadministered with methotrexate in patients with active rheumatoid arthritis: the PLANETRA study. Ann Rheum Dis 2013;72:1613–1620.

13 Danese S, Fiorino G, Michetti P: Viewpoint: knowledge and viewpoints on biosimilar monoclonal antibodies among members of the European Crohn's and Colitis Organization. J Crohns Colitis 2014;8:1548–1550.

14 Danese S, Gomollon F: ECCO position statement: the use of biosimilar medicines in the treatment of inflammatory bowel disease (IBD). J Crohns Colitis 2013;7:586–589.

15 Argüelles-Arias F, Barreiro-de-Acosta M, Carballo F, Hinojosa J, Tejerina T: Joint position statement by 'Sociedad Espana de Patología Digestiva (Spanish Society of Gastroenterology) and 'Sociada Espanola de Farmacologia' (Spanish Society of Pharmacology) on biosimilar therapy for inflammatory bowel disease. Rev Esp Enferm Dig (Madrid) 2013;105: 37–32.

16 Feagan BG, Choquette D, Ghosh S, Gladman DD, Ho V, Meibohm B, et al: The challenge of indication extrapolation for infliximab biosimilars. Biologicals 2014; 42:177–183.

17 Fiorino G, Girolomoni G, Lapadula G, Orlando A, Danese S, Olivieri I: The use of biosimilars in immune-mediated disease: a joint Italian Society of Rheumatology (SIR), Italian Society of Dermatology (SIDeMaST), and Italian Group of Inflammatory Bowel Disease (IG-IBD) position paper. Autoimmun Rev 2014;13:751–755.

18 Lee H: Is extrapolation of the safety and efficacy data in one indication to another appropriate for biosimilars? AAPS J 2014;16:22–26.

19 Hlavaty T, Letkovsky J: Biosimilars in the therapy of inflammatory bowel diseases. Eur J Gastroenterol Hepatol 2014; 26:581–587.

20 Weise M, Bielsky MC, De Smet K, Ehmann F, Ekman N, Giezen TJ, et al: Biosimilars: what clinicians should know. Blood 2012;120:5111–5117.

21 Gecse KB, Khanna R, van den Brink GR, Ponsioen CY, Löwenberg M, Jairath V, et al: Biosimilars in IBD: hope or expectation? Gut 2013;62:803–807.

22 Moum B, Lundin KE: Biotilsvarende legemidler ved inflammatorisk tarmsykdom. Tidsskr Nor Legeforen 2014;134: 819–820.

23 Brodszky V, Baji P, Balogh O, Pentek M: Budget impact analysis of biosimilar infliximab (CT-P13) for the treatment of rheumatoid arthritis in six Central and Eastern European countries. Eur J Health Econ 2014;15(suppl 1):S65–S71.

24 McCamish M, Woollett G: The continuum of comparability extends to biosimilarity: how much is enough and what clinical data are necessary? Clin Pharmacol Ther 2013;93:315–317.

25 Dranitsaris G, Dorward K, Hatzimichael E, Amir E: Clinical trial design in biosimilar drug development. Invest New Drugs 2013;31:479–487.

26 Committee for Medicinal Products for Human Use (CHMP): Guideline on immunogenicity assessment of monoclonal antibodies intended for in vivo clinical use, 2012. http://www.ema.europa.eu/docs/en_GB/document_library/Scientific_guideline/2012/06/WC500128688.pdf (accessed May 17, 2015).

27 Ebbers HC, Crow SA, Vulto AG, Schellekens H: Interchangeability, immunogenicity and biosimilars. Nat Biotechnol 2012;30:1186–1190.

28 Calvo B, Zuniga L: EU's new pharmacovigilance legislation: considerations for biosimilars. Drug Saf 2014;37:9–18.

29 Casadevall N, Edwards IR, Felix T, Graze PR, Litten JB, Strober BE, et al: Pharmacovigilance and biosimilars: considerations, needs and challenges. Expert Opin Biol Ther 2013;13:1039–1047.

30 Ramanan S, Grampp G: Drift, evolution, and divergence in biologics and biosimilars manufacturing. BioDrugs 2014;28: 363–372.

Mark Ainsworth, MD, PhD, DMSc
Department of Gastroenterology, Copenhagen University Hospital at Herlev
Herlev Ringvej 75
DK–2730 Herlev (Denmark)
E-Mail mark.ainsworth@regionh.dk

Rogler G, Herfarth H, Hibi T, Nielsen OH (eds): Anti-Tumor Necrosis Factor Therapy in Inflammatory Bowel Disease.
Front Gastrointest Res. Basel, Karger, 2015, vol 34, pp 113–118 (DOI: 10.1159/000381581)

Potential Concerns and Questions

Gerhard Rogler

Division of Gastroenterology and Hepatology and Zurich Center for Integrative Human Physiology, University of Zurich, Zurich, Switzerland

Abstract

Biosimilars are biological products that are very similar, but not identical, to an originator product. For anti-TNF biosimilars for inflammatory bowel disease treatment, a number of concerns have been raised by pharmacologists and gastroenterologists with respect to the evaluation of biosimilarity, product stability, production condition stability, biosimilar name, extrapolation of indications, traceability, interchangeability and pharmacovigilance. These points will be discussed in this review. There are several questions that have not been satisfactorily answered so far, leading to different regulatory guidelines in Europe (European Medicines Agency), the USA (Food and Drug Administration), Canada and other countries. For clinicians, it will be important to have knowledge about these concerns to make reasonable patient-oriented decisions in the upcoming confusing market of biosimilars for established anti-TNF antibodies.

Introduction

In the field of inflammatory bowel disease, biosimilar products to Infliximab are the first approved monoclonal antibody biosimilars. Substances called Remsima® (Celltrion), Inflectra® (Hospira and Alvogen) and Flammegis® (Egis) are biosimilars to Remicade® that have come into the market [1–3]. Current development is underway to establish biosimilars to adalimumab (Humira®). However, there are several concerns and questions that have to be addressed despite the fact that the first biosimilar biologicals are already used in clinical practice [4–7]. First, the evaluation of biosimilarity is still a matter of debate. Does a clinical trial in just one indication together with biochemical and pharmacokinetic characterization already prove biosimilarity? Is interchangeability more important? Which indications can be extrapolated and how? Another point of concern is reference product stability. Furthermore, the biosimilar name (the international nonproperty name; INN) is still a matter of debate. The final point to be addressed in discussions about biosimilars is pharmacovigilance. The knowledge about these points in private practice is low. Awareness of those problems, however, is necessary to avoid treatment mistakes and damage to the patient.

Evaluation of Biosimilarity

There is certainly a difference in evaluating and ensuring biosimilarity between simple peptides or proteins and therapeutic antibodies. Whereas simple peptides and proteins with the same amino acid structure certainly should have the same pharmacological behavior, it is much more difficult to directly copy antibodies [8–12]. Two antibodies with the same amino acid sequence that have been produced in different expression systems or cell lines will have a different glycosylation pattern [13]. After the 'simple' cellular process of the generation of the amino acid chain via translation from mRNA, modifications are introduced into the amino acid chain, and its physicochemical characteristics are dependent on the system in which the antibody is produced [13]. Important modifications that are induced by the expression system are, as mentioned, glycosylation, fucosylation, sialylation and disulfide shuffling. Analytical methods to determine such modifications have been developed in recent years [14–17]. In the guidelines on 'similar biological medicinal products containing monoclonal antibody – nonclinical and clinical issues' published by the European Medicines Agency (EMA), a stepwise comparability exercise is requested and recommended [18]. According to this document, the definition of comparability will depend on similar physicochemical characteristics and biological activity to the reference product, comparable pharmacodynamics and pharmacokinetics, comparable preclinical toxicology results and, finally, clinical trial results. However, whereas there is agreement on most of the requirements for the analytical methods needed to provide preclinical evidence for biosimilarity, different regulatory agencies have different opinions about the requested evidence from clinical trials for biosimilarity (see below).

The assessment report for Remsima® shows that there is high similarity with respect to amino acid analysis, peptide mapping by liquid chromatography mass spectrometry, analysis of post-translational modifications, N-terminal and C-terminal sequencing and heavy and light chain mass determination [19]. Furthermore, disulfide bond localization, the determination of free sulfhydryl groups, secondary and tertiary structure analysis and (calorimetric) analysis of the stability of higher-order structures provided similar results compared to Remicade®. To further characterize both antibodies, aggregate content and monomeric purity analyses, electrophoretic mobility shift assays under nonreducing and reducing conditions, SDS-PAGE analysis, analysis of C-terminal lysine variability, and product deamination and oxidation were examined [19]. No significant differences were found in any of the mentioned analyses.

To further address the above mentioned concerns about post-translational modifications, glycosylation analysis was carried out to investigate site-specific glycosylation, the monosaccharide content of neutral and amino sugars, N-linked glycans, and the absence of O-linked glycans. Furthermore, oligosaccharide profiling and sialic acid analysis were done. This shows the efforts that are necessary to demonstrate molecular biosimilarity. However, biologicals may change over time due to production changes (see below), and so far, there is no guarantee that those changes will always be made for both the originator and the biosimilar.

For Remsima®, comparable binding to human TNFα was shown by ELISA and surface plasmon resonance [19]. Furthermore, there was comparable binding to membrane-bound TNF based on cell-based ELISAs. There was a lack of affinity to human TNFβ. Comparable affinity for human tissues and to mouse, rat, canine, porcine and rhesus monkey TNF were also confirmed. Comparable neutralization of TNFα in vitro was shown, as well as comparable induction of apoptosis [19]. Further, suppression of cytokine secretion in epithelial cell lines, C1q binding, toxicity and FC receptor binding were compared. However, the question of the extent to which comparability is requested is still a matter of debate. Is it really a 15% margin relative to the comparator, or should the margin that is requested for comparability approval be narrower? There are arguments on both sides.

With respect to the pharmacokinetic profile, Park et al. showed that the mean serum concentrations of Remsima® are almost identical to those of the reference drug if 5 mg per kg bodyweight were given [20, 21]. Also, with respect to safety, no significantly different signs were determined [20, 21]. Remsima® was analyzed in rheumatic diseases, and its efficacy was very comparable. However, the question again arises, for which indications does similar efficacy need to be shown to be sure that it is acceptable to extrapolate this finding to other diseases.

Reference Product Stability

Biologics, especially monoclonal antibodies, evolve over time. No batch of any biological, including the reference product, is identical to the previous one [22]. This nonidentity between batches is a normal feature of biotechnology that has to be controlled by tight specifications of the critical attributes of the products. For approved products such as Remicade®, in the meantime, more than 30 changes in the manufacturing process have been approved by regulatory agencies. A biological that is biosimilar at a certain point during the production process might undergo

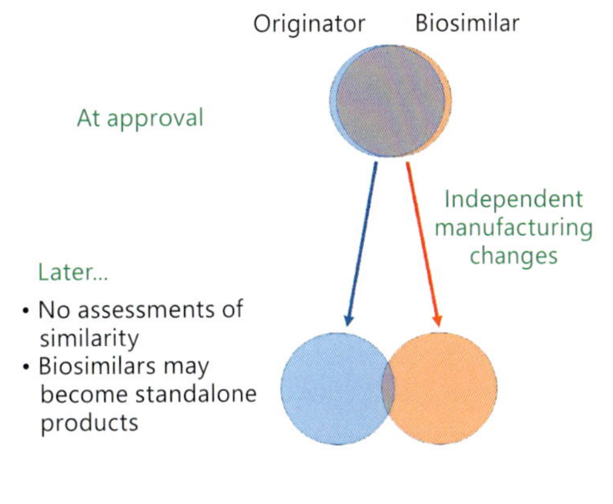

Fig. 1. Potential impact of manufacturing changes on biosimilars (adapted from P. Michetti, Lausanne).

manufacturing changes that are different from those of the originator. After a certain number of manufacturing changes, the biosimilarity of both products may be questionable. This may be overcome in the future by regulations with respect to manufacturing changes. Perhaps biosimilars will need to undergo the same manufacturing changes as have been approved for the originator. One certain problem is that later on in the clinical development of a biosimilar product, no assessments of similarity will be necessary. This may lead at the end to a situation in which biosimilars may become standalone products, as the overlap between activities is reduced (fig. 1).

Also, manufacturing processes may dramatically influence the side effects of a certain product. In the experience with erythropoietin, a change in manufacturing had a dramatic impact on the incidence of antibody-mediated pure red cell aplasia. A change in manufacturing (the introduction of a new syringe with uncoated rubber stoppers for subcutaneous use) led to the release of polysorbate from those stoppers, which acted as an immunological adjuvant to trigger an immune response to erythropoietin [23]. Such manufacturing changes will of course be product-specific and will need to be tightly controlled.

Biosimilar Name

The INN for a biosimilar product is still a matter of debate. At the moment, different regulatory agencies have a different opinion about the INN. Can a biosimilar to Infliximab also be called Infliximab? The EMA stated in September 2013 that for the biosimilar, an INN identical to the originator can be used. The Food and Drug Administration in their draft statement had no statement about the name (February 2012). In Australia, it has been suggested that 'Sim' should always precede the name of the biosimilar. In Switzerland, it was suggested that the biosimilar name should be creative or the INN linked to the company name, like 'Infliximab-Celltrion'. In a European Crohn's and Colitis Organization survey, most organization members had the opinion that a biosimilar monoclonal antibody should have a different INN than its originator to avoid confusion and to avoid the mix-up of products or the interpretation of these products as being identical.

Extrapolation of Indications

Different regulatory agencies have different opinions on the requests that should be made to extrapolate indications. These regulations are based on the thinking that the goal of biosimilar development is to demonstrate biosimilarity, not clinical benefit. A clinical benefit should have been already established for the reference product. The comprehensive stepwise comparability exercise followed to approve a biosimilar is much more sensitive to the detection of differences between a biosimilar and the reference product than to equivalence in clinical trial results. At the moment, the regulation requirements include at least one clinical study showing bioequivalence. Regulatory agencies think that more clinical trials will not add to the value of the evaluation. Based on clinical trials in rheumatoid arthritis, the EMA granted full extrapolation of indications to the Remicade® biosimilar CT-P13 (Remsima®/Inflectra®). This may be seen differently by other regulatory agencies. It appears that Health Canada did not approve full extrapolation of indications for Remsima®/Inflectra® and that for each disease, different studies will be necessary. Another question is the extent to which a biosimilar is allowed to be different from the originator. At the moment, for clinical trials, this margin is usually considered to be 15%. However, as some biologicals only reach remission rates of 18–25% in a disease such as ulcerative colitis, a difference of 15% has a huge impact on the treatment. In the extreme, this could mean that remission rates of 4% for the biosimilar versus 18% for the originator would still be considered to be acceptable which obviously is clinically nonsense.

Interchangeability/Pharmacovigilance

According to the Food and Drug Administration, interchangeability means that the biosimilar and the reference product are expected to produce the same effect in any given patient. If this is the case, the risk of switching or alternating between a biosimilar and a reference product should be not greater than the risk of using the reference product several times. This then could mean that interchangeable biological products may be substituted at the pharmacy without the intervention of the health care provider. This concept, interestingly, is fully integrated into the USA Biologics Price Competition and Innovation Act of 2009. The concept is not supported by Health Canada or Swissmedic because of potential changes in the reference product and the biosimilar over time with later manufacturing evolution as mentioned above. The European Union demands that a full risk management plan needs to be established that is in accordance with current legislation regarding pharmacovigilance guidelines that are developed for newly approved biosimilars. Overall, it seems that the European Union does not approve easy interchangeability between a biosimilar and a reference product. The different regulations outlined above that have been implemented by different regulatory agencies may impact the process of biosimilar approval in different countries. They also, however, represent a risk for patients who live in different countries and under different regulatory agencies. They may not be aware of the differences, for example, with respect to the exchangeability of biosimilars.

Conclusions and Future Directions

The facts outlined above indicate that there are still a number of open questions with respect to the approval and the use of biosimilars in inflammatory bowel disease. Hopefully, a number of those questions will be solved in the near future to avoid confusion of patients and treating doctors. Regulatory agencies are still discussing how to handle those questions, and the solutions so far are not uniform. An extrapolation of indications is accepted by the EMA but not by the Canadian agencies. Some biosimilar producers will perform trials in the respective indications, but others will not.

It will be a challenge for gastroenterological societies in the respective countries to provide their members with an unbiased view and information on this topic and to establish guidelines for the interchange of compounds and for tracing different biosimilars.

References

1 Beck A, Reichert JM: Approval of the first biosimilar antibodies in Europe: a major landmark for the biopharmaceutical industry. mAbs 2013;5:621–623.
2 McKeage K: A review of CT-P13: an infliximab biosimilar. BioDrugs 2014;28:313–321.
3 Rinaudo-Gaujous M, Paul S, Tedesco ED, Genin C, Roblin X, Peyrin-Biroulet L: Review article: biosimilars are the next generation of drugs for liver and gastrointestinal diseases. Aliment Pharmacol Ther 2013;38:914–924.
4 Feagan BG, Choquette D, Ghosh S, Gladman DD, Ho V, Meibohm B, Zou G, Xu Z, Shankar G, Sealey DC, Russell AS: The challenge of indication extrapolation for infliximab biosimilars. Biologicals 2014;42:177–183.
5 Fiorino G, Danese S: The biosimilar road in inflammatory bowel disease: the right way? Best Pract Res Clin Gastroenterol 2014;28:465–471.
6 Hlavaty T, Letkovsky J: Biosimilars in the therapy of inflammatory bowel diseases. Eur J Gastroenterol Hepatol 2014;26:581–587.
7 Vermeer NS, Spierings I, Mantel-Teeuwisse AK, Straus SM, Giezen TJ, Leufkens HG, Egberts TC, De Bruin ML: Traceability of biologicals: present challenges in pharmacovigilance. Expert Opin Drug Saf 2015;14:63–72.
8 Chow SC, Endrenyi L, Lachenbruch PA, Mentre F: Scientific factors and current issues in biosimilar studies. J Biopharm Stat 2014;24:1138–1153.
9 Chugh PK, Roy V: Biosimilars: current scientific and regulatory considerations. Curr Clin Pharmacol 2014;9:53–63.
10 Chow SC, Wang J, Endrenyi L, Lachenbruch PA: Scientific considerations for assessing biosimilar products. Stat Med 2013;32:370–381.
11 O'Connor A, Rogge M: Nonclinical development of a biosimilar: the current landscape. Bioanalysis 2013;5:537–544.
12 Tsiftsoglou AS, Ruiz S, Schneider CK: Development and regulation of biosimilars: current status and future challenges. BioDrugs 2013;27:203–211.
13 Kozlowski S, Woodcock J, Midthun K, Sherman RB: Developing the nation's biosimilars program. New Engl J Med 2011;365:385–388.
14 Vashist SK: Effect of antibody modifications on its biomolecular binding as determined by surface plasmon resonance. Anal Biochem 2012;421:336–338.
15 Stackhouse N, Miller AK, Gadgil HS: A high-throughput UPLC method for the characterization of chemical modifications in monoclonal antibody molecules. J Pharm Sci 2011;100:5115–5125.
16 Yan B, Valliere-Douglass J, Brady L, Steen S, Han M, Pace D, Elliott S, Yates Z, Han Y, Balland A, Wang W, Pettit D: Analysis of post-translational modifications in recombinant monoclonal antibody IgG1 by reversed-phase liquid chromatography/mass spectrometry. J Chromatogr A 2007;1164:153–161.
17 Blake RC 2nd, Li X, Yu H, Blake DA: Covalent and noncovalent modifications induce allosteric binding behavior in a monoclonal antibody. Biochemistry 2007;46:1573–1586.
18 Committee for Medicinal Products for Human Use (CHMP): Guideline on similar biological medicinal products containing monoclonal antibodies – non-clinical and clinical issues, 2012. http://www.ema.europa.eu/docs/en_GB/document_library/Scientific_guideline/2012/06/WC500128686.pdf (accessed June 2014).
19 Committee for Medicinal Products for Human Use (CHMP): Assessment report: Remsima, 2013. http://www.ema.europa.eu/docs/en_GB/document_library/EPAR_-_Public_assessment_report/human/002576/WC500151486.pdf (accessed June 2014).

20 Park W, Hrycaj P, Jeka S, Kovalenko V, Lysenko G, Miranda P, Mikazane H, Gutierrez-Urena S, Lim M, Lee YA, Lee SJ, Kim H, Yoo DH, Braun J: A randomised, double-blind, multicentre, parallel-group, prospective study comparing the pharmacokinetics, safety, and efficacy of CT-P13 and innovator infliximab in patients with ankylosing spondylitis: the PLANETAS study. Ann Rheum Dis 2013;72:1605–1612.

21 Park W, Jaworski J, Brzezicki J, Gnylorybov A, Kadinov V, Goecke Sariego I, Abud-Mendoza C, Otero Escalante WJ, Kang SW, Andersone D, Blanco F, Yoo DH, Ahn C, Kim HU, Braun J: A randomised, double-blind, parallel-group, phase-1 study comparing the pharmacokinetics, safety and efficacy of CT-P13 and infliximab in patients with active ankylosing spondylitis: 54 week results from the PLANETAS study. Ann Rheum Dis 2013;72(suppl 3):516.

22 Schneider CK: Biosimilars in rheumatology: the wind of change. Ann Rheum Dis 2013;72:315–318.

23 Boven K, Stryker S, Knight J, Thomas A, van Regenmortel M, Kemeny DM, Power D, Rossert J, Casadevall N: The increased incidence of pure red cell aplasia with an eprex formulation in uncoated rubber stopper syringes. Kidney Int 2005;67:2346–2353.

Gerhard Rogler, MD, PhD
Division of Gastroenterology and Hepatology, University Hospital Zurich
Rämistrasse 100
CH–8091 Zurich (Switzerland)
E-Mail gerhard.rogler@usz.ch

Rogler G, Herfarth H, Hibi T, Nielsen OH (eds): Anti-Tumor Necrosis Factor Therapy in Inflammatory Bowel Disease.
Front Gastrointest Res. Basel, Karger, 2015, vol 34, pp 119–125 (DOI: 10.1159/000381583)

Psoriasis-Like Lesions and Skin Reactions

Hans H. Herfarth[a] • Millie D. Long[a] • Christopher Sayed[b]

[a]Department of Medicine, Division of Gastroenterology and Hepatology, and [b]Department of Dermatology, University of North Carolina, Chapel Hill, N.C., USA

Abstract

The clinical identification and classification of anti-TNF therapy-associated dermatological side effects present an increasing clinical challenge for gastroenterologists treating patients with inflammatory bowel diseases. In addition to skin hypersensitivity reactions and infectious complications, the new onset of paradoxical inflammation of the skin and other organs can occur in patients on anti-TNF therapy. The inflammatory bowel disease literature reports an increasing prevalence of paradoxical psoriasis. Less often, anti-TNF-induced lupus-like drug reactions with concomitant cutaneous pathologies occur after the initiation of anti-TNF therapy. The following review will focus on psoriatic lesions and other skin complications that may occur during anti-TNF therapy.

Introduction

In large single center cohorts, anti-TNF-associated dermatological adverse effects, including infectious complications of the skin, have been reported in 22–62% of inflammatory bowel disease (IBD) patients treated with anti-TNF agents (table 1) [1, 2]. At around 2007, several years following the worldwide introduction of infliximab as the first anti-TNF agent in IBD therapy, a new onset of autoimmune skin pathologies occurring in tandem with anti-TNF therapy began to be increasingly described in the IBD literature [3–6]. This obvious delay in time suggests either an overall low incidence or the onset of lesions only after prolonged treatment periods, which have not been captured in the limited time frames of clinical trials. The underlying mechanisms of the *de novo* development of psoriatic lesions during anti-TNF therapy have not been completely elucidated. The inflammatory process is currently best described as 'paradoxical inflammation' occurring in patients on anti-TNF therapy that has been initiated to treat an inflammatory condition such as rheumatoid arthritis (RA) or IBD. Aside from psoriasis, paradoxical inflammation clinically presents as polyarthralgia, *de novo* IBD, uveitis and/or scleritis, a demyelinating central nervous system disorder and sarcoidosis [7].

Table 1. Skin pathologies associated with anti-TNF therapy

Skin infections
Psoriasis
Allergic hypersensitivity and injection site reactions
Cutaneous lupus
Localized infections
Eczema
Alopecia
Melanoma and nonmelanoma skin cancers

Paradoxical Psoriasis and Eczematous Eruptions after Initiation of Anti-TNF Therapy

The prevalence of anti-TNF therapy-induced psoriasiform skin lesions in IBD has been reported to range from 2 to 10% in patients treated with this drug class [1, 8–12]. Due to a lack of large prospective studies, the incidence of this paradoxical adverse reaction has not yet been determined. Paradoxical psoriasis is not a phenomenon unique to IBD patients but has been described in patients with every condition who have been treated with anti-TNF agents, including RA and ankylosing spondylitis [13]. Interestingly, other than an increased risk of cutaneous infections, other dermatological side effects of anti-TNF therapy, such as paradoxical psoriasis, have not been reported in IBD patients participating in prospective placebo-controlled trials.

The pathophysiology of paradoxical psoriasis has not been completely elucidated. All currently available anti-TNF agents (infliximab, adalimumab, certolizumab, golimumab, and etanercept) have been found to instigate psoriasiform skin reactions [3, 10, 14]. Thus, despite the slightly different mechanisms of action of certolizumab and etanercept compared to those of adalimumab, infliximab and golimumab, a class effect is likely. Histologically, anti-TNF-induced 'paradoxical' psoriasis appears identical to 'typical' psoriasis, and no reproducible clinical predictor for the development of the lesions has been identified to date. For example, lupus-associated antibodies (anti-nuclear antibodies (ANAs) and anti-double-stranded (ds) DNA antibodies) have been found at identical frequencies in patients on anti-TNF therapy with or without anti-TNF-induced psoriasis [8]. A genetic predisposition is probable because disease-modifying effects of IL-23R, IL-23A and IL-12B gene variants have been recently described [8, 15]. Currently, it is postulated that anti-TNF therapy may lead to an imbalance in the pro-inflammatory cutaneous milieu characterized by infiltrating interferon-gamma-expressing Th1 lymphocytes and increased numbers of IL-17A/IL-22-expressing Th17 cells [5]. Another hypothesis proposes that there is an imbalance of TNF and IFN-alpha as a consequence of the uncontrolled release of IFN-alpha by dermal plasmacytoid dendritic cells after TNF blockade [16, 17].

Clinically, the cutaneous lesions have been most frequently reported as nonspecific psoriasiform eruptions (56%), followed by classic plaque-type psoriasis (21%) and pustular-type psoriasis (4%) [3] (figure 1 and figure 2). The most frequent sites of these skin lesions are the limbs, followed by the trunk and scalp. In some series, palmoplantar pustulosis and scalp psoriasis associated with alopecia have been reported in a substantial number of patients [18]. Additional subgroups of patients exist with a guttate pattern of psoriasis [3]. Typically, affected patients do not report a previous history of psoriasis or an atopic predisposition. Whereas some studies have claimed that anti-TNF-induced psoriasis is more common in women, others have not found a gender difference [1, 3, 9].

The time between anti-TNF administration and the development of psoriatic lesions is extremely variable and has been reported as early as 1 month after the start of anti-TNF therapy in patients with RA [19]. However, it seems that IBD psoriasiform lesions do not usually develop during the induction regimen, they more commonly

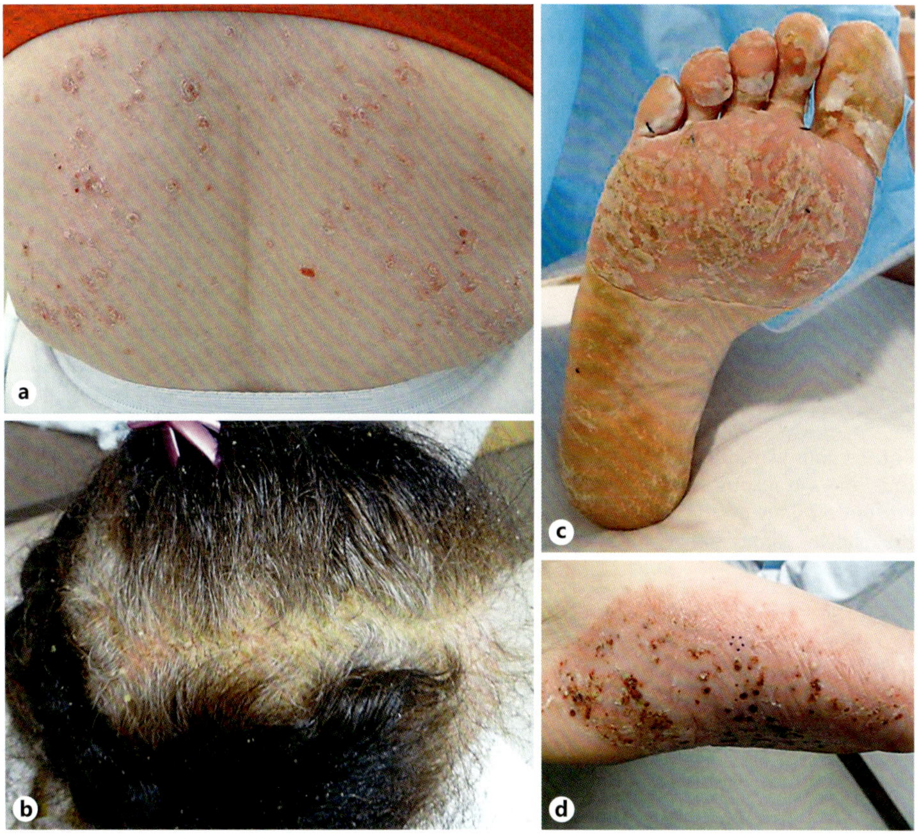

Fig. 1. Varied presentations of anti-TNF-Induced psoriasis. **a** Widespread, erythematous, scaly plaques of common plaque psoriasis on the trunk. **b** Scalp psoriasis with thick, adherent, compact scales distributed diffusely throughout the scalp. **c** Plantar psoriasis with thick, peeling scales, painful fissures and a few scattered pustules. **d** Palmoplantar pustulosis with deep-seated pustules on an erythematous base.

appear several months after treatment initiation during the maintenance phase of anti-TNF therapy [1, 9, 10, 12].

The most obvious action in response to the development of lesions is to halt the anti-TNF therapy. The decision to stop therapy should be made by a team-based assessment, involving a dedicated dermatologist, the treating gastroenterologist and the patient. Still, stopping anti-TNF therapy only leads to the complete resolution of symptoms in around 30% of patients [3]. Many mild cases can be successfully maintained on anti-TNF therapy with additional topical steroid therapy. Several small series have reported the efficacy of switching to another anti-TNF agent, the addition of methotrexate to anti-TNF therapy or a switch to an anti IL-12/23 approach with ustekinumab [9, 10, 20, 21]. Switching the patient to another anti-TNF agent may reduce the severity of the psoriasis, and around 50–60% of patients can be maintained on a second anti-TNF agent, but due to a lack of prospective data, the degree of improvement in the psoriatic lesions is difficult to assess [9, 10]. The efficacy of adding methotrexate to anti-TNF therapy has been described in a small

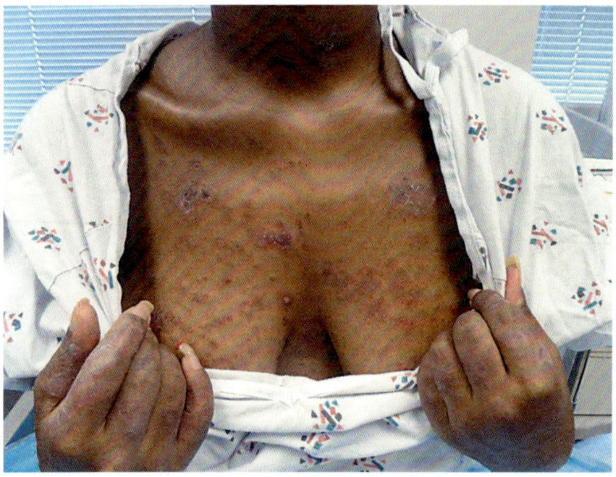

Fig. 2. Lupus-like eruption. Photo-distributed, erythematous and violaceous annular plaques with scales and crusted erosions on the central chest and hands. Note the relative sparing of the interphalangeal joints.

number of patients and seems to have only limited therapeutic success [10, 21]. In patients with severe paradoxical psoriasis, a switch to ustekinumab, which also has proven efficacy in the treatment of psoriasis, seems to yield the best therapeutic results [20]. However, the ustekinumab efficacy data are only based on a few case reports and one small study [8, 22]. In this study, a German group reported a 100% response rate in 9 patients with severe psoriasiform lesions and/or anti-TNF antibody-induced alopecia on ustekinumab.

Allergic Skin Reactions and Infections

Both IgE- and non-IgE-mediated injection site reactions have been described with the use of injectable anti-TNF agents [23]. In placebo-controlled trials, 20% of patients treated with adalimumab developed injection site reactions (erythema and/or itching, hemorrhage, pain or swelling) compared to 14% of patients receiving placebo [24]. The rate of injection site reactions was 6% in patients treated with golimumab compared with 2% in patients in the control group [25]. Currently, no incidence numbers of injection site reactions are available for certolizumab [26].

Local infections have been reported in up to 1.5% of patients exposed to biologics [27]. Apart from anti-TNF therapy, cofactors, such as comorbidities and the concomitant administration of immunosuppressive medications, contribute to the incidences of viral, bacterial and fungal infections in IBD patients. Herpes zoster has often been associated with anti-TNF therapy, but interestingly, in a recent study of a large cohort of >33,000 patients initiated on anti-TNF therapy, no higher risk of herpes zoster was found in the patients on anti-TNF therapy compared to those on nonbiologic treatment regimens [28].

The treatment of local reactions and infections depends on the cause, severity and extent. Most local allergic reactions can be treated with supportive and preventive measures, such as cool packs, topical corticosteroids and the rotation of injection sites.

Drug-Induced Lupus Erythematosus and Lupus-Like Syndrome

Many systemic and/or organ-specific autoimmune diseases have been associated with the use of biological agents [13]. The incidence of drug-induced lupus erythematosus (DILE) in post-marketing studies of RA has been estimated to be around 0.2%, whereas no such numbers are available for IBD [13]. In a cohort of 500 and 125 patients with IBD treated at the Mayo Clinic and at a tertiary center in Belgium, 3 (0.6%) and 2 (1.6%) patients, respectively, developed DILE [29, 30]. However, incidence rates of 6.9% for DILE have also been reported [31]. This condition occurs significantly more often in female than in male patients [31–33]. There are currently no standard diagnostic criteria for DILE, and in many cases, patients do not fulfill the American College of Rheumatology criteria for systemic lupus erythematosus (SLE). The four most common features (arthritis, serositis, ANAs and anti-histone antibodies) can be assessed, but DILE often present with cutaneous rashes, arthralgia, myalgia or general malaise and fever. For the diagnosis of DILE, symptoms must have begun after the initiation of a drug treatment and must resolve upon discontinuation of that treatment [34]. Recently, a Spanish registry analyzed 140 reported cases of SLE, of which specific SLE criteria were detailed in only 97 [33]. A total of 40% patients fulfilled 4 or more criteria, 21% fulfilled 3 criteria and 29% exhibited 2 or less criteria.

It is important to note that the existence of autoantibodies alone is not sufficient to diagnose DILE. Increased prevalences of ANAs as well as dsDNA have been described for infliximab, adalimumab, etanercept and golimumab [25, 35, 36]. The highest prevalence of ANA of around 44–57% has been reported for infliximab therapy [30, 37]. Of ANA-positive patients, 15–30% also have detectable dsDNA. The rate of ANA formation in the CLASSIC-II trial of adalimumab was 19%, and the rates in clinical trails of certolizumab have ranged from 1 to 8% [38–40]. There are currently no ANA data available from the golimumab ulcerative colitis trials, but in phase 3 trials of RA, psoriatic arthritis and ankylosing spondylitis through 1 year of follow-up, 4.0% of Simponi-treated patients were newly ANA-positive, whereas the presence of anti-dsDNA antibodies at 1 year of follow-up was uncommon in patients who were anti-dsDNA-negative at baseline [25, 41, 42]. Several studies of RA have also demonstrated that the development of ANA has no effect on anti-TNF treatment efficacy [43].

The induction of DILE by anti-TNF agents has been viewed as a class effect, but patients with this condition and those who need continuing anti-TNF therapy might benefit from a switch to certolizumab [44]. Also, the successful switch from infliximab to adalimumab has been described [31, 32, 45]. However, the continuous monitoring of clinical symptoms and autoantibody status is indicated because they both can worsen after the switch.

Conclusions and Future Directions

The prevalence of dermatological pathologies seems to be increasing, and paradoxical psoriasis in particular is now a well-known adverse effect of anti-TNF therapy. Prospective studies should be conducted at IBD centers, focusing on the elucidation of the pathophysiologies of these cutaneous side effects and the development and validation of specific treatment algorithms.

References

1 Cleynen I, Vermeire S: Paradoxical inflammation induced by anti-TNF agents in patients with IBD. Nat Rev Gastroenterol Hepatol 2012;9:496–503.

2 Baumgart DC, Grittner U, Steingraber A, et al: Frequency, phenotype, outcome, and therapeutic impact of skin reactions following initiation of adalimumab therapy: experience from a consecutive cohort of inflammatory bowel disease patients. Inflamm Bowel Dis 2011;17:2512–2520.

3 Denadai R, Teixeira FV, Steinwurz F, et al: Induction or exacerbation of psoriatic lesions during anti-TNF-alpha therapy for inflammatory bowel disease: a systematic literature review based on 222 cases. J Crohns Colitis 2013;7:517–524.

4 Torres J, Buche S, Delaporte E, et al: Skin side effects of inflammatory bowel disease therapy. Inflamm Bowel Dis 2013;19:1086–1098.

5 Niess JH, Danese S: Anti-TNF and skin inflammation in IBD: a new paradox in gastroenterology? Gut 2014;63:533–535.

6 Moran GW, Lim AW, Bailey JL, et al: Review article: dermatological complications of immunosuppressive and anti-TNF therapy in inflammatory bowel disease. Aliment Pharmacol Ther 2013;38:1002–1024.

7 Fiorino G, Danese S, Pariente B, et al: Paradoxical immune-mediated inflammation in inflammatory bowel disease patients receiving anti-TNF-alpha agents. Autoimmun Rev 2014;13:15–19.
8 Tillack C, Ehmann LM, Friedrich M, et al: Anti-TNF antibody-induced psoriasiform skin lesions in patients with inflammatory bowel disease are characterised by interferon-gamma-expressing Th1 cells and IL-17A/IL-22-expressing Th17 cells and respond to anti-IL-12/IL-23 antibody treatment. Gut 2014;63:567–577.
9 Cullen G, Kroshinsky D, Cheifetz AS, et al: Psoriasis associated with anti-tumour necrosis factor therapy in inflammatory bowel disease: a new series and a review of 120 cases from the literature. Aliment Pharmacol Ther 2011;34:1318–1327.
10 Afzali A, Wheat CL, Hu JK, et al: The association of psoriasiform rash with anti-tumor necrosis factor (anti-TNF) therapy in inflammatory bowel disease: a single academic center case series. J Crohns Colitis 2014;8:480–488.
11 Rahier JF, Buche S, Peyrin-Biroulet L, et al: Severe skin lesions cause patients with inflammatory bowel disease to discontinue anti-tumor necrosis factor therapy. Clin Gastroenterol Hepatol 2010;8:1048–1055.
12 Guerra I, Algaba A, Perez-Calle JL, et al: Induction of psoriasis with anti-TNF agents in patients with inflammatory bowel disease: a report of 21 cases. J Crohns Colitis 2012;6:518–523.
13 Perez-Alvarez R, Perez-de-Lis M, Ramos-Casals M, et al: Biologics-induced autoimmune diseases. Curr Opin Rheumatol 2013;25:56–64.
14 Soto Lopes MS, Trope BM, Rochedo Rodriguez MP, et al: Paradoxical reaction to golimumab: tumor necrosis factor alpha inhibitor inducing psoriasis pustulosa. Case Rep Dermatol 2013;5:326–331.
15 Sherlock ME, Walters T, Tabbers MM, et al: Infliximab-induced psoriasis and psoriasiform skin lesions in pediatric Crohn disease and a potential association with IL-23 receptor polymorphisms. J Pediatr Gastroenterol Nutr 2013;56:512–518.
16 Nestle FO, Conrad C, Tun-Kyi A, et al: Plasmacytoid predendritic cells initiate psoriasis through interferon-alpha production. J Exp Med 2005;202:135–143.
17 Collamer AN, Battafarano DF: Psoriatic skin lesions induced by tumor necrosis factor antagonist therapy: clinical features and possible immunopathogenesis. Semin Arthritis Rheum 2010;40:233–240.
18 Shmidt E, Wetter DA, Ferguson SB, et al: Psoriasis and palmoplantar pustulosis associated with tumor necrosis factor-alpha inhibitors: the Mayo Clinic experience, 1998 to 2010. J Am Acad Dermatol 2012;67:e179–e185.
19 Harrison MJ, Dixon WG, Watson KD, et al: Rates of new-onset psoriasis in patients with rheumatoid arthritis receiving anti-tumour necrosis factor alpha therapy: results from the British Society for Rheumatology Biologics Register. Ann Rheum Dis 2009;68:209–215.
20 Schmitt J, Rosumeck S, Thomaschewski G, et al: Efficacy and safety of systemic treatments for moderate-to-severe psoriasis: meta-analysis of randomized controlled trials. Br J Dermatol 2014;170:274–303.
21 Buisson A, Cuny JF, Barbaud A, et al: Methotrexate for psoriasiform lesions associated with anti-tumour necrosis factor therapy in inflammatory bowel disease. Aliment Pharmacol Ther 2012;35:1178–1180.
22 Mihaly E, Szekely H, Herszenyi L, et al: Letter: dermatological complications with therapy for inflammatory bowel disease. Aliment Pharmacol Ther 2014;39:232–233.
23 Murdaca G, Spano F, Puppo F: Selective TNF-alpha inhibitor-induced injection site reactions. Expert Opin Drug Saf 2013;12:187–193.
24 U.S. Food and Drug Administration: Adalimumab – FDA full prescribing information, 2014. http://www.fda.gov/safety/medwatch/safetyinformation/ucm194134.htm (accessed July 20, 2014).
25 U.S. Food and Drug Administration: Golimumab – FDA full prescribing information, 2014. http://www.fda.gov/safety/medwatch/safetyinformation/ucm351838.htm (accessed July 20, 2014).
26 U.S. Food and Drug Administration: Certolizumab pegol – FDA full prescribing information, 2014. http://www.fda.gov/safety/medwatch/safetyinformation/ucm327828.htm (accessed July 20, 2014).
27 Kerbleski JF, Gottlieb AB: Dermatological complications and safety of anti-TNF treatments. Gut 2009;58:1033–1039.
28 Winthrop KL, Baddley JW, Chen L, et al: Association between the initiation of anti-tumor necrosis factor therapy and the risk of herpes zoster. JAMA 2013;309:887–895.
29 Colombel JF, Loftus EV Jr, Tremaine WJ, et al: The safety profile of infliximab in patients with Crohn's disease: the Mayo clinic experience in 500 patients. Gastroenterology 2004;126:19–31.
30 Vermeire S, Noman M, Van Assche G, et al: Autoimmunity associated with anti-tumor necrosis factor alpha treatment in Crohn's disease: a prospective cohort study. Gastroenterology 2003;125:32–39.
31 Yanai H, Shuster D, Calabrese E, et al: The incidence and predictors of lupus-like reaction in patients with IBD treated with anti-TNF therapies. Inflamm Bowel Dis 2013;19:2778–2786.
32 Subramanian S, Yajnik V, Sands BE, et al: Characterization of patients with infliximab-induced lupus erythematosus and outcomes after retreatment with a second anti-TNF agent. Inflamm Bowel Dis 2011;17:99–104.
33 Ramos-Casals M, Roberto Perez A, Diaz-Lagares C, et al: Autoimmune diseases induced by biological agents: a double-edged sword? Autoimmun Rev 2010;9:188–193.
34 Vedove CD, Del Giglio M, Schena D, et al: Drug-induced lupus erythematosus. Arch Dermatol Res 2009;301:99–105.
35 Ramos-Casals M, Brito-Zeron P, Soto MJ, et al: Autoimmune diseases induced by TNF-targeted therapies. Best Pract Res Clin Rheumatol 2008;22:847–861.
36 Bardazzi F, Odorici G, Virdi A, et al: Autoantibodies in psoriatic patients treated with anti-TNF-alpha therapy. J Dtsch Dermatol Ges 2014;12:401–406.
37 Beigel F, Schnitzler F, Paul Laubender R, et al: Formation of antinuclear and double-strand DNA antibodies and frequency of lupus-like syndrome in anti-TNF-alpha antibody-treated patients with inflammatory bowel disease. Inflamm Bowel Dis 2011;17:91–98.
38 Sandborn WJ, Feagan BG, Stoinov S, et al: Certolizumab pegol for the treatment of Crohn's disease. N Engl J Med 2007;357:228–238.

39 Sandborn WJ, Hanauer SB, Rutgeerts P, et al: Adalimumab for maintenance treatment of Crohn's disease: results of the CLASSIC II trial. Gut 2007;56:1232–1239.
40 Schreiber S, Khaliq-Kareemi M, Lawrance IC, et al: Maintenance therapy with certolizumab pegol for Crohn's disease. N Engl J Med 2007;357:239–250.
41 Sandborn WJ, Feagan BG, Marano C, et al: Subcutaneous golimumab induces clinical response and remission in patients with moderate-to-severe ulcerative colitis. Gastroenterology 2014;146:85–95.
42 Sandborn WJ, Feagan BG, Marano C, et al: Subcutaneous golimumab maintains clinical response in patients with moderate-to-severe ulcerative colitis. Gastroenterology 2014;146:96–109.
43 Atzeni F, Talotta R, Salaffi F, et al: Immunogenicity and autoimmunity during anti-TNF therapy. Autoimmun Rev 2013,12.703–708.
44 Verma HD, Scherl EJ, Jacob VE, et al: Anti-nuclear antibody positivity and the use of certolizumab in inflammatory bowel disease patients who have had arthralgias or lupus-like reactions from infliximab or adalimumab. J Dig Dis 2011;12:379–383.
45 Wetter DA, Davis MD: Lupus-like syndrome attributable to anti-tumor necrosis factor alpha therapy in 14 patients during an 8-year period at Mayo Clinic. Mayo Clin Proc 2009;84:979–984.

Hans H. Herfarth, MD, PhD
Department of Medicine, Division of Gastroenterology and Hepatology
University of North Carolina, Bioinformatics Bldg., CB#7080
Chapel Hill, NC, 27599 (USA)
E-Mail hherf@med.unc.edu

Rogler G, Herfarth H, Hibi T, Nielsen OH (eds): Anti-Tumor Necrosis Factor Therapy in Inflammatory Bowel Disease.
Front Gastrointest Res. Basel, Karger, 2015, vol 34, pp 126–131 (DOI: 10.1159/000381590)

The Elicitation of Rheumatic Symptoms at Vascular Sites

Matthias Geyer · Ulf Müller-Ladner

Justus-Liebig-University Giessen, Internal Medicine and Rheumatology, Kerckhoff-Klinik, Department of Rheumatology and Clinical Immunology, Bad Nauheim, Germany

Abstract

The use of pharmacological agents is a key issue of therapeutic medicine. For more than a decade, TNF-α inhibitors have been prescribed for a growing number of conditions in different disciplines covering gastroenterology, as well as for several rheumatic disorders. The risks and side effects of TNF-α inhibitors comprise serious infections caused by latent disease reactivation or *de novo* disease acquisition, potential malignancies, neurological conditions and skin and other single- or even varying multi-organ involvement with partially severe courses. At least for multi-organ involvement, vascular inflammation at different sites of the organism may represent a common link. This can cause a versatile complexity of symptoms, and the 'rheumatic' kind of symptoms seem to be the most diverse. However, drug-induced vasculitides turn out to be controllable as long as they are recognized in time and are treated adequately. However, there are still two questions to be answered regarding autoimmune reactions. First, do 'induced' vasculitides and underlying disease pertain to the identical, i.e. simultaneous, pathogenic mechanism? Second, could key players with pivotal immunological roles prove to be false targets since several therapeutics used for the treatment of cytokine-associated disorders could act in an opposing manner?

Introduction

Apart from the many other risks and side effects discussed elsewhere, the application of TNF-blocking agents, which are currently widely used potent immunomodulators, may evoke or mimic certain rheumatologic conditions. When reflecting potential 'rheumatic' entities or 'rheumatology' in general, it is primarily the joints that will usually come to most of the people's mind, primarily due to the widespread association of 'rheumatology' with disorders of the musculoskeletal system. This is clinically justifiable and reflects the picture of a rheumatologist's daily clinical practice. It is, however, only half the truth because the disturbances of systemic inflammation might pertain to not only articular but also 'classic' internal organ systems such as the heart, lung, liver, kidney or digestive tract as well as to the vasculature per se and the skin. Joint affection does not always need to be present and, if it is present, does not necessarily represent the leading symptom – even if drug-induced.

The most frequent sites of affection in this context are the skin and its blood vessels. The total vasculature, however, serves as a kind of guiding system on the route to the potential involvement of different further organs, with inflammatory reactions most frequently affecting small blood vessels and thus triggering dermal, articular, pulmonary and renal irritations. While the focus discussed within the other chapters of this section will consist in the dermatologic and serologic events leading to psoriasiform and other localized skin lesions or lupus-like syndrome, the topic herein, in contrast, will emphasize some typical vasculitic side effects that may occur upon anti-TNF therapy.

Drug-Induced Vasculitic Syndromes: Entities of Their Own?

The current evidence for the association of anti-TNF agents with the development of vasculitis is based on several case reports describing typical and well-known vasculitides such as Henoch-Schönlein purpura [1–4] or cutaneous leukocytoclastic vasculitis [5]. This is not restricted to the therapy of inflammatory bowel disease but includes different rheumatologic diseases that these agents are approved for [1–9]. While these vasculitic disorders are usually not associated with the formation of antineutrophil cytoplasmic antibodies (ANCAs), but rather are characterized by the formation of immune complexes, some other systematic reviews have highlighted drug-induced vasculitides as an independent group of manifestations that, most importantly, display an association with ANCAs [10, 11]. How can such discrepancies be overcome? On one hand, the resolution lies in the fact that nearly all of these clinical case reports date back to years prior to the release of the current revised classification system of the Chapel Hill Consensus Conference addressing the nomenclature of vasculitides in 2012 [12]. Even more importantly, on the other hand, it is legitimate to handle the confusing terminological aspects in that field with care and to sometimes doubt the diagnoses proposed within these earlier case descriptions because there is ambiguity in clinical correlations and even in the interpretation of these diseases as a primary or secondary form. Although all cases were assumed to originate potentially from medication and thus represent side effects, it remains a possibility that the underlying inflammatory (e.g. bowel) disease itself might have led to the interpretation of vascular inflammation as a (known) vasculitic syndrome [11].

Essential Terminological Aspects and Classification

In general, there are – in short – cutaneously limited and other single-organ vasculitides as well as systemic forms grouped according to their site of origination into small, medium or large vessel inflammatory disorders. Drug-induced vasculitides usually pertain to small blood vessels. According to the current classification, vasculitis that is most likely induced by a pharmacological agent should – due to its probable etiology – be regarded as 'drug-associated immune complex vasculitis' or 'drug-associated ANCA-associated vasculitis' [12].

While 'leukocytoclastic' refers to the histopathological aspect, this adjective is still clinically used as a synonym for immune complex-mediated vasculitides [13], even though it should be avoided with the exception of its use in the term 'cutaneous leukocytoclastic vasculitis' [12, 14]. In any case, the 'leukocytoclastic' character of immune complex-mediated vasculitides is histologically reflected by perivascular immunoglobulin (Ig) deposits. Entities with IgG and IgM deposition are often called 'hypersensitivity', 'allergic', or 'necrotizing' vasculitis, although such terms already should have been avoided according to the Chapel Hill Consensus Conference of 1994, as the majority of patients with this syndrome should instead be diagnosed with microscopic polyangiitis or cutaneous leukocytoclastic vasculitis [14]. They may, however, indeed have a necrotizing disease course despite their pauci-immune character. By contrast, if IgA deposition is found, systemic 'IgA vasculitis' such as Henoch-Schönlein purpura is most likely present, showing a worse course than with IgG or IgM and presenting in both children and adults [13]. Finally, a 'leukocytoclastic' vasculitis can also represent both the initial and an accompanying feature of systemic ANCA-associated vasculitis [15].

Pathogenic Mechanisms

The detailed pathogenesis of drug-associated vasculitides has still not been fully elucidated, but multifactorial events including immune complex formation are suspected. Immune complexes are able to interact with endothelial cells and complement factors. As a consequence, kinin and anaphylatoxin production can be observed. This may initiate the phase of vascular inflammation, in which neutrophils are directed to the vascular site via complement-derived chemoattractant substances [16]. Neutrophil activation through their Fcγ receptors by immune complexes causes the release of inflammatory products such as myeloperoxidase (MPO) from their granules, which, in turn, can also directly convert the drug into cytotoxic products [10, 17]. This effect, as well as drug-modified MPO, could spread the immune response to other autoantigens, resulting in epitope spreading and immunogenic transformation of neutrophil proteins, e.g. targeting T cells, which may activate B cells to produce ANCAs [17]; therefore, ANCA production does not contradict the presence of drug-induced vasculitides. In this context, neutrophil apoptosis might also play a role since neutrophil apoptosis is associated with the translocation of cytoplasmic antigens to the cell surface, which then induces the production of ANCAs [18]. ANCAs, again, are able to bind to membrane-bound antigens, causing a vicious cycle by cross-linking MPO or proteinase 3 with Fcγ receptors. Additionally, the activation of platelets can result in microvascular ischemia, thus potentially exacerbating the pre-existing tissue damage [16].

Clinical Signs and Symptoms

Cutaneously and subcutaneously restricted forms of vasculitides are quite common as side effects of the administration of drugs including TNF inhibitors, whereas systemic syndromes might only develop in a small number of patients who are treated for a long period of time [19]. The clinical manifestations of drug-associated vasculitis may be similar to those of primary vasculitides, but drug-associated vasculitis usually shows a milder course. There are several nonspecific symptoms, including malaise, fever and, eventually, weight loss. Arthralgia, e.g. that of the ankles, knees or elbows, and myalgia are quite common, but these symptoms usually do not develop into evident arthritis or myositis [10]. However, the exacerbation to life-threatening vasculitis with specific organ involvement might also develop, particularly when the causative agent continues to be used [20]. This usually affects the kidney, leading to proteinuria, hematuria, and elevated serum creatinine levels in certain circumstances, e.g. rapidly progressive glomerulonephritis as a rare complication, and the lung, leading to intra-alveolar hemorrhages resulting in cough, dyspnea and hemoptysis as components of acute respiratory distress syndrome or interstitial pneumonia [10, 11, 21, 22]. Renal affection is not a prerequisite, but if it occurs, up to one-third of patients may progress to end-stage organ failure [23]. Nevertheless, even though it might develop after several months of treatment with TNF inhibitors [1], classical IgA vasculitis appears to remain a rare complication. Of note, in the majority of cases, cutaneous vasculitic manifestations occur within 3 months after initiating anti-TNF therapy.

Diagnostic Testing

Diagnosing drug-induced vasculitis is complicated by insufficient recognition of relevant symptoms and by a variable interval between the initiation of medication and the onset of vasculitic clues. Thus, a thorough drug history encompassing several months prior to the presentation of the patient with symptoms is obligatory. Other conditions mimicking or associated with vasculitis should be excluded, especially infections, malignancies and other defined types of vasculitis [10]. Although there are no specific laboratory markers to distinguish drug-induced vasculitis from other autoimmune disorders, some tests may facilitate the diagnosis and indicate the related organ involvement. These parameters mainly include white blood count, erythrocyte sedimentation rate, and the C-reactive protein, creatinine and urea levels [10]. Of note, patients suspected for drug-induced vasculitis frequently show multispecific ANCAs [24]. Antihistone and antiphospholipid antibodies can also be observed [10, 25], while anti-dsDNA antibodies appear to be less frequent [26]. Urine evaluation may uncover hematuria and proteinuria [20]. Plain chest radiography or sometimes – if necessary – high-resolution computed tomography is indicated to elucidate pulmonary symptoms [27]. Finally, tissue biopsies from skin lesions or renal or lung tissues are recommended on an individual basis to provide a definitive diagnosis of vasculitis, to determine the disease severity and to exclude other diseases [20, 28]. Histology may demonstrate IgA and C3 complement factor deposits in the blood vessel wall, especially when investigated by immunofluorescence. For example, in skin samples obtained from patients with overt cutaneous vasculitis, IgA deposition is predictive of associated renal and gastrointestinal organ involvement [13].

Treatment Options

As a primary approach, the withdrawal of the medication suspected to be the causative agent constitutes the ultimate and adequate procedure to clarify the clinical situation. Of note, positive seroconversion to the presence of autoantibodies alone is not a sufficient reason to discontinue the precipitating drug since the development of a clinically relevant vasculitic syndrome in the minority of patients with positive ANCA is not a compelling consequence [10, 28]. If it occurs, however, then withdrawal might prove to be sufficient in the majority of cases when only nonspecific symptoms are present, often resulting in dramatic resolution of clinical manifestations and avoiding the need for further immunosuppressive treatment [1, 21]. Apart from that and depending on the individual severity of organ involvement, resolution of clinical symptoms occurs within 1–4 weeks [24], when immunosuppressive drugs with or without systemic corticosteroids are required as a supportive mode of action [1, 10, 11]. Cyclophosphamide, azathioprine and mycophenolate mofetil, however, are restricted to situations of critical organ failure and are nevertheless usually limited to induction therapy without a need for maintenance [10]. Only in rare cases with persistent alterations, this might also become necessary to avoid chronic organ failure.

Conclusions and Future Directions

Pharmacological therapy including anti-TNF medication rarely leads to vasculitic or other autoimmune complications. Despite possible clinical and diagnostic testing to facilitate the diagnosis, it may not be trivial to distinguish in (academic) detail the kind of disease that a patient presenting with the tentative diagnosis of (drug-induced) vasculitis is suffering from. However, the awareness of corresponding symptoms by physicians is essential to avoid any delay and to start adequate treatment to alleviate and clear the symptoms and to prevent chronic disease.

Because several autoimmune disorders induced by biological therapies may be treated with alternative agents or other substances targeting specific constituents of the immune system within an obscure circle of paradox immune responses in some cases, we have to face another chicken-or-egg causality dilemma. It is therefore of utmost importance to further elucidate whether currently known (auto)immune diseases could perhaps incorporate aspects of otherwise identified clinical features that lead to different diagnoses despite belonging to the same disorder; that is to say, to which extent also vasculitic manifestations may be due to either drug use or are part of the underlying condition the drug was initially used for [29, 30]. This is especially true for TNF-α based on its pivotal role in health and disease [31]. For the future, it remains a complex challenge when and how novel insights into pathogenic pathways and newly gathered knowledge on molecular processes might hopefully contribute to broadly unravel some more 'biological' (!) secrets that we are still reflecting on in the field of autoimmunity right now.

References

1 Rahman FZ, Takhar GK, Roy O, Shepherd A, Bloom SL, McCartney SA: Henoch-Schönlein purpura complicating adalimumab therapy for Crohn's disease. World J Gastrointest Pharmacol Ther 2010;1:119–122.

2 Nobile S, Catassi C, Felici L: Herpes zoster infection followed by Henoch-Schönlein purpura in a girl receiving infliximab for ulcerative colitis. J Clin Rheumatol 2009;15:101.

3 Lee A, Kasama R, Evangelisto A, Elfenbein B, Falasca G: Henoch-Schönlein purpura after etanercept therapy for psoriasis. J Clin Rheumatol 2006;12:249–251.

4 Duffy TN, Genta M, Moll S, Martin PY, Gabay C: Henoch-Schönlein purpura following etanercept treatment of rheumatoid arthritis. Clin Exp Rheumatol 2006;24:S106.

5 Mohan N, Edwards ET, Cupps TR, Slifman N, Lee JH, Siegel JN, Braun MM: Leukocytoclastic vasculitis associated with tumor necrosis factor-alpha blocking agents. J Rheumatol 2004;31:1955–1958.

6 Ramos-Casals M, Brito-Zeron P, Cuadrado MJ, Khamashta MA: Vasculitis induced by tumor necrosis factor-targeted therapies. Curr Rheumatol Rep 2008;10:442–448.

7 Ramos-Casals M, Brito-Zeron P, Munoz S, Soria N, Galiana D, Bertolaccini L, Cuadrado MJ, Khamashta MA: Autoimmune diseases induced by TNF-targeted therapies: analysis of 233 cases. Medicine (Baltimore) 2007;86:242–251.

8 Saint Marcoux B, De Bandt M, (CRI) Club Rhumatismes et Inflammation: Vasculitides induced by TNF-alpha antagonists: a study in 39 patients in France. Joint Bone Spine 2006;73:710–713.

9 De Bandt M, Saint-Marcoux B: Tumour necrosis factor alpha blockade and the risk of vasculitis. Ann Rheum Dis 2006;65:1534–1535.

10 Radić M, Martinović Kaliterna D, Radić J: Drug-induced vasculitis: a clinical and pathological review. Neth J Med 2012;70:12–17.

11 Simms R, Kipgen D, Dahill S, Marshall D, Rodger RS: ANCA-associated renal vasculitis following anti-tumor necrosis factor alpha therapy. Am J Kidney Dis 2008;51:e11–e14.

12 Jennette JC, Falk RJ, Bacon PA, Basu N, Cid MC, Ferrario F, Flores-Suarez LF, Gross WL, Guillevin L, Hagen EC, Hoffman GS, Jayne DR, Kallenberg CGM, Lamprecht P, Langford CA, Luqmani RA, Mahr AD, Matteson EL, Merkel PA, Ozen S, Pusey CD, Rasmussen N, Rees AJ, Scott DGI, Specks U, Stone JH, Takahashi K, Watts RA: 2012 revised International Chapel Hill Consensus Conference Nomenclature of Vasculitides. Arthritis Rheum 2013;65:1–11.

13 Alalwani M, Billings SD, Gota CE: Clinical significance of immunoglobulin deposition in leukocytoclastic vasculitis: a 5-year retrospective study of 88 patients at Cleveland clinic. Am J Dermatopathol 2014;36:723–729.

14 Jennette JC, Falk RJ, Andrassy K, Bacon PA, Churg J, Gross WL, Hagen EC, Hoffman GS, Hunder GG, Kallenberg CG, Mccluskey RT, Sinico RA, Rees AJ, Van Es LA, Waldherr R, Wiik A, Seruminstitut S: Nomenclature of systemic vasculitides. Proposal of an international consensus conference. Arthritis Rheum 1994;37:187–192.
15 Daoud MS, Gibson LE, DeRemee RA, Specks U, El-Azhary RA, Su WP: Cutaneous Wegener's granulomatosis: clinical, histopathologic and immunopathologic features of thirty patients. J Am Acad Dermatol 1994;31:605–612.
16 Stone JH, Murali MR: Case 10–2013: a 30-year-old man with fever, myalgias, arthritis, and rash. N Engl J Med 2013; 368:1239–1245.
17 Jiang X, Khursigara G, Rubin RL: Transformation of lupus-inducing drugs to cytotoxic products by activated neutrophils. Science 1994;266:810–813.
18 Ralston DR, Marsh CB, Lowe MP, Wewers MD: Antineutrophil cytoplasmic antibodies induce monocyte IL-8 release. Role of surface proteinase-3, alpha1-antitrypsin, and Fcgamma receptors. J Clin Invest 1997;100:1416–1424.
19 Vasoo S: Drug-induced lupus: an update. Lupus 2006;15:757–761.
20 Cuellar ML: Drug-induced vasculitis. Curr Rheumatol Rep 2002;4:55–59.
21 Doyle MK, Cuellar ML: Drug-induced vasculitis. Expert Opin Drug Saf 2003;2: 401–409.
22 John R, Herzenberg AM: Renal toxicity of therapeutic drugs. J Clin Pathol 2009; 62:505–515.
23 Saulsbury FT: Clinical update: Henoch-Schönlein purpura. Lancet 2007;369: 976–978.
24 Wiik A: Drug-induced vasculitis. Curr Opin Rheumatol 2008;20:35–39.
25 Hemmati I, Kur J: Adalimumab-associated antiphospholipid syndrome: a case report and review of the literature. Clin Rheumatol 2013;32:1095–1098.
26 Atzeni F, Turiel M, Capsoni F, Doria A, Meroni P, Sarzi-Puttini P: Autoimmunity and anti-TNF-alpha agents. Ann N Y Acad Sci 2005;1051:559–569.
27 Lee JY, Chung JH, Lee YJ, Park SS, Kim SY, Koo HK, Lee JH, Lee CT, Yoon HI: Propylthiouracil-induced nonspecific interstitial pneumonia. Chest 2011;139: 687–690.
28 Merkel PA: Drug-induced vasculitis. Rheum Dis Clin North Am 2001;27: 849–862.
29 Perez-Alvarez R, Perez-de-Lis M, Ramos-Casals M, BIOGEAS study group: Biologics-induced autoimmune diseases. Curr Opin Rheumatol 2013;25:56–64.
30 Viguier M, Richette P, Bachelez H, Wendling D, Aubin F: Paradoxical adverse effects of anti-TNF-alpha treatment: onset or exacerbation of cutaneous disorders. Expert Rev Clin Immunol 2009;5:421–431.
31 Sfikakis PP: The first decade of biologic TNF antagonists in clinical practice: lessons learned, unresolved issues and future directions. Curr Dir Autoimmun 2010;11:180–210.

Matthias Geyer, MD
Department of Rheumatology and Clinical Immunology, Kerckhoff-Klinik
Benekestrasse 2–8
DE–61231, Bad Nauheim (Germany)
E-Mail m.geyer@kerckhoff-klinik.de

Rogler G, Herfarth H, Hibi T, Nielsen OH (eds): Anti-Tumor Necrosis Factor Therapy in Inflammatory Bowel Disease.
Front Gastrointest Res. Basel, Karger, 2015, vol 34, pp 132–137 (DOI: 10.1159/000381592)

Serum Reaction, Lupus-Like Syndrome

Fabian Schnitzler

Department of Medicine II – Grosshadern, Ludwig-Maximilians-University (LMU), Munich, Germany

Abstract

The induction of autoimmunity due to the development of antinuclear antibodies, anti-double-stranded DNA antibodies or anti-histone antibodies is common in patients with inflammatory bowel disease treated with anti-TNF therapies. However, anti-TNF drug-induced lupus is a relatively rare disease entity, occurring in a minority of up to 2% of these patients. A diagnosis of anti-TNF drug-induced lupus is likely for patients presenting with symptoms including arthralgia, myalgia, fever, serositis, nephritis, vasculitis and dermatological rash occurring at least 1 month after the start of anti-TNF treatment followed by an improvement of symptoms within days/weeks of drug discontinuation. Typical laboratory findings include the detection of autoantibodies against double-stranded DNA, nuclear proteins or histones, hypocomplementemia, leukopenia and thrombocytopenia. Once the diagnosis of drug-induced lupus is established, a change in therapeutic management has to be addressed. In patients with severe symptoms, the initiation of corticosteroid and/or immunosuppressive therapy is often necessary. Patients with severe joint involvement and massive arthralgia may benefit from starting methotrexate treatment as an alternative to thiopurine treatment. Since autoimmunity induced by anti-TNF therapies seems to be a class-wide effect of all available anti-TNF therapies and given the controversial experiences reported in the literature after adjustment to a second-line anti-TNF therapy, a switch to another anti-TNF therapy should be addressed carefully. With the approval of vedolizumab for the treatment of Crohn's disease and ulcerative colitis, a new substance class of biological therapies is available for the treatment of inflammatory bowel disease, and this class of drugs could be a good treatment option, especially in those patients who develop lupus-like syndrome during anti-TNF treatment.

Introduction

Anti-TNF therapies with infliximab, adalimumab and golimumab have been proven in clinical trials to alleviate the inflammatory bowel disease (IBD) course by rapidly inducing and maintaining clinical remission and mucosal healing in IBD patients [1–8]. In moderate to severe forms of IBD, these biological therapies are indispensable for therapeutic management of IBD. Especially during long-term treatment with anti-TNF agents, various side effects including infections, malignancies, demyelinating disease, aplastic anemia, congestive heart failure, and induction of autoimmune conditions may occur [9–13]. Moreover, the prevalence of dermatological complications is increasing with injection site reactions, cutaneous manifestations of infusion reactions, cutaneous infections, nonmelanoma skin cancer, and psoriasiform skin lesions [9, 11, 13].

Anti-TNF therapies may induce autoimmunity due to the formation antinuclear antibodies (ANAs), anti-double-stranded DNA (dsDNA) antibodies, and other antibodies (e.g. anti-histone antibodies, anti-cardiolipin antibodies, anti-phospholipid antibodies) [14–17]. Autoimmunity may manifest in the long term during anti-TNF treatment as serum reaction and symptoms of lupus-like syndrome, including fever, lymphadenopathy, arthralgia, cutaneous eruptions, gastrointestinal disturbances and serositis. These effects often necessitate the discontinuation of anti-TNF therapy [12]. For the first time, classical drug-induced lupus (DIL) was described in 1945 in patients following treatment with sulfadiazine, which resulted in the development of symptoms consistent with lupus erythematosus [18, 19]. Since then, DIL has been recognized as a subset of lupus-related diseases. Procainamide is the commonly implicated involved drug in the epidemiology of DIL [18, 19]. To date, more than 80 medications have been associated with the development of DIL, and especially, anti-TNF therapies may induce DIL (anti-TNF DIL) despite their use to treat autoimmune disorders [18–20].

No stringent criteria for the diagnosis of anti-TNF DIL have been established to date, but the diagnosis of anti-TNF DIL is almost certain based on the following clinical and laboratory findings [18–31]: treatment with the suspected drug for at least 1 month, usually longer; typical clinical symptoms/organ manifestations of arthralgia, myalgia, fever, serositis, nephritis, vasculitis and dermatological rash.

Laboratory Findings

Laboratory findings include antibodies against nuclear proteins, dsDNA, or histones, hypocomplementemia, leukopenia and thrombocytopenia followed by an improvement of symptoms within days/weeks of drug discontinuation. It is estimated that up to 2% of patients treated with anti-TNF drugs will develop symptoms consistent with anti-TNF DIL [14, 19, 32].

Pathogenesis of Anti-TNF Drug-Induced Lupus

The underlying mechanism resulting in a subsequent induction of autoantibodies during treatment with anti-TNF therapies is not yet understood [20]. Interestingly, differences in the potential to induce lupus like symptoms have been reported for the different anti-TNF therapies [22]. A recently published clinical trial compared the risk of DIL in patients with rheumatic diseases who had been treated with the monoclonal anti-TNF therapies infliximab or adalimumab or the soluble TNF receptor-2- immunoglobulin hybrid molecule etanercept [22]. Importantly, the relative risk to induce lupus-like syndrome was comparable between infliximab (OR 10.97) and adalimumab (OR 9.03) but was lower for the soluble TNF receptor-based compound etanercept (OR 4.02) [22]. The pathophysiology of anti-TNF therapy-induced autoimmunity resulting in the development of symptoms of lupus-like syndrome seems to be complex, including increased apoptosis of predominantly inflammatory cells induced by anti-TNF agents and impaired clearance of nuclear waste [22]. The major groups of autoantibodies are directed against antigens presented by apoptotic cells, such as ANAs, anti-dsDNA antibodies or anti-phospholipid autoantibodies [33–36]. Several hypotheses have been proposed to explain the underlying mechanisms by which anti-TNF therapies induce autoimmunity [20]. One aspect of this mechanism may be due to an accumulation of nucleosomes from apoptotic cells, thereby inducing autoantibody production in susceptible patients [20]. Patients exposed to anti-TNF treatment have a higher risk of infectious complications, which may trigger autoimmunity via the activation of lymphocytes to induce the production of autoantibodies, particularly ANA formation [20, 22, 37]. Under physiological conditions, IFN-α can be downregulated by TNF [38]. Thus, the blockade of TNF by anti-TNF drugs may result in increased release of IFN-α [39] in impaired autoimmune conditions with the development of lupus like symptoms. Another mechanism may involve the suppression of Th1 responses by anti-TNF agents, likely causing an increased Th2 response, improved B cell survival and subsequent induction of autoantibody synthesis [22, 40]. Interestingly, other anti-TNF therapy-induced effects such as psoriasiform skin lesions have also been attributed to increased IFN-α levels [13]. Anti-TNF DIL differs from the described classical DIL caused by drugs such as sulfadiazine or procainamide [20]. Glomerulonephritis or vascular manifestations are more common in anti-TNF agent-induced lupus, and cutaneous involvement is seen more frequently in anti-TNF DIL than in classical DIL [20].

Classical DIL is usually not associated with autoantibodies targeting dsDNA, extractable nuclear antigens or with complement consumption, whereas up to 90% of patients with anti-TNF DIL will develop anti-dsDNA antibodies, and half of these patient will have antibodies against extractable nuclear antigens and decreased serum complement levels [20]. Classical DIL is characterized by the presence of ANAs and anti-histone antibodies, whereas in anti-TNF DIL, low anti-histone antibody titers are seen [19]. A potential predisposition for allergic reactions in the presence of an autoimmune condition seems plausible but is not yet proven [20]. The diagnosis of anti-TNF DIL is sometimes difficult, probably because of symptoms of the underlying autoimmune disease (e.g. IBD or rheumatic disorder), mimicking symptoms caused by the side effects of anti-TNF therapy.

Clinical Presentation of Anti-TNF Drug-Induced Lupus

Clinically, the diagnosis of DIL or serum sickness is mostly established based on the characteristic or suggestive symptoms occurring during anti-TNF therapy and the resolution of symptoms after withdrawal of anti-TNF therapy.

Prevention of Autoimmunity in Patients Treated with Anti-TNF Therapies
A possible association between the formation of ANAs and anti-dsDNA antibodies and antibodies directed against TNF-α agents with subsequent loss of the anti-TNF therapy response is not yet clearly understood [32]. Furthermore, the role of concomitant immunosuppressive therapy in the formation of autoantibodies and the occurrence of symptoms of anti-TNF DIL have not yet been clearly defined. The recently published Study of Biologic and Immunomodulator Naive Patients in Crohn's Disease (SONIC) and SUCCESS trials prospectively compared the efficacy and safety of infliximab and azathioprine monotherapy with their combination therapy for Crohn's disease and ulcerative colitis, respectively [41, 42]. In both clinical trials, the proportion of IBD patients receiving combination therapy with infliximab plus azathioprine and developing antibodies against infliximab was lower compared with that of anti-TNF monotherapy with infliximab through a one-year follow-up. This suggests a protective role of concomitant immunosuppressive therapy

in the development of antibodies against infliximab in patients with IBD [41, 42]. However, the formation of ANAs and dsDNA antibodies was not addressed. In daily clinical practice, risk stratification is advisable when using concomitant immunosuppressive treatment in anti-TNF drug-treated patients given the potential side effects of combination therapy.

Treatment of Anti-TNF Drug-Induced Lupus

As the number of patients with IBD receiving anti-TNF therapies continues to increase, the diagnosis and management of anti-TNF DIL will become an increasingly important challenge. The treatment of anti-TNF DIL first requires the withdrawal of anti-TNF treatment and, in patients with severe symptoms, the initiation of corticosteroid and/or immunosuppressive therapy. In patients with severe joint involvement with massive arthralgia, methotrexate may be a good alternative to thiopurines such as azathioprine or 6-mercaptopurine [32]. Autoimmunity induced by anti-TNF therapies in patients with IBD seems to be a class-wide effect, and given the controversial experiences reported in the literature after a switch to a second-line anti-TNF therapy following the occurrence of lupus-like syndromes, a switch to another anti-TNF therapy should be addressed carefully [32, 43–45]. However, good results have been reported for switching to certolizumab after anti-TNF DIL under infliximab [46]. However, apparently, anti-TNF DIL has been described for all currently available anti-TNF drugs [20, 47, 48]. Since the approval of vedolizumab in Europe in May 2014 for the treatment of Crohn's disease and ulcerative colitis, a new substance class of biological therapies are available for the treatment of IBD [49, 50]. Vedolizumab is a monoclonal antibody that binds to integrin α4β7, thereby blocking the α4β7 integrin-MADCAM-1 interaction and resulting in gut-selective anti-inflammatory activity. This drug has been shown to be effective in patients with moderate to severe IBD in whom anti-TNF treatment failed [49, 50]. In particular, vedolizumab can be considered as further therapeutic option for those patients who develop lupus-like syndromes. A systematic pre-treatment serologic evaluation before the start of an anti-TNF therapy to predict the occurrence of anti-TNF DIL cannot be recommended in general, as no predictors for the development of anti-TNF DIL have yet been identified in patients naïve to anti-TNF therapies [20]. In patients with a history of lupus-like syndrome, e.g. with rash, fever or positive ANA titers, a thorough pre-treatment serologic evaluation should be considered to aid in the interpretation of the clinical and laboratory evaluation of patients with new signs of DIL during anti-TNF treatment [20].

Conclusion and Future Directions

In conclusion, the induction of autoimmunity due to the development of ANAs and anti-dsDNA antibodies in patients with IBD treated with anti-TNF therapies is common, while anti-TNF DIL is a relatively rare disease entity, occurring in a minority of up to 2% of these patients during anti-TNF therapy. In clinical practice, rapid recognition and interpretation of typical associated symptoms and laboratory findings such as a triad of arthralgia, detection of anti-dsDNA antibodies and high ANA titers, along with other symptoms like rash, erythema, myalgia, or elevation of liver enzymes in patients treated with anti-TNF-α antagonists is of great importance. Moreover, the diagnosis of anti-TNF DIL should be established when other differential diagnoses are excluded, and the therapeutic consequences need to be taken into account. A switch to vedolizumab may be considered for IBD patients in whom the anti-TNF treatment needs to be discontinued due to the development of lupus-like syndromes although the clinical experiences are scarce.

References

1 Sandborn WJ, Feagan BG, Marano C, Zhang H, Strauss R, et al: Subcutaneous golimumab induces clinical response and remission in patients with moderate-to-severe ulcerative colitis. Gastroenterology 2014;146:85–95; quiz e14–e85.

2 Sandborn WJ, Feagan BG, Marano C, Zhang H, Strauss R, et al: Subcutaneous golimumab maintains clinical response in patients with moderateto-severe ulcerative colitis. Gastroenterology 2014; 146:96–109.e1.

3 Rutgeerts P, Sandborn WJ, Feagan BG, Reinisch W, Olson A, et al: Infliximab for induction and maintenance therapy for ulcerative colitis. N Engl J Med 2005; 353:2462–2476.

4 Sandborn WJ, van Assche G, Reinisch W, Colombel JF, D'Haens G, et al: Adalimumab induces and maintains clinical remission in patients with moderate-to-severe ulcerative colitis. Gastroenterology 2012;142:257–265.e1–e3.

5 Sands BE, Blank MA, Patel K, van Deventer SJ, Study AI: Long-term treatment of rectovaginal fistulas in Crohn's disease: response to infliximab in the ACCENT II Study. Clin Gastroenterol Hepatol 2004;2:912–920.

6 Colombel JF, Sandborn WJ, Rutgeerts P, Enns R, Hanauer SB, et al: Adalimumab for maintenance of clinical response and remission in patients with Crohn's disease: the CHARM trial. Gastroenterology 2007;132:52–65.

7 Hanauer SB, Feagan BG, Lichtenstein GR, Mayer LF, Schreiber S, et al: Maintenance infliximab for Crohn's disease: the ACCENT I randomised trial. Lancet 2002;359:1541–1549.

8 Reinisch W, Sandborn WJ, Hommes DW, D'Haens G, Hanauer S, et al: Adalimumab for induction of clinical remission in moderately to severely active ulcerative colitis: results of a randomised controlled trial. Gut 2011;60: 780–787.

9 Van Assche G, Lewis JD, Lichtenstein GR, Loftus EV, Ouyang Q, et al: The London position statement of the World Congress of Gastroenterology on Biological Therapy for IBD with the European Crohn's and Colitis Organisation: safety. Am J Gastroenterol 2011; 106:1594–1602; quiz 1593, 1603.

10 Burmester GR, Panaccione R, Gordon KB, McIlraith MJ, Lacerda AP: Adalimumab: long-term safety in 23 458 patients from global clinical trials in rheumatoid arthritis, juvenile idiopathic arthritis, ankylosing spondylitis, psoriatic arthritis, psoriasis and Crohn's disease. Ann Rheum Dis 2013;72:517–524.

11 Fidder H, Schnitzler F, Ferrante M, Noman M, Katsanos K, et al: Long-term safety of infliximab for the treatment of inflammatory bowel disease: a singlecentre cohort study. Gut 2009;58:501–508.

12 Schnitzler F, Fidder H, Ferrante M, Noman M, Arijs I, et al: Long-term outcome of treatment with infliximab in 614 patients with Crohn's disease: results from a single-centre cohort. Gut 2009;58:492–500.

13 Tillack C, Ehmann LM, Friedrich M, Laubender RP, Papay P, et al: Anti- TNF antibody-induced psoriasiform skin lesions in patients with inflammatory bowel disease are characterised by interferon-gamma-expressing Th1 cells and IL-17A/IL-22-expressing Th17 cells and respond to anti-IL-12/IL-23 antibody treatment. Gut 2014;63:567–577.

14 Vermeire S, Noman M, Van Assche G, Baert F, Van Steen K, et al: Autoimmunity associated with anti-tumor necrosis factor alpha treatment in Crohn's disease: a prospective cohort study. Gastroenterology 2003;125:32–39.

15 Jonsdottir T, Forslid J, van Vollenhoven A, Harju A, Brannemark S, et al: Treatment with tumour necrosis factor alpha antagonists in patients with rheumatoid arthritis induces anticardiolipin antibodies. Ann Rheum Dis 2004;63:1075–1078.

16 Charles PJ, Smeenk RJ, De Jong J, Feldmann M, Maini RN: Assessment of antibodies to double-stranded DNA induced in rheumatoid arthritis patients following treatment with infliximab, a monoclonal antibody to tumor necrosis factor alpha: findings in open-label and randomized placebo-controlled trials. Arthritis Rheum 2000;43:2383–2390.

17 Eriksson C, Engstrand S, Sundqvist KG, Rantapaa-Dahlqvist S: Autoantibody formation in patients with rheumatoid arthritis treated with anti-TNF alpha. Ann Rheum Dis 2005;64:403–407.

18 Antonov D, Kazandjieva J, Etugov D, Gospodinov D, Tsankov N: Drug-induced lupus erythematosus. Clin Dermatol 2004;22:157–166.

19 Katz U, Zandman-Goddard G: Drug-induced lupus: an update. Autoimmun Rev 2010;10:46–50.

20 Costa MF, Said NR, Zimmermann B: Drug-induced lupus due to anti-tumor necrosis factor alpha agents. Semin Arthritis Rheum 2008;37:381–387.

21 Piga M, Chessa E, Ibba V, Mura V, Floris A, et al: Biologics-induced autoimmune renal disorders in chronic inflammatory rheumatic diseases: systematic literature review and analysis of a monocentric cohort. Autoimmun Rev 2014;13:873–879.

22 Moulis G, Sommet A, Lapeyre-Mestre M, Montastruc JL, Association Francaise des Centres Regionaux de Pharmaco-Vigilance: Is the risk of tumour necrosis factor inhibitorinduced lupus or lupus-like syndrome the same with monoclonal antibodies and soluble receptor? A case/non-case study in a nationwide pharmacovigilance database. Rheumatology (Oxford) 2014;53:1864–1871.

23 van Rijthoven AW, Bijlsma JW, Canninga-van Dijk M, Derksen RH, van Roon JA: Onset of systemic lupus erythematosus after conversion of infliximab to adalimumab treatment in rheumatoid arthritis with a pre-existing anti-dsDNA antibody level. Rheumatology (Oxford) 2006;45:1317–1319.

24 Stokes MB, Foster K, Markowitz GS, Ebrahimi F, Hines W, et al: Development of glomerulonephritis during anti-TNF-alpha therapy for rheumatoid arthritis. Nephrol Dial Transplant 2005; 20:1400–1406.

25 Perez-Garcia C, Maymo J, Lisbona Perez MP, Almirall Bernabe M, Carbonell Abello J: Drug-induced systemic lupus erythematosus in ankylosing spondylitis associated with infliximab. Rheumatology (Oxford) 2006;45:114–116.

26 Klapman JB, Ene-Stroescu D, Becker MA, Hanauer SB: A lupus-like syndrome associated with infliximab therapy. Inflamm Bowel Dis 2003;9:176–178.

27 Favalli EG, Sinigaglia L, Varenna M, Arnoldi C: Drug-induced lupus following treatment with infliximab in rheumatoid arthritis. Lupus 2002;11:753–755.

28 Elkayam O, Caspi D: Infliximab induced lupus in patients with rheumatoid arthritis. Clin Exp Rheumatol 2004;22: 502–503.
29 Chadha T, Hernandez JE: Infliximab-related lupus and associated valvulitis: a case report and review of the literature. Arthritis Rheum 2006;55:163–166.
30 Benucci M, Li Gobbi F, Fossi F, Manfredi M, Del Rosso A: Drug-induced lupus after treatment with infliximab in rheumatoid arthritis. J Clin Rheumatol 2005; 11:47–49.
31 De Bandt M, Sibilia J, Le Loet X, Prouzeau S, Fautrel B, et al: Systemic lupus erythematosus induced by anti-tumour necrosis factor alpha therapy: a French national survey. Arthritis Res Ther 2005;7:R545–R551.
32 Beigel F, Schnitzler F, Paul Laubender R, Pfennig S, Weidinger M, et al: Formation of antinuclear and double-strand DNA antibodies and frequency of lupus-like syndrome in anti-TNF-alpha antibody-treated patients with inflammatory bowel disease. Inflamm Bowel Dis 2011;17:91–98.
33 Aringer M, Smolen JS: The role of tumor necrosis factor-alpha in systemic lupus erythematosus. Arthritis Res Ther 2008; 10:202.
34 Ferraccioli GF, Assaloni R, Di Poi E, Gremese E, De Marchi G, et al: Rescue of combination therapy failures using infliximab, while maintaining the combination or monotherapy with methotrexate: results of an open trial. Rheumatology (Oxford) 2002;41:1109–1112.
35 Casciola-Rosen L, Rosen A, Petri M, Schlissel M: Surface blebs on apoptotic cells are sites of enhanced procoagulant activity: implications for coagulation events and antigenic spread in systemic lupus erythematosus. Proc Natl Acad Sci U S A 1996;93:1624–1629.
36 Utz PJ, Hottelet M, Schur PH, Anderson P: Proteins phosphorylated during stress-induced apoptosis are common targets for autoantibody production in patients with systemic lupus erythematosus. J Exp Med 1997;185:843–854.
37 Chang C, Gershwin ME: Drugs and autoimmunity – a contemporary review and mechanistic approach. J Autoimmun 2010;34:J266–J275.
38 Palucka AK, Blanck JP, Bennett L, Pascual V, Banchereau J: Cross-regulation of TNF and IFN-alpha in autoimmune diseases. Proc Natl Acad Sci U S A 2005; 102:3372–3377.
39 Aringer M, Smolen JS: Therapeutic blockade of TNF in patients with SLE promising or crazy? Autoimmun Rev 2012;11:321–325.
40 Via CS, Shustov A, Rus V, Lang T, Nguyen P, et al: In vivo neutralization of TNF-alpha promotes humoral autoimmunity by preventing the induction of CTL. J Immunol 2001;167:6821–6826.
41 Colombel JF, Sandborn WJ, Reinisch W, Mantzaris GJ, Kornbluth A, et al: Infliximab, azathioprine, or combination therapy for Crohn's disease. N Engl J Med 2010;362:1383–1395.
42 Panaccione R, Ghosh S, Middleton S, Marquez JR, Scott BB, et al: Combination therapy with infliximab and azathioprine is superior to monotherapy with either agent in ulcerative colitis. Gastroenterology 2014;146:392–400.e3.
43 Kocharla L, Mongey AB: Is the development of drug-related lupus a contraindication for switching from one TNF alpha inhibitor to another? Lupus 2009; 18:169–171.
44 Spillane AP, Xia Y, Sniezek PJ: Drug-induced lupus erythematosus in a patient treated with adalumimab. J Am Acad Dermatol 2007;56:S114–S116.
45 Havel J, Aboutalebi S, Doughty L, Wirges M: Development of systemic lupus erythematosus in a patient with rheumatoid arthritis following treatment conversion of infliximab to adalimumab. J Drugs Dermatol 2008;7:796–798.
46 Subramanian S, Yajnik V, Sands BE, Cullen G, Korzenik JR: Characterization of patients with infliximab-induced lupus erythematosus and outcomes after retreatment with a second anti-TNF agent. Inflamm Bowel Dis 2011;17:99–104.
47 Brunasso AM, Aberer W, Massone C: New onset of dermatomyositis/polymyositis during anti-TNF-alpha therapies: a systematic literature review. ScientificWorldJournal 2014;2014:179180.
48 Williams VL, Cohen PR: TNF alpha antagonist-induced lupus-like syndrome: report and review of the literature with implications for treatment with alternative TNF alpha antagonists. Int J Dermatol 2011;50:619–625.
49 Sandborn WJ, Feagan BG, Rutgeerts P, Hanauer S, Colombel JF, et al: Vedolizumab as induction and maintenance therapy for Crohn's disease. N Engl J Med 2013;369:711–721.
50 Feagan BG, Rutgeerts P, Sands BE, Hanauer S, Colombel JF, et al: Vedolizumab as induction and maintenance therapy for ulcerative colitis. N Engl J Med 2013;369:699–710.

Fabian Schnitzler, MD
Department of Medicine II – Grosshadern, Ludwig-Maximilians University (LMU) Munich
DE–81377 Munich (Germany)
E-Mail fabian.schnitzler@med.uni-muenchen.de

Rogler G, Herfarth H, Hibi T, Nielsen OH (eds): Anti-Tumor Necrosis Factor Therapy in Inflammatory Bowel Disease.
Front Gastrointest Res. Basel, Karger, 2015, vol 34, pp 138–142 (DOI: 10.1159/000381593)

Risk of Non-Hematologic Malignancy with Anti-TNF Therapy in Inflammatory Bowel Diseases

Animesh Jain[a] · Hans H. Herfarth[b] · Millie D. Long[b]

[a]Department of Medicine, Division of Gastroenterology and Hepatology, Johns Hopkins University, Baltimore, Md., and [b]Department of Medicine, Division of Gastroenterology and Hepatology, University of North Carolina at Chapel Hill, Chapel Hill, N.C., USA

Abstract

Anti-tumor necrosis factor-alpha (anti-TNF) therapy has been demonstrated to be efficacious in the treatment of inflammatory bowel diseases. The use of anti-TNF agents has therefore increased over the past decade. While anti-TNF therapy is associated with significant benefits, there are also co-existing risks. Multiple studies have shown no increase in the overall malignancy risk in association with this therapy. However, two specific types of nonhematologic malignancy, skin cancer and cervical cancer, may be associated with anti-TNF agent use. The following review will summarize data on the nonhematologic malignancy risk associated with the use of anti-TNF agents, discuss important components of risk communication with patients, and identify recommended preventive measures for patients initiating this therapy.

Introduction

As clinical experience with anti-tumor necrosis factor-alpha (anti-TNF) therapy has grown, so has awareness regarding the potential complications of these agents. While much of the data have focused on hematologic malignancies, such as lymphoma or myeloproliferative disorders, additional data on the increased risk of nonhematologic malignancies due to the immunosuppressive effects of anti-TNF agents are also of importance.

Determining the precise risk of malignancy attributable to anti-TNF therapy, however, remains challenging on many fronts. Patients treated with anti-TNF agents typically have more aggressive disease, and they have often been treated with other classes of medications, including aminosalicylates and thiopurines. There is also a concern that inflammatory bowel diseases (IBDs) lead to an increased malignancy risk due to ongoing chronic inflammation. Hence, in clinical studies, it is challenging to differentiate the malignancy risk attributed to anti-TNF agents from that due to underlying inflammatory diseases or other medications, particularly thiopurines. Moreover, most studies are not specifically designed to examine malignancy risk attributed to anti-TNF agents. In many cases, we are left to infer the risk from studies that are observational in nature and may have a short follow-up period that is not adequate to determine long-term malignancy risk.

Multiple studies reassuringly have shown no increase in overall malignancy risk associated with anti-TNF therapy in IBD patients [1–8]. However, some studies have suggested that there is an increased malignancy risk specifically for nonmelanoma skin cancer (NMSC), melanoma, and cervical cancer/dysplasia. In this chapter, we discuss the emerging and sometimes conflicting evidence regarding these nonhematologic malignancies, with an emphasis on practical points for clinicians.

Skin Cancer

Non-Melanoma Skin Cancer

Individuals with IBD are at increased risk of NMSC. The incidence of NMSC among patients with IBD has been estimated to be 733 per 100,000 patient-years compared to 447 per 100,000 patient-years in an age-matched non-IBD population [9]. There is mounting evidence that NMSC risk is strongly associated with thiopurine use in IBD. A 2010 nested case control study demonstrated an increased risk of NMSC in IBD patients with both the recent (≤90 days) and persistent (>365 days) use of thiopurines [9]. Subsequent studies have included a large prospective French cohort study and a separate large nested case control study, both of which have confirmed an increased risk of NMSC in patients treated with thiopurines [10, 11]. Importantly, even after discontinuation of the thiopurine, the increased risk of NMSC persists. This continuation of risk is likely related to prior photo-toxic damage that occurred while on the drug [10].

Data regarding anti-TNF therapy and NMSC are more limited. A nested case control study by Long et al. did show an elevated risk of NMSC in Crohn's disease (CD) patients with >365 days of anti-TNF therapy exposure (OR = 2.18, 95% CI 1.07–4.46) [9]. A more recent study pooled data from nearly 1,600 patients treated with adalimumab in CD clinical trials. The authors found no elevated risk of NMSC with adalimumab monotherapy, but they did observe an increased risk of NMSC associated with combination therapy with adalimumab and other immunosuppressants (standardized incidence ratio (SIR) = 4.59, 95% CI 2.51–7.70 compared to the general population, and SIR = 3.46, 95% CI 1.08–11.06 compared to adalimumab monotherapy) [4]. There has been no statistically significant evidence of an increased risk of NMSC in ulcerative colitis (UC) patients treated with anti-TNF therapy, although fewer patients with UC have been treated with anti-TNF agents at the time that these prior studies were conducted. Data from rheumatoid arthritis populations have also shown an increased risk of NMSC in association with anti-TNF use (relative risk 2.02, 95% CI 1.11–3.95) [12], albeit concomitant and prior use of immunosuppressive agents, such as methotrexate, likely contributed to this increase.

Melanoma

A recent meta-analysis showed a significantly increased incidence of melanoma in IBD patients of 27.5 cases per 100,000 patient-years compared to 21.0 cases per 100,000 patient-years expected in the general population [13]. However, data in support of a link between anti-TNF therapy and melanoma risk are more limited because melanoma is a relatively rare form of skin cancer. In a 2012 nested case control study of 209 IBD patients with melanoma matched to 823 control patients, exposure to anti-TNF therapy was found to be associated with increased melanoma risk (OR = 1.88, 95% CI 1.08–3.29). When patients were stratified by disease subtype, this trend held for CD (OR = 1.94, 95% CI 1.03–3.68) but not for UC (OR = 1.73, 95% CI 0.53–5.63) [11]. There was no association between thiopurine use and melanoma. A similar trend of increased melanoma risk with anti-TNF therapy in rheumatoid arthritis patients has been shown; in a 2011 meta-analysis, the pooled relative risk estimate for melanoma was 1.79 (95% CI 0.92–2.67) [14].

Skin Cancer Prevention

Current guidelines do not specifically address skin cancer screening and prevention strategies in the IBD population. Given the apparent increased risk of melanoma and NMSC in certain subsets of immunosuppressed IBD patients, attention to skin cancer prevention is an important topic in this population [15]. Wearing sun-protective clothing, finding shade during peak sun hours, and using broad-spectrum sunscreens should be recommended to IBD patients [16]. While annual skin examination is not currently a standard practice in IBD populations, it is recommended by various organ transplant societies due to the ongoing immunosuppressant use and increased skin cancer risk of transplant recipients [17, 18]. Skin examinations should be considered in IBD populations, and prompt evaluation by a dermatologist should be recommended for any IBD patient with a concerning skin lesion.

Cervical Cancer

While data from organ transplant patients have shown a link between immunosuppression and cervical dysplasia [19–21], the impact of IBD on cervical dysplasia and cancer remains less clear. A total of four case control studies have investigated this topic. Early case control studies conducted in 2006 and 2008 suggested an overall increased incidence of cervical dysplasia in IBD patients, while two larger subsequent case control studies showed no such relationship [22–25].

The role of immunosuppression and cervical dysplasia is even less clear in IBD patients. In a small study performed by Kane et al., women with IBD exposed to at least 6 months of immunosuppressant therapy (corticosteroids, thiopurines, methotrexate, and/or infliximab) had an increased risk of cervical dysplasia [23]. A larger study conducted in Manitoba, Canada showed an increased risk of cervical dysplasia only in women with IBD exposed to both corticosteroids and immunosuppressants (thiopurines, methotrexate, cyclosporine, and/or infliximab) [24]. Two other case control studies showed no link between immunosuppression and cervical dysplasia or cancer in women with IBD [22, 25].

None of the aforementioned studies were powered to isolate the effects of individual immunosuppressant medications, and all of the studies included relatively small numbers of patients on anti-TNF therapy. With the limited data at this time, it is hard to make any firm conclusions. It appears that immunosuppressive medications, especially combination therapy, may increase the risk of cervical dysplasia, but the specific role of anti-TNF therapy cannot be determined.

Cervical Cancer Screening and Prevention

Current United States guidelines suggest screening for cervical cancer in women starting at the age of 21 using Pap smears every 3 years until the age of 65 [26]. Optionally, screening can be extended to every 5 years if performed along with human papillomavirus testing in women aged 30–65. However, these most recent guidelines do not apply to women who are immunocompromised, such as those who have undergone solid organ transplantation [26]. Given that only 70% of women with IBD receive cervical cancer screening at the appropriate intervals [27], gastroenterologists should take active roles in promoting adequate cervical cancer screening in IBD patients. Moreover, human papillomavirus vaccination (Gardasil) has been shown to be efficacious in women with IBD on immunosuppression, without any evidence of the exacerbation of the IBD [28]. This vaccine is recommended in all women aged 9–26 in the US. These preventive measures are likely the most critical for women on combination therapy with anti-TNF agents and other immunosuppressive medications.

Summary

We have reviewed the key evidence of the increased risks of various nonhematologic malignancies in IBD patients treated with non-hematologic anti-TNF therapy. Although the data are limited, anti-TNF therapy does appear to be associated with an increased risk of melanoma, particularly in CD patients. Anti-TNF therapy also likely plays a role in NMSC risk in patients on combination therapy with other immunosuppressants, such as thiopurines. There are also multiple studies showing a link between thiopurine use alone and increased NMSC risk. There are limited data demonstrating a connection between immunosuppression in general and cervical dysplasia, and the data are too few to draw any conclusions on the specific role of anti-TNF therapy.

The limitations of the current studies and the nuances of the results obtained have left clinicians with no clear, straightforward direction for managing patients. Collectively, the data show at most small increases in the risks of skin cancer and perhaps cervical dysplasia. These risks are likely the greatest in patients on combination therapy with anti-TNF and other immunosuppressive agents. When clinicians present data to patients on the risks of these agents, doing so in a fashion that clearly demonstrates both the absolute risks and the benefits of therapy can aid in clinical decision making. When presenting data on risks, it is better to present data on absolute risks with common denominators (such as 'X' per 10,000), use visual aids when possible, and give perspectives on other diseases and life risk factors. Information presented in this format is easier for patients to understand [29, 30].

The malignancy risks of anti-TNF therapy are likely outweighed by the clinical benefits in most IBD patients. Clinicians can help to mitigate the risks of anti-TNF therapy by following the appropriate preventive measures that have been outlined (fig. 1).

- Counsel on sun protection via sun protective clothing and/or regular sunscreen use
- Consider full skin examinations in for at-risk patients
- Advocate adherence to cervical cancer screening for women at recommended intervals
- Offer human papillomavirus vaccination to women aged 9–26

Fig. 1. Preventive measures associated with malignancy risk in inflammatory bowel disease patients on anti-TNF and other immunosuppressive therapies.

References

1 Nyboe Andersen N, Pasternak B, Basit S, et al: Association between tumor necrosis factor-alpha antagonists and risk of cancer in patients with inflammatory bowel disease. JAMA 2014;311:2406–2413.

2 Lichtenstein GR, Feagan BG, Cohen RD, et al: Drug therapies and the risk of malignancy in Crohn's disease: results from the TREAT Registry. Am J Gastroenterol 2014;109:212–223.

3 Williams CJ, Peyrin-Biroulet L, Ford AC: Systematic review with meta-analysis: malignancies with anti-tumour necrosis factor-alpha therapy in inflammatory bowel disease. Aliment Pharmacol Ther 2014;39:447–458.

4 Osterman MT, Sandborn WJ, Colombel JF, et al: Increased risk of malignancy with adalimumab combination therapy, compared with monotherapy, for Crohn's disease. Gastroenterology 2014;146:941–949.

5 Lichtenstein GR, Rutgeerts P, Sandborn WJ, et al: A pooled analysis of infections, malignancy, and mortality in infliximab- and immunomodulator-treated adult patients with inflammatory bowel disease. Am J Gastroenterol 2012;107:1051–1063.

6 Biancone L, Petruzziello C, Orlando A, et al: Cancer in Crohn's disease patients treated with infliximab: a long-term multicenter matched pair study. Inflamm Bowel Dis 2011;17:758–766.

7 Fidder H, Schnitzler F, Ferrante M, et al: Long-term safety of infliximab for the treatment of inflammatory bowel disease: a single-centre cohort study. Gut 2009;58:501–508.

8 Caspersen S, Elkjaer M, Riis L, et al: Infliximab for inflammatory bowel disease in Denmark 1999–2005: clinical outcome and follow-up evaluation of malignancy and mortality. Clin Gastroenterol Hepatol 2008;6:1212–1217; quiz 1176.

9 Long MD, Herfarth HH, Pipkin CA, et al: Increased risk for non-melanoma skin cancer in patients with inflammatory bowel disease. Clin Gastroenterol Hepatol 2010;8:268–274.

10 Peyrin-Biroulet L, Khosrotehrani K, Carrat F, et al: Increased risk for nonmelanoma skin cancers in patients who receive thiopurines for inflammatory bowel disease. Gastroenterology 2011; 141:1621–1628.e1–e5.

11 Long MD, Martin CF, Pipkin CA, et al: Risk of melanoma and nonmelanoma skin cancer among patients with inflammatory bowel disease. Gastroenterology 2012;143:390–399.e1.

12 Askling J, Fahrbach K, Nordstrom B, et al: Cancer risk with tumor necrosis factor alpha (TNF) inhibitors: meta-analysis of randomized controlled trials of adalimumab, etanercept, and infliximab using patient level data. Pharmacoepidemiol Drug Saf 2011;20:119–130.

13 Singh S, Nagpal SJ, Murad MH, et al: Inflammatory bowel disease is associated with an increased risk of melanoma: a systematic review and meta-analysis. Clin Gastroenterol Hepatol 2014; 12:210–218.

14 Mariette X, Matucci-Cerinic M, Pavelka K, et al: Malignancies associated with tumour necrosis factor inhibitors in registries and prospective observational studies: a systematic review and meta-analysis. Ann Rheum Dis 2011;70:1895–1904.

15 Long MD, Kappelman MD, Pipkin CA: Nonmelanoma skin cancer in inflammatory bowel disease: a review. Inflamm Bowel Dis 2011;17:1423–1427.

16 Wang SQ, Balagula Y, Osterwalder U: Photoprotection: a review of the current and future technologies. Dermatol Ther 2010;23:31–47.

17 Hofbauer GF, Anliker M, Arnold A, et al: Swiss clinical practice guidelines for skin cancer in organ transplant recipients. Swiss Med Wkly 2009;139:407–415.

18 Kasiske BL, Vazquez MA, Harmon WE, et al: Recommendations for the outpatient surveillance of renal transplant recipients. American Society of Transplantation. J Am Soc Nephrol 2000; 11(suppl 15):S1–S86.

19 Kay S, Frable WJ, Hume DM: Cervical dysplasia and cancer developing in women on immunosuppression therapy for renal homotransplantation. Cancer 1970;26:1048–1052.

20 Collett D, Mumford L, Banner NR, et al: Comparison of the incidence of malignancy in recipients of different types of organ: a UK Registry audit. Am J Transplant 2010;10:1889–1896.

21 Madeleine MM, Finch JL, Lynch CF, et al: HPV-related cancers after solid organ transplantation in the United States. Am J Transplant 2013;13:3202–3209.

22 Bhatia J, Bratcher J, Korelitz B, et al: Abnormalities of uterine cervix in women with inflammatory bowel disease. World J Gastroenterol 2006;12:6167–6171.

23 Kane S, Khatibi B, Reddy D: Higher incidence of abnormal Pap smears in women with inflammatory bowel disease. Am J Gastroenterol 2008;103:631–636.

24 Singh H, Demers AA, Nugent Z, et al: Risk of cervical abnormalities in women with inflammatory bowel disease: a population-based nested case-control study. Gastroenterology 2009;136:451–458.

25 Lees CW, Critchley J, Chee N, et al: Lack of association between cervical dysplasia and IBD: a large case-control study. Inflamm Bowel Dis 2009;15:1621–1629.

26 Committee on Practice Bulletins–Gynecology: ACOG Practice Bulletin Number 131: screening for cervical cancer. Obstet Gynecol 2012;120:1222–1238.

27 Long MD, Porter CQ, Sandler RS, et al: Suboptimal rates of cervical testing among women with inflammatory bowel disease. Clin Gastroenterol Hepatol 2009;7:549–553.

28 Jacobson DL, Bousvaros A, Ashworth L, et al: Immunogenicity and tolerability to human papillomavirus-like particle vaccine in girls and young women with inflammatory bowel disease. Inflamm Bowel Dis 2013;19:1441–1449.

29 Peters E, Hibbard J, Slovic P, et al: Numeracy skill and the communication, comprehension, and use of risk-benefit information. Health Aff (Millwood) 2007;26:741–748.

30 Fagerlin A, Ubel PA, Smith DM, et al: Making numbers matter: present and future research in risk communication. Am J Health Behav 2007;31(suppl 1): S47–S56.

Millie D. Long, MD, MPH
Department of Medicine, Division of Gastroenterology and Hepatology, University of North Carolina
Bioinformatics Bldg., CB#7080
Chapel Hill, NC 27599 (USA)
E-Mail millie_long@med.unc.edu

Rogler G, Herfarth H, Hibi T, Nielsen OH (eds): Anti-Tumor Necrosis Factor Therapy in Inflammatory Bowel Disease.
Front Gastrointest Res. Basel, Karger, 2015, vol 34, pp 143–146 (DOI: 10.1159/000381594)

Risk of Lymphoma

Masakazu Nagahori • Mamoru Watanabe

Department of Gastroenterology and Hepatology, Tokyo Medical and Dental University, Tokyo, Japan

Abstract

Inflammatory bowel disease patients who are treated with anti-TNF therapy in combination with thiopurines seem to have an increased risk of developing lymphoma. However, the risk associated with anti-TNF therapy itself is considered to be negligible. The clear benefit of this effective treatment is likely to outweigh several risks, including lymphoma, in most patients.

Introduction

Through its efficacy with an improved probability of mucosal healing, anti-TNF therapy has significantly changed treatment goals for inflammatory bowel disease (IBD) patients. The therapeutic efficacy of this therapy has been clearly shown in both Crohn's disease (CD) and ulcerative colitis patients in meta-analyses of randomized double-blinded placebo-controlled trials [1, 2]. However, several safety issues, especially the potential risk of lymphoma, have not yet been resolved, limiting its use mainly to patients who are refractory to conventional therapies. The association between anti-TNF therapy and the development of lymphoma was first investigated in rheumatoid arthritis patients [3]. Among the IBD treatments, thiopurines, which are commonly used along with anti-TNF therapy, have been shown to increase the risk of developing malignant lymphoma in IBD patients [4].

Main Points

Epidemiological Studies to Investigate Lymphoma Risk Due to Anti-TNF Therapy
Two meta-analyses have been published to evaluate the risk of anti-TNF treatment in adult IBD patients. Peyrin-Biroulet et al. have analyzed 21 placebo-controlled trials enrolling 5,356 CD patients and have concluded that there is no difference in the frequency of malignancies, including lymphoma, between the groups [5].

Another meta-analysis examined the risk of lymphoma associated with a combination of anti-TNF and immunomodulator therapies in patients with CD [6]. They included twenty-six studies involving 8,905 patients with 21,178 patient-years of follow-up (PYF). These studies included nine randomized controlled trials, three cohort studies and 14 case series of consecutive patients. A total of 13 lymphoma cases were observed, yielding a rate of 6.1 non-Hodgkin lymphomas (NHLs) per 10,000 patient-years. When compared with the expected rate of NHL determined from the Surveillance Epidemiology and End Results (SEER) cancer registry data (1.9 per 10,000 patient-years), the standardized incidence ratio (SIR) was calculated to be 3.23 (95% CI: 1.5–6.9). On the other hand, when compared with the observed rate of NHL in CD patients receiving immunomodulator therapy alone reported by Kandiel et al. (3.6 per 10,000 patient-years), the SIR was 1.7 (95% CI: 0.5–7.1) [4]. Furthermore, most of the 13 lymphoma patients were being treated or had been previously treated with immunomodulators.

Analysis of the five-year follow-up of the Crohn's Therapy, Resource, Evaluation, and Assessment Tool (TREAT) registry showed similar incidence rates of lymphoma in an infliximab (IFX)-treated group (0.05 per 100 patient-years) and an other-treatments-only group (0.05 per 100 patient-years), which did not significantly differ from that in the background SEER population [7].

A population-based study to evaluate the safety of IFX treatment was conducted among 11 medical centers in Stockholm County between 1999 and 2001, comprising 217 IBD patients treated with IFX [8]. Three lymphoma cases were observed and resulted in an annual incidence of 1.5%, whereas that in Stockholm County was only 0.115%.

A retrospective Mayo Clinic study was performed to investigate the safety profile of IFX treatment in 500 consecutive CD patients [9]. The patients received a median of 3 infusions, and the median follow-up time was 17 months. A 70-year-old male patient developed NHL after 3 infusions of IFX along with azathioprine. Although pelvic lymphadenopathy had been noted before IFX treatment, it was judged to be related to the treatment due to the rapid progression of the lymphoma.

Recently, a German IBD single-center cohort was retrospectively investigated to reveal the risk of malignancies associated with anti-TNF therapy alone and with thiopurine therapy [10]. Among 666 IBD patients who were exposed to thiopurine and/or anti-TNF therapy, 404 (61%) were treated with anti-TNF therapy with or without thiopurines (the TNF+ group). The median follow-up time was significantly shorter for the patients treated with thiopurines alone (TP group), with a median of 68 weeks, compared with those in the TNF+ group, with a median of 140 weeks. Lymphoma was observed in 4 patients in the TP group and one in the TNF+ group. A male patient with CD developed hepatosplenic T-cell lymphoma (HSTCL) at age 58 and in addition, he had been treated with thiopurines for 60 months.

A recent meta-analysis evaluated the risk of lymphoma associated with anti-TNF therapy in pediatric IBD patients (≤18 years), evaluating 5,528 patients with 9,516 PYF in 65 studies [11]. A total of 84% of the patients had CD, and IFX was used to treat 90% of them. Seventy-four percent of the included studies had a mean per patient follow-up period of shorter than 2 years. Two patients developed lymphoma, one with Hodgkin and another with non-Hodgkin (B cell) type, resulting in an absolute rate of 2.1 per 10,000 PYF. The rate of lymphoma was numerically lower than that seen in pediatric IBD patients treated with thiopurine monotherapy (SIR, 0.47; $p = 0.48$; 95% CI: 0.03–6.44) and that determined in adult IBD patients treated with anti-TNF therapy (SIR, 0.34; $p = 0.14$; 95% CI: 0.04–1.51). Unfortunately, the risk of HSTCL could not be evaluated because no patients developed it in this patient population.

The Kaiser Permanente IBD registry data (1996–2009) were used to evaluate the lymphoma risk among 16,023 IBD patients [12]. Over an average follow-up time of 5.8 years, 48 patients developed lymphoma. Compared with the general Kaiser Permanente population, the standardized incidence rate ratios (SIRRs) were 0.3 (95% CI: 0.2–0.4) among past and 1.4 (95% CI: 1.2–2.7) among current users of thiopurine. For the anti-TNF users (with or without thiopurine), the SIRRs were 5.5 (95% CI: 4.5–6.6) among past and

4.4 (95% CI: 3.4–5.4) among current users. On the other hand, the SIRR was 1.0 (95% CI: 0.96–1.1) among the IBD patients who had not been treated with thiopurine or anti-TNF therapy. Naturally, we could not determine the contribution of anti-TNF therapy to the increased rate of lymphoma because of the concomitant thiopurine treatment received by the anti-TNF users.

In a population-based study conducted in Denmark, 651 IBD patients who were treated with IFX from 1999 to 2005 were evaluated, with a median follow-up period of 29.1 months [13]. Among them, 4 patients were diagnosed with cancer during the follow-up period. However, no lymphoma case was observed.

In a multi-center matched pair study that compared the cancer rate among CD patients treated with IFX and those who had never been treated with IFX who were matched for sex, age, CD site, follow-up duration, immunosuppressant use, and CD duration, no differences were observed between the groups in a median follow-up period of 6 years [14]. Among 404 patients who had been exposed to IFX, only one case of leukemia and one case of Hodgkin's lymphoma were observed.

Hepatosplenic T-Cell Lymphoma

HSTCL is a very uncommon but exclusively aggressive and fatal subtype of extranodal lymphoma. Patients may present with fever, weight loss, abdominal pain, weakness, and significant splenomegaly without lymphadenopathy. Kotlyar et al. reported a case series of 36 patients with IBD complicated by HSTCL, 20 of whom received both IFX and thiopurine and 16 of whom received thiopurine alone [15]. Only 2 female patients were included. Among 30 patients with known ages, 27 were younger than 35 years old. Because the development of HSTCL has not been reported among IBD patients who have been treated with anti-TNF monotherapy, the discontinuation of thiopurine might well be considered in patients receiving combination therapy, particularly in young male patients.

Risk Interpretation and Better Communication

To interpret the lymphoma risk associated with anti-TNF therapy among IBD patients, we must determine the possible association between IBD itself and lymphoma, which is still controversial. In a Manitoba population-based study investigating the cancer risk of IBD patients compared with individuals without IBD who were matched for year, age, gender, and postal area of residence, the incidence rate ratio of lymphoma was elevated only in male CD patients (3.63; 95% CI: 1.53–8.62) [16]. We must also know the possible role of protopathic bias to interpret the lymphoma risk. When IBD patients develop symptoms such as fever and fatigue, these symptoms could be wrongly attributed to an IBD flare-up rather than a complication of lymphoma, and anti-TNF medication could be administered.

How to effectively communicate lymphoma risk to patients should also be mentioned here. To overcome difficulties, several recommendations have been made for clear communication [17]. Vague descriptive words, such as rare and common, should not be used. When presenting data, it is better to use multiple formats, including numbers and graphs. When numbers are presented, consistent numbers should be used. Absolute risks, not relative risks, should be presented, without using the number needed to harm. To avoid using a small percentage, such as 0.06%, a frequency (6 of 10,000) should be presented.

Finally, to help providers and patients to make a shared decision of an alternative treatment option, such as anti-TNF monotherapy or combination therapy (with thiopurines), several easy-to-use tools have been made, and one of which is presented in 'Option Grids' (http://www.optiongrid.org/).

Conclusions and Future Directions

Overall, anti-TNF treatment itself does not seem to be associated with an increased risk of lymphoma among IBD patients. However, we still cannot be sure whether the efficacy of combination therapy with thiopurines outweighs the potential risk of lymphoma in each IBD patient who is treated with anti-TNF therapy.

References

1 Peyrin-Biroulet L, Deltenre P, de Suray N, Branche J, Sandborn WJ, Colombel JF: Efficacy and safety of tumor necrosis factor antagonists in Crohn's disease: meta-analysis of placebo-controlled trials. Clin Gastroenterol Hepatol 2008;6: 644–653.

2 Lawson MM, Thomas AG, Akobeng AK: Tumour necrosis factor alpha blocking agents for induction of remission in ulcerative colitis. Cochrane Database Syst Rev 2006;3:CD005112.

3 Leombruno JP, Einarson TR, Keystone EC: The safety of anti-tumour necrosis factor treatments in rheumatoid arthritis: meta and exposure-adjusted pooled analyses of serious adverse events Ann Rheum Dis 2009;68:1136–1145.

4 Kandiel A, Fraser AG, Korelitz BI, Brensinger C, Lewis JD: Increased risk of lymphoma among inflammatory bowel disease patients treated with azathioprine and 6-mercaptopurine. Gut 2005;54:1121–1125.

5 Peyrin-Biroulet L, Deltenre P, de Suray N, Branche J, Sandborn WJ, Colombel JF: Efficacy and safety of tumor necrosis factor antagonists in Crohn's disease: meta-analysis of placebo-controlled trials. Clin Gastroenterol Hepatol 2008;6: 644–653.

6 Siegel CA, Marden SM, Persing SM, Larson RJ, Sands BE: Risk of lymphoma associated with combination anti-tumor necrosis factor and immunomodulator therapy for the treatment of Crohn's disease: a meta-analysis Clin Gastroenterol Hepatol 2009;7:874–881.

7 Lichtenstein GR, Feagan BG, Cohen RD, Salzberg BA, Diamond RH, Langholff W, Londhe A, Sandborn WJ: Drug therapies and the risk of malignancy in Crohn's disease: results from the TREAT™ Registry. Am J Gastroenterol 2014;109:212–223.

8 Ljung T, Karlén P, Schmidt D, Hellström PM, Lapidus A, Janczewska I, Sjöqvist U, Löfberg R: Infliximab in inflammatory bowel disease: clinical outcome in a population based cohort from Stockholm County. Gut 2004;53:849–853.

9 Colombel JF, Loftus EV Jr, Tremaine WJ, Egan LJ, Harmsen WS, Schleck CD, Zinsmeister AR, Sandborn WJ: The safety profile of infliximab in patients with Crohn's disease: the Mayo clinic experience in 500 patients. Gastroenterology 2004;126:19–31.

10 Beigel F, Steinborn A, Schnitzler F, Tillack C, Breiteneicher S, John JM, Van Steen K, Laubender RP, Göke B, Seiderer J, Brand S, Ochsenkühn T: Risk of malignancies in patients with inflammatory bowel disease treated with thiopurines or anti-TNF alpha antibodies Pharmacoepidemiol. Drug Saf 2014;23: 735–744.

11 Dulai PS, Thompson KD, Blunt HB, Dubinsky MC, Siegel CA: Risks of serious infection or lymphoma with anti-tumor necrosis factor therapy for pediatric inflammatory bowel disease: a systematic review. Clin Gastroenterol Hepatol 2014; 12:1443–1451.

12 Herrinton LJ, Liu L, Weng X, Lewis JD, Hutfless S, Allison JE: Role of thiopurine and anti-TNF therapy in lymphoma in inflammatory bowel disease. Am J Gastroenterol 2011;106:2146–2153.

13 Caspersen S, Elkjaer M, Riis L, Pedersen N, Mortensen C, Jess T, Sarto P, Hansen TS, Wewer V, Bendtsen F, Moesgaard F, Munkholm P; Danish Crohn Colitis Database: Infliximab for inflammatory bowel disease in Denmark 1999–2005: clinical outcome and follow-up evaluation of malignancy and mortality. Clin Gastroenterol Hepatol 2008;6:1212–1217.

14 Biancone L, Petruzziello C, Orlando A, Kohn A, Ardizzone S, Daperno M, Angelucci E, Castiglione F, D'Incà R, Zorzi F, Papi C, Meucci G, Riegler G, Sica G, Rizzello F, Mocciaro F, Onali S, Calabrese E, Cottone M, Pallone F: Cancer in Crohn's Disease patients treated with infliximab: a long-term multicenter matched pair study. Inflamm Bowel Dis 2011;17:758–766.

15 Kotlyar DS, Osterman MT, Diamond RH, Porter D, Blonski WC, Wasik M, Sampat S, Mendizabal M, Lin MV, Lichtenstein GR: A systematic review of factors that contribute to hepatosplenic T-cell lymphoma in patients with inflammatory bowel disease. Clin Gastroenterol Hepatol 2011;9:36–41.

16 Bernstein CN, Blanchard JF, Kliewer E, Wajda A: Cancer risk in patients with inflammatory bowel disease: a population-based study. Cancer 2001;91:854–862.

17 Siegel CA: Review article: explaining risks of inflammatory bowel disease therapy to patients. Aliment Pharmacol Ther 2011;33:23–32.

Mamoru Watanabe
Department of Gastroenterology and Hepatology
Tokyo Medical and Dental University, 1–5–45 Yushima Bunkyo-ku
〒113–8519 Tokyo (Japan)
E-Mail mamoru.gast@tmd.ac.jp

Rogler G, Herfarth H, Hibi T, Nielsen OH (eds): Anti-Tumor Necrosis Factor Therapy in Inflammatory Bowel Disease.
Front Gastrointest Res. Basel, Karger, 2015, vol 34, pp 147–151 (DOI: 10.1159/000381595)

Risk of Serious Infection

Makoto Naganuma

Center for Diagnostic and Therapeutic Endoscopy, School of Medicine, Keio University, Tokyo, Japan

Abstract

Anti-TNF therapy is effective for inducing and maintaining remission in both pediatric Crohn's disease and ulcerative colitis patients; however, adverse effects, such as serious infection and lymphoma, are of concern. A recent study has indicated that anti-TNFα therapy in patients aged ≥50 years is associated with significantly increased rates of serious infections; therefore, physicians should pay careful attention to detect the development of infections in elderly patients treated with this therapy. Patients with inflammatory bowel disease (IBD) should be considered for the five following vaccines: the varicella zoster, human papillomavirus, influenza, hepatitis B, and pneumococcal vaccines. Because IBD patients often fail to recognize whether they have previously had a vaccine-preventive illness, such as varicella zoster virus infection, antibodies for varicella zoster virus should be measured as early as possible after diagnosis of IBD, and vaccination might be considered for patients who do not have antibodies before anti-TNFα agents are used.

Introduction

Opportunistic infections are caused by the lack of an appropriate innate immune response [1]. Acquired immune deficiency syndrome [2] and chemotherapy-induced neutropenia [3] have been associated with increased incidences of these opportunistic infections.

Anti-TNF therapy has been shown to be an effective treatment option for inducing and maintaining remission in both Crohn's disease (CD) and ulcerative colitis (UC) patients. Inflammatory cytokines, such as TNFα, play a pivotal role in inducing the apoptosis of infected cells [4]. Thus, the most concerning adverse events of this therapy include serious infections associated with use of anti-TNFα agents. A previous study has indicated that the use of a combination of immunosuppressants is associated with an increased risk of opportunistic infections [5]. Furthermore, tuberculosis (TB) has occurred in some patients treated with biologics. In this issue, serious infections caused by anti-TNFα therapy and the measures used to manage these infections are described.

Incidence of Infections in Anti-TNFα Users with Inflammatory Bowel Disease

Recently, pooled analysis has been performed of infections in infliximab and immunomodulator-treated patients with inflammatory bowel disease

(IBD) [6]. In this study, the incidence of infections was determined in 5 clinical trials involving the efficacy and safety of infliximab (ACCENT I, ACCENT II, SONIC, ACT 1, and ACT 2). Almost half (50.1%) of UC patients who were treated with infliximab had at least one infection, and this incidence of serious infection was significantly higher than that in the placebo group. Interestingly, the incidence of infections was comparable between the infliximab-treated CD patients and placebo-treated patients. The rates of serious infections were 5.4% for the UC patients and 4.5% for the CD patients. This rate was also comparable between the infliximab-treated and placebo-treated patients [6]. Conversely, other studies have indicated that anti-TNFα therapy is associated with a significantly increased rate of serious infections [5, 7, 8]. The use of infliximab has been associated with increased odds (odds ratio 4.4) of developing opportunistic infections [5] compared to no use of this agent. The TREAT registry showed an increased risk of serious infections with anti-TNFα therapy in CD patients, although this risk was less than that for corticosteroid-treated patients [7]. A recent meta-analysis of all published data from randomized controlled trials involving IBD has demonstrated a 2-fold increased risk of opportunistic infections with anti-TNFα therapy [8]. The incidences of serious infections in IBD patients treated with anti-TNFα agents are summarized in table 1.

Table 1. The incidences of serious infections in patients with IBD treated with anti-TNFα agents

Author's name	Disease	Anti-TNFα agent	
		duration of treatment	incidence of serious infection, %
Hanauer	CD	IFX, 54 W	3.6
Rutgeerts	CD	IFX, 48 W	0.0
Sandborn	UC	IFX, 54 W	3.9
Colombel	CD	ADA, 56 W	2.7
Sandborn	CD	ADA, 56 W	3.4
Schreiber	CD	CTZ, 24 W	2.8

CD = Crohn's disease; UC = ulcerative colitis; IFX = infliximab; ADA = adalimumab; CTZ = certolizumab.

A state of dysregulated immune function contributes to an increased risk of infections in the elderly population [9]. A recent study has indicated that the risk of opportunistic infections is greater in IBD patients who are older than 50 years of age [5]. Our group also has demonstrated that an age of ≥50 years is an independent risk factor for the development of opportunistic infections in these patients [10]. Regarding the risks associated with anti-TNFα agents in elderly patients, higher rates of severe infections and mortality were found in IBD patients older than 65 years of age treated with these agents compared with younger patients [11]. Although the elderly population has not been defined, physicians should pay close attention to the risk of infection when an anti-TNF agent is used to treat a patient who is ≥50 years of age.

Therapies using combinations of immunomodulators for IBD are associated with an incremental increase in the relative risk of opportunistic infections [5, 6]. However, there is no evidence of an increased risk of serious infections in patients treated with the combination of an anti-TNFα agent and thiopurine [6, 12].

Tuberculosis

TNF plays a critical role in the maintenance of granulomas, which are necessary for patients to contain *Mycobacterium tuberculosis* infections [13]. Careful screening for TB should be conducted, particularly in IBD patients who have been prescribed steroids, thiopurines, and biologics [13]. In fact, the reactivation of latent TB in patients treated with anti-TNFα agents is increased and is more severe than that in the background population [14]. Suspected TB could be excluded prior to the use of biologics by a careful

Table 2. List of vaccines that should be given to patients with inflammatory bowel disease

Varicella zoster virus vaccine
Human papilloma virus vaccine
Influenza vaccine
Hepatitis B vaccine
Pneumococcal vaccine

evaluation using a method such as a chest X-ray, tuberculin skin test, or interferon-γ release assay (QuantiFERON-TB test). Tuberculin skin testing may not be useful in patients with IBD because it may show negative results for patients who have used corticosteroids and other immunosuppressants.

Treatment with isoniazid for 6–9 months is performed as chemoprophylaxis for TB. In cases in which there is latent TB and active IBD, anti-TNFα therapy should be delayed for at least 3 weeks after starting chemotherapy, except in cases of greater clinical urgency and with specialist advice [14].

Viral Infection

TNFα also plays a major role in the containment of chronic viral infections. To prevent viral infections, vaccination is recommended for those that are vaccine-preventive. Table 2 indicates that every patient with IBD should be considered for receiving five vaccines [14]. Acute hepatitis has occurred in patients with evidence of hepatitis B surface antigen positivity who have received an anti-TNFα agent [15, 16]. Furthermore, the reactivation of hepatitis B virus (HBV) has occurred in patients with evidence of quiescent infection (anti-HBs positivity and/or anti-HBc positivity) [13]. Thus, physicians should pay careful attention to detect the reactivation of viral infections, such as HBV, when anti-TNFα agents are given. Before, during, and for at least 12 months after immunomodulator treatment has ceased, patients who are hepatitis B surface antigen-positive should receive potent anti-viral agents [14]. Patients with evidence of quiescent infection should be monitored for evidence of HBV replication intermittently over the course of therapy, although there is no consensus on the frequency of monitoring required [13].

The use of anti-TNFα agents has also been linked to the reactivation of varicella zoster virus (VZV) infection. Patients on immunomodulators have been shown to have an increased risk of zoster in a case-controlled study [17, 18]. A recent study showed that varicella was fatal in five of 20 infected IBD patients [19]. VZV meningitis associated with anti-TNFα agents has been reported in patients with CD who have been treated with adalimumab [20]. Thus, the risk of varicella zoster infection should be cautioned in IBD patients, especially in those treated with anti-TNFα agents. While a recent study has suggested that even during TNFα therapy, the VZV vaccine can be given safely and effectively [21], a recent guideline has recommended that seronegative immunocompetent patients with IBD should receive two doses of varicella vaccine and should complete the course at least 3 weeks before being started on any immunomodulators [22].

Conclusion and Future Direction

Obviously, anti-TNFα agents are among the most promising and effective treatments for IBD patients, although a previous study has indicated that their use is associated with an increased risk of opportunistic infections. However, the use of these agents should not be delayed due to this increased risk. Before anti-TNFα treatment, screening for infections should be performed, and appropriate chemoprophylaxis should be given, if necessary.

Live vaccines are best given before the introduction of immunomodulator therapy because

IBD patients on immunomodulators/biologics should not receive live vaccination unless they have discontinued the use of these agents. After an anti-TNFα agent is discontinued, the risk of an infusion reaction is increased when it is re-administered. It may therefore be reasonable for physicians to check whether IBD patients have antibodies for live attenuated vaccines before they administer immunomodulators/biologics. Recently, our group has reported that the seronegative rates for varicella zoster/chickenpox, measles, and rubella are relatively high. The seronegative incidence rates for at least 1 virus and 2 viruses in patients on biologics were 49% and 21%, respectively [23]. However, almost 40% of IBD patients did not remember having previous varicella zoster, rubella, measles, or mumps infections. These results indicate that physicians should be aware that these patients often fail to recognize that they have previously had these infections [23]. The respective antibodies should be measured as early as possible after the diagnosis of IBD, and vaccination might be considered for patients who do not have antibodies before thiopurine/biologics are used.

References

1 Viget N, Vernier-Massouille G, Salmon-Ceron D, et al: Opportunistic infections in patients with inflammatory bowel disease: prevention and diagnosis. Gut 2008;57:549–558.

2 Hammer SM: Clinical practice: management of newly diagnosed HIV infection. N Engl J Med 2005;353:1702–1710.

3 Crawford J, Dale DC, Lyman GH: Chemotherapy-induced neutropenia: risks, consequences, and new directions for its management. Cancer 2004;100:228–237.

4 Kollas G, Kontoyiannis D: Role of TNF/TNFR in autoimmunity: specific TNF receptor blockade may be advantageous to anti-TNF treatments. Cytokine Growth Factor Rev 2002;13:315–321.

5 Toruner M, Loftus EV Jr, Harmsen WS, et al: Risk factors for opportunistic infections in patients with inflammatory bowel disease. Gastroenterology 2008;134:929–936.

6 Lichtenstein GR, Rutgeerts P, Sandborn WJ, et al: A pooled analysis of infections, malignancy, and mortality in infliximab- and immunomodulator-treated adult patients with inflammatory bowel disease. Am J Gastroenterol 2012;107:1051–1063.

7 Lichtenstein GR, Feagan BG, Cohen RD, et al: Serious infection and mortality in patients with Crohn's disease: more than 5 years of follow-up in the TREAT registry. Am J Gastroenterol 2012;107:1409–1422.

8 Ford AC, Peyrin-Biroulet L: Opportunistic infections with anti-tumor necrosis factor-alpha therapy in inflammatory bowel disease: meta-analysis of randomized controlled trials. Am J Gastroenterol 2013;108:1268–1276.

9 Castle SC: Clinical relevance of age-related immune dysfunction. Clin Infect Dis 2000;31:578–585.

10 Naganuma M, Kunisaki R, Yoshimura N, et al: A prospective analysis of the incidence of and risk factors for opportunistic infections in patients with inflammatory bowel disease. J Gastroenterol 2013;48:595–600.

11 Cottone M, Kohn A, Daperno M, et al: Advanced age is an independent risk factor for severe infections and mortality in patients given anti-tumor necrosis factor therapy for inflammatory bowel disease. Clin Gastroenterol Hepatol 2011;9:30–35.

12 Colombel JF, Sandborn WJ, Reinisch W, et al: Infliximab, azathioprine, or combination therapy for Crohn's disease. N Engl J Med 2010;362:1383–1395.

13 Targownik LE, Bernstein CN: Infectious and malignant complications of TNF inhibitor therapy in IBD. Am J Gastroenterol 2013;108:1835–1842.

14 Rahier JF, Magro F, Abreu C, et al: Second European evidence-based consensus on the prevention, diagnosis and management of opportunistic infections in inflammatory bowel disease. J Crohns Colitis 2014;8:443–468.

15 Ueno Y, Tanaka S, Shimamoto M, et al: Infliximab therapy for Crohn's disease in a patient with chronic hepatitis B. Dig Dis Sci 2005;50:163–166.

16 Ojiro K, Naganuma M, Ebinuma H, et al: Reactivation of hepatitis B in a patient with Crohn's disease treated using infliximab. J Gastroenterol 2008;43:397–3401.

17 Gupta G, Lautenbach E, Lewis JD: Incidence and risk factors for herpes zoster among patients with inflammatory bowel disease. Clin Gastroenterol Hepatol 2006;4:1483–1490.

18 Winthrop KL, Baddley JW, Chen L, et al: Association between the initiation of anti-tumor necrosis factor therapy and the risk of herpes zoster. JAMA 2013;309:887–895.

19 Cullen G, Baden RP, Cheifetz AS: Varicella zoster virus infection in inflammatory bowel disease. Inflamm Bowel Dis 2012;18:2392–2403.

20 Ma C, Walters B, Fedorak RN: Varicella zoster meningitis complicating combined anti-tumor necrosis factor and corticosteroid therapy in Crohn's disease. World J Gastroenterol 2013;19:3347–3351.

21 Zhang J, Xie F, Delzell E, et al: Association between vaccination for herpes zoster and risk of herpes zoster infection among older patients with selected immune-mediated diseases. JAMA 2012;308:43–49.

22 Marin M, Guris D, Chaves SS, Schmid S, Seward JF: Prevention of varicella: recommendations of the Advisory Committee on Immunization Practices (ACIP). MMWR Recomm Rep 2007;56:1–40.

23 Naganuma M, Nagahori M, Fujii T, et al: Poor recall of prior exposure to varicella zoster, rubella, measles, or mumps in patients with IBD. Inflamm Bowel Dis 2013;19:418–422.

Makoto Naganuma, MD, PhD
Center for Diagnostic and Therapeutic Endoscopy, School of Medicine, Keio University
35 Shinanomachi, Shinjuku-ku
Tokyo 160–8582 (Japan)
E-Mail nagamakoto@z7.keio.jp

Rogler G, Herfarth H, Hibi T, Nielsen OH (eds): Anti-Tumor Necrosis Factor Therapy in Inflammatory Bowel Disease.
Front Gastrointest Res. Basel, Karger, 2015, vol 34, pp 152–158 (DOI: 10.1159/000381596)

Risk of Post-Operative Infections with Anti-TNF Therapy

Benjamin L. Cohen

Dr. Henry D. Janowitz Division of Gastroenterology, Icahn School of Medicine at Mount Sinai, New York, N.Y., USA

Abstract

Anti-TNF therapy is the current standard of care for moderate to severe Crohn's disease and ulcerative colitis. However, despite advancements in immunosuppressive therapy, many patients will require surgery during their disease course. Patients are often exposed to immunosuppressive therapy peri-operatively, leading to concern about possible increased risks of infectious complications. While studies have established the infectious risk associated with steroids and the general safety of thiopurines, the effect of pre-operative anti-TNF on post-operative complications in inflammatory bowel disease is controversial. This chapter reviews current knowledge regarding anti-TNF and the risk of post-operative infections and proposes potential management strategies.

Introduction

Between 20 and 30% of subjects with ulcerative colitis (UC) and approximately two-thirds of subjects with Crohn's disease (CD) will require surgery at some point during their disease course. Current therapies for inflammatory bowel disease (IBD) focus on immunosuppression, and recent studies have shown combination therapy using both anti-TNF agents and thiopurines to be the most effective therapy for both moderate to severe UC and CD [1, 2]. Despite the use of more effective therapies, the risk of needing surgery remains high in the biologic era [3, 4]. Data from referral center cohorts have shown that up to 50% of patients are exposed to anti-TNF agents prior to their first surgery [5].

TNF plays an integral role in immune function through its effects on the differentiation of monocytes into macrophages, neutrophil recruitment, and the creation of granulomas, and it is therefore thought that use of anti-TNF agents may predispose patients to increased infections [6]. A 5-year follow-up of the large Crohn's Therapy, Resource, Evaluation, and Assessment Tool (TREAT) Registry has shown that factors independently associated with serious infections include moderate to severe disease activity (hazard ratio (HR) = 2.24, 95% CI = 1.57–3.19; $p < 0.001$), narcotic analgesic treatment (HR = 1.98, 95% CI = 1.44–2.73; $p < 0.001$), prednisone therapy (HR = 1.57, 95% CI = 1.17–2.10; $p = 0.002$), and infliximab treatment (HR = 1.43, 95% CI = 1.11–1.84; $p = 0.006$) [7]. However, the overall risk of serious infection associated with anti-TNF in IBD has been shown to be small when pooling randomized controlled trials and prospective cohorts (OR 1.28, 95% CI 0.67–2.44), and it is unclear to what extent the risk is modified by both disease activity and concomitant use of other immunosuppressives [6, 8].

While studies have established the infectious risk associated with pre-operative corticosteroid use [9–11] and the general safety of thiopurines [9, 10, 12], the effect of pre-operative anti-TNF on post-operative complications in IBD is controversial. Animal studies have shown a significant decrease in wound healing tensile strength as well as colonic anastomosis tensile strength in rats treated with infliximab [13, 14]. These observations imply an increased post-operative risk of infection in the setting of anti-TNF therapy. Contradictory to these findings, other studies have found elevated TNF-α present in chronic venous leg ulcers [15]. Investigators have proposed that low levels of TNF-α may promote wound healing via increased macrophage growth factor production and that a high concentration may instead impair wound healing by suppressing production and increasing degradation of extracellular matrix proteins [16, 17].

Studies of Peri-Operative Anti-TNF in Crohn's Disease

Nine single-center retrospective studies [12, 18–25], three multi-center retrospective studies [26–28], and one population-based retrospective study [29] assessing post-operative complications in CD had been published as of 2014. Ten of the studies failed to show that infliximab infused within 8–12 weeks of intra-abdominal CD surgery increased the risk of major post-operative complications, including infection [12, 18–23, 26, 27, 29]. The Mayo Clinic reported the experience of 370 CD patients undergoing abdominal surgery from 2005 to 2008 [22]. The authors defined anti-TNF exposure as pre-operative dosing within 8 weeks or post-operative dosing within 30 days of surgery. The respective rates of overall post-operative complications (27.9 vs. 30.1%, p = 0.63) and intra-abdominal infection (5.0 vs. 7.2%, p = 0.44) were similar in anti-TNF-exposed (n = 119) and unexposed patients. However, extra-abdominal septic complications were not included in the infection analysis, and an association with anti-TNF exposure may have been missed.

In contrast, an analysis of a retrospective series of 389 patients undergoing ileocolonic resection for CD at the Cleveland Clinic found that infliximab use within 3 months prior to surgery (n = 60) is associated with increased rates of post-operative sepsis (20 vs. 9.7%, p = 0.024), abscess (10.0 vs. 4.3%, p = 0.1) and hospital readmission (20 vs. 9.4%, p = 0.019) [30]. Diverting stoma was found to be potentially protective against infectious complications. More recently, Syed et al. reported that pre-operative use of anti-TNF within 8 weeks of surgery (n = 150) at a large referral center was an independent predictor of overall infectious (OR 2.43, 95% CI 1.18–5.03) and surgical site (OR 1.96, 95% CI 1.02–3.77) complications in CD surgery.

Nørgard et al. performed a population-based study of CD using nationwide registries in Denmark to assess the risk of post-operative complications due to anti-TNF therapy [29]. The study compared 30- and 60-day complication rates between CD patients undergoing intestinal resection who were exposed to anti-TNF within 12 weeks of surgery (n = 214) and unexposed patients. No difference was seen in the rate of post-operative death, reoperation, anastomotic leak, or percutaneous drainage between the groups. Subgroup analysis found that exposure to anti-TNF within 14 days of surgery did not confer greater risk than more distant exposure did.

Interpretation of the current literature on CD is complicated by low sample sizes; selection bias; and heterogeneity in the definition of anti-TNF exposure, the definition of infectious complications, the types of surgeries analyzed, and the inclusion of other potential confounding factors for post-operative infection. Despite the fact that most individual studies of anti-TNF association with post-operative infection in CD have not identified a significant relationship, four meta-analyses of the available studies have shown a small increased risk of post-operative complications and infection [31–34], whereas one showed no risk [35].

Studies of Peri-Operative Anti-TNF in Ulcerative Colitis

The data regarding post-surgical complications in UC subjects receiving infliximab prior to surgery are also conflicting. Ten single-center retrospective cohort studies have explored the subject, with six showing no significant association [36–45]. A review of 151 ileal pouch-anal anastomosis (IPAA) or subtotal colectomies for refractory UC at Cedars-Sinai did not find any difference in post-operative complications following anti-TNF exposure [40]. Similarly, review of 141 patients undergoing colectomy for UC in Leuven, Belgium, found that moderate- to high-dose corticosteroids (OR 5.19, 95% CI 1.72–15.66) and restorative proctocolectomy without defunctioning ileostomy (OR 6.45, 95% CI 2.12–19.64), but not anti-TNF exposure, were independent predictors of short-term post-operative infectious complications [45].

Conversely, a retrospective review of the Mayo Clinic experience with total proctocolectomy and IPAA for UC found that anti-TNF exposure was the only factor independently associated with infectious complications (OR 3.5, 95% CI 1.6–7.5) in 301 patients (47 exposed to anti-TNF) [44]. A review of the Cleveland Clinic experience with 588 patients (167 exposed to anti-TNF) undergoing either initial subtotal colectomy with end ileostomy (3-stage) or total proctocolectomy with IPAA (2-stage) for medically refractory colitis since Food and Drug Administration approval of infliximab in 2005 [41]. Complications within 30 days of the procedure (including leak, sepsis, and wound infection) did not differ with anti-TNF exposure for either 2-stage or 3-stage procedures. However, the rates of pelvic sepsis within 1 year of surgery were significantly higher in anti-TNF-exposed patients undergoing a 2-stage procedure compared with unexposed patients (HR 2.62, 95% CI 1.11–6.15). No difference was seen for 3-stage procedures. The authors concluded that the pouch should be constructed after subtotal colectomy as a three-stage process in anti-TNF-exposed UC patients undergoing restorative proctocolectomy.

All but one single-center study included fewer than 50 anti-TNF-exposed patients. However, a large population-based study from Denmark by Nørgard et al. compared 30- and 60-day complication rates between 199 anti-TNF-exposed and 1,027 unexposed UC patients undergoing colectomy. No difference was seen in the rate of post-operative death, reoperation, anastomotic leak, or percutaneous drainage between the groups. A 2012 meta-analysis of available studies, involving 2,933 UC patients undergoing abdominal surgery, did not find a significant association between pre-operative infliximab therapy and early infectious or noninfectious post-operative complications [46]. As in CD, the included studies were very heterogeneous due to differences in the definitions of infection and noninfectious complications, the types of surgery, and the availability of data on other potentially confounding risk factors.

Studies of Peri-Operative Anti-TNF in Combined Crohn's Disease and Ulcerative Colitis

Multiple centers have reviewed CD and UC surgeries together in an attempt to increase sample size and power [47–51]. Krane et al. included 142 patients exposed to infliximab within 12 weeks of elective laparoscopic resection and found no difference in complications (25.3 vs. 24.5%, p = 0.93), infections (12 vs. 11.2%, p = 0.92), or anastomotic leak (5.2 vs. 2.9%, p = 0.69) between anti-TNF-exposed and unexposed patients [47]. Rates remained similar between UC and CD.

Waterman et al. performed a retrospective case-control study comparing 195 anti-TNF-exposed patients with 278 matched controls and found no difference in most post-operative outcomes, including infections [48]. However, patients on combination therapy with anti-TNF agents and thiopurines had significantly increased frequencies of wound infections (p = 0.0045) and urinary tract infections (p = 0.0007). The influence of the time interval between the last anti-TNF dose and surgery was examined, and no difference in the complication rate related to wound healing between receiving anti-TNF within 14 days or 15–30 days of surgery or greater than 30 days from surgery (23 vs. 15 vs. 21%, p = 0.51) was found.

Measuring Peri-Operative Anti-TNF Exposure and Management Recommendations

Published studies on the association of anti-TNF with post-operative infection have been plagued by variable definitions of anti-TNF exposure, ranging from 8 weeks to 6 months pre-operatively. However, pharmacokinetic analyses of infliximab in IBD have reported that the half-life is between 7 and 18.5 days, suggesting that these retrospective studies may not have measured true drug exposure [52–54]. Waterman et al. attempted to examine exposure to anti-TNF based on the presence of detectable infliximab levels within 2 months of surgery in a subset of 19 patients, but only a trend toward increased wound infections (3/10 in exposed patients vs. 0/9 in unexposed patients, p = 0.21) was seen. Studies presented in abstract form have suggested increased complications in CD surgeries, but not in UC surgeries, in patients with detectable anti-TNF levels at the time of surgery [55, 56].

There are no standard recommendations for peri-operative anti-TNF management, despite its increased use. Medication washout may be considered in select cases prior to elective surgery to minimize risk. However, disease flares during a washout period may further complicate surgery and must be considered [57]. Experts have proposed timing elective CD surgeries mid-interval for infliximab to prevent pre-operative disease flares and allow for on-time anti-TNF continuation 4 weeks post-operatively [20]. Clinical scenarios in which anti-TNF may provide limited benefit, such as stricturing CD, pose the opportunity for a washout period [57]. However, IBD surgery is often performed on an urgent or semi-urgent basis. Strategies to minimize known risk factors for post-operative complications, such as use of surgical wound protectors [58], correction of nutritional deficiency [59, 60], post-operative glycemic control [61], and targeted anti-microbial prophylaxis [62], should be used.

Summary

Anti-TNF agents are increasingly used for the treatment of IBD, but patients often still require surgery. While the infectious risk of peri-operative corticosteroids is clear, the association of anti-TNF agents with post-operative complications, such as anastomotic leak/abscess, sepsis, pneumonia, peritonitis, and wound infection, is still widely debated. The existing literature consists primarily of retrospective single-center studies and meta-analyses subject to bias and confounding, given the inability to accurately ascertain the severity and duration of illness, malnutrition, and the type and duration of exposure to antibiotics and immune-suppressing medications. The sample sizes of single-center studies are also often too small to identify significant differences in outcomes and to adjust for confounders. Interpretation of the current literature on the safety of peri-operative anti-TNF exposure is further complicated by heterogeneity in the definitions used for infectious complications, the types of surgeries analyzed, and the definition of anti-TNF exposure. Large prospective studies using drug levels to define exposure are needed to clarify the risk and to guide peri-operative management of anti-TNF agents.

References

1 Colombel JF, Sandborn WJ, Reinisch W, et al: Infliximab, azathioprine, or combination therapy for Crohn's disease. N Engl J Med 2010;362:1383–1395.
2 Panccione R, Ghosh S, Middleton S, et al: Infliximab, azathioprine, or infliximab plus azathioprine for treatment of moderate to severe ulcerative colitis: the UC Success Trial. Gastroenterology 2011;140:S134.
3 Bouguen G, Peyrin-Biroulet L: Surgery for adult Crohn's disease: what is the actual risk? Gut 2011;60:1178–1181.
4 Danese S, Fiocchi C: Ulcerative colitis. N Engl J Med 2011;365:1713–1725.
5 Peyrin-Biroulet L, Oussalah A, Williet N, et al: Impact of azathioprine and tumour necrosis factor antagonists on the need for surgery in newly diagnosed Crohn's disease. Gut 2011;60:930–936.
6 Targownik LE, Bernstein CN: Infectious and malignant complications of TNF inhibitor therapy in IBD. Am J Gastroenterol 2013;108:1835–1842, quiz 1843.
7 Lichtenstein GR, Feagan BG, Cohen RD, et al: Serious infection and mortality in patients with Crohn's disease: more than 5 years of follow-up in the TREAT™ registry. Am J Gastroenterol 2012;107:1409–1422.
8 Singh JA, Wells GA, Christensen R, et al: Adverse effects of biologics: a network meta-analysis and Cochrane overview. Cochrane Database Syst Rev 2011;2:CD008794.
9 Aberra FN, Lewis JD, Hass D, et al: Corticosteroids and immunomodulators: postoperative infectious complication risk in inflammatory bowel disease patients. Gastroenterology 2003;125:320–327.
10 Mahadevan U, Loftus EV Jr, Tremaine WJ, et al: Azathioprine or 6-mercaptopurine before colectomy for ulcerative colitis is not associated with increased postoperative complications. Inflamm Bowel Dis 2002;8:311–316.
11 Reding R, Michel LA, Donckier J, et al: Surgery in patients on long-term steroid therapy: a tentative model for risk assessment. Br J Surg 1990;77:1175–1178.
12 Colombel JF, Loftus EV, Tremaine WJ, et al: Early postoperative complications are not increased in patients with Crohn's disease treated perioperatively with infliximab or immunosuppressive therapy. Am J Gastroenterol 2004;99:878–883.
13 Lopes JV, Freitas LA, Marques RD, et al: Analysis of the tensile strength on the healing of the abdominal wall of rats treated with infliximab. Acta Cir Bras 2008;23:441–446.
14 de Oliveira PG, Soares EG, Aprilli F: Influence of misoprostol, a synthetic prostaglandin E1 analog, on the healing of colonic anastomoses in rats. Dis Colon Rectum 1994;37:660–663.
15 Cowin AJ, Hatzirodos N, Rigden J, et al: Etanercept decreases tumor necrosis factor-alpha activity in chronic wound fluid. Wound Repair Regen 2006;14:421–426.
16 Barrientos S, Stojadinovic O, Golinko MS, et al: Growth factors and cytokines in wound healing. Wound Repair Regen 2008;16:585–601.
17 Hession MT, Gottlieb AB: Perioperative management of tumor necrosis factor antagonists in patients with psoriasis and other inflammatory disorders. J Dermatolog Treat 2011;22:90–101.
18 Bafford AC, Powers S, Ha C, et al: Immunosuppressive therapy does not increase operative morbidity in patients with Crohn's disease. J Clin Gastroenterol 2013;47:491–495.
19 Uchino M, Ikeuchi H, Matsuoka H, et al: Risk factors for surgical site infection and association with infliximab administration during surgery for Crohn's disease. Dis Colon Rectum 2013;56:1156–1165.
20 Kasparek MS, Bruckmeier A, Beigel F, et al: Infliximab does not affect postoperative complication rates in Crohn's patients undergoing abdominal surgery. Inflamm Bowel Dis 2012;18:1207–1213.
21 Canedo J, Lee SH, Pinto R, et al: Surgical resection in Crohn's disease: is immunosuppressive medication associated with higher postoperative infection rates? Colorectal Dis 2011;13:1294–1298.
22 Nasir BS, Dozois EJ, Cima RR, et al: Perioperative anti-tumor necrosis factor therapy does not increase the rate of early postoperative complications in Crohn's disease. J Gastrointest Surg 2010;14:1859–1866.
23 Marchal L, D'Haens G, Van Assche G, et al: The risk of post-operative complications associated with infliximab therapy for Crohn's disease: a controlled cohort study. Aliment Pharmacol Ther 2004;19:749–754.
24 Syed A, Cross RK, Flasar MH: Anti-tumor necrosis factor therapy is associated with infections after abdominal surgery in Crohn's disease patients. Am J Gastroenterol 2013;108:583–593.
25 Appau KA, Fazio VW, Shen B, et al: Use of infliximab within 3 months of ileocolonic resection is associated with adverse postoperative outcomes in Crohn's patients. J Gastrointest Surg 2008;12:1738–1744.
26 Myrelid P, Marti-Gallostra M, Ashraf S, et al: Complications in surgery for Crohn's disease after preoperative antitumour necrosis factor therapy. Br J Surg 2014;101:539–545.

27 El-Hussuna A, Andersen J, Bisgaard T, et al: Biologic treatment or immunomodulation is not associated with postoperative anastomotic complications in abdominal surgery for Crohn's disease. Scand J Gastroenterol 2012;47:662–668.

28 Serradori T, Germain A, Scherrer ML, et al: The effect of immune therapy on surgical site infection following Crohn's Disease resection. Br J Surg 2013;100:1089–1093.

29 Nørgård BM, Nielsen J, Qvist N, et al: Pre-operative use of anti-TNF-α agents and the risk of post-operative complications in patients with Crohn's disease – a nationwide cohort study. Aliment Pharmacol Ther 2013;37:214–224.

30 Appau KA, Fazio VW, Shen B, et al: Use of infliximab within 3 months of ileocolonic resection is associated with adverse postoperative outcomes in Crohn's patients. J Gastrointest Surg 2008;12:1738–1744.

31 Ahmed Ali U, Martin ST, Rao AD, et al: Impact of preoperative immunosuppressive agents on postoperative outcomes in Crohn's disease. Dis Colon Rectum 2014;57:663–674.

32 Yang ZP, Hong L, Wu Q, et al: Preoperative infliximab use and postoperative complications in Crohn's disease: a systematic review and meta-analysis. Int J Surg 2014;12:224–230.

33 El-Hussuna A, Krag A, Olaison G, et al: The effect of anti-tumor necrosis factor alpha agents on postoperative anastomotic complications in Crohn's disease: a systematic review. Dis Colon Rectum 2013;56:1423–1433.

34 Kopylov U, Ben-Horin S, Zmora O, et al: Anti-tumor necrosis factor and postoperative complications in Crohn's disease: systematic review and meta-analysis. Inflamm Bowel Dis 2012;18:2404–2413.

35 Rosenfeld G, Qian H, Bressler B: The risks of post-operative complications following pre-operative infliximab therapy for Crohn's disease in patients undergoing abdominal surgery: a systematic review and meta-analysis. J Crohns Colitis 2013;7:868–877.

36 Uchino M, Ikeuchi H, Matsuoka H, et al: Infliximab administration prior to surgery does not increase surgical site infections in patients with ulcerative colitis. Int J Colorectal Dis 2013;28:1295–1306.

37 Bregnbak D, Mortensen C, Bendtsen F: Infliximab and complications after colectomy in patients with ulcerative colitis. J Crohns Colitis 2012;6:281–286.

38 Gainsbury ML, Chu DI, Howard LA, et al: Preoperative infliximab is not associated with an increased risk of short-term postoperative complications after restorative proctocolectomy and ileal pouch-anal anastomosis. J Gastrointest Surg 2011;15:397–403.

39 Coquet-Reinier B, Berdah SV, Grimaud JC, et al: Preoperative infliximab treatment and postoperative complications after laparoscopic restorative proctocolectomy with ileal pouch-anal anastomosis: a case-matched study. Surg Endosc 2010;24:1866–1871.

40 Schluender SJ, Ippoliti A, Dubinsky M, et al: Does infliximab influence surgical morbidity of ileal pouch-anal anastomosis in patients with ulcerative colitis? Dis Colon Rectum 2007;50:1747–1753.

41 Gu J, Remzi FH, Shen B, et al: Operative strategy modifies risk of pouch-related outcomes in patients with ulcerative colitis on preoperative anti-tumor necrosis factor-α therapy. Dis Colon Rectum 2013;56:1243–1252.

42 Eshuis EJ, Al Saady RL, Stokkers PC, et al: Previous infliximab therapy and postoperative complications after proctocolectomy with ileum pouch anal anastomosis. J Crohns Colitis 2013;7:142–149.

43 Mor IJ, Vogel JD, da Luz Moreira A, et al: Infliximab in ulcerative colitis is associated with an increased risk of postoperative complications after restorative proctocolectomy. Dis Colon Rectum 2008;51:1202–1207; discussion 1207–1210.

44 Selvasekar CR, Cima RR, Larson DW, et al: Effect of infliximab on short-term complications in patients undergoing operation for chronic ulcerative colitis. J Am Coll Surg 2007;204:956–962.

45 Ferrante M, D'Hoore A, Vermeire S, et al: Corticosteroids but not infliximab increase short-term postoperative infectious complications in patients with ulcerative colitis. Inflamm Bowel Dis 2009;15:1062–1070.

46 Yang Z, Wu Q, Wang F, et al: Meta-analysis: effect of preoperative infliximab use on early postoperative complications in patients with ulcerative colitis undergoing abdominal surgery. Aliment Pharmacol Ther 2012;36:922–928.

47 Krane MK, Allaix ME, Zoccali M, et al: Preoperative infliximab therapy does not increase morbidity and mortality after laparoscopic resection for inflammatory bowel disease. Dis Colon Rectum 2013;56:449–457.

48 Waterman M, Xu W, Dinani A, et al: Preoperative biological therapy and short-term outcomes of abdominal surgery in patients with inflammatory bowel disease. Gut 2013;62:387–394.

49 Regadas FSP, Pinto RA, Murad-Regadas SM, et al: Short-term outcome of infliximab and other medications on patients with inflammatory bowel disease undergoing ileostomy reversal. Colorectal Dis 2011;13:555–560.

50 Rizzo G, Armuzzi A, Pugliese D, et al: Anti-TNF-alpha therapies do not increase early postoperative complications in patients with inflammatory bowel disease. An Italian single-center experience. Int J Colorectal Dis 2011;26:1435–1444.

51 Kunitake H, Hodin R, Shellito PC, et al: Perioperative treatment with infliximab in patients with Crohn's disease and ulcerative colitis is not associated with an increased rate of postoperative complications. J Gastrointest Surg 2008;12:1730–1736.

52 Klotz U, Teml A, Schwab M: Clinical pharmacokinetics and use of infliximab. Clin Pharmacokinet 2007;46:645–660.

53 Ternant D, Aubourg A, Magdelaine-Beuzelin C, et al: Infliximab pharmacokinetics in inflammatory bowel disease patients. Ther Drug Monit 2008;30:523–529.

54 Ali T, Yun L, Rubin DT: Risk of post-operative complications associated with anti-TNF therapy in inflammatory bowel disease. World J Gastroenterol 2012;18:197–204.

55 Lau CC, Dubinsky M, Melmed GY, et al: Higher preoperative serum biologic levels are associated with postoperative complications in Crohn's disease patients. Gastroenterology 2013;144:S190.

56 Lau CC, Dubinsky M, Melmed GY, et al: Preoperative serum biologic levels do not impact postoperative outcomes in ulcerative colitis. Gastroenterology 2013;144:S189–S190.

57 Sorrentino D, Fogel S, Van den Bogaerde J: Surgery for Crohn's disease and anti-TNF agents: the changing scenario. Expert Rev Gastroenterol Hepatol 2013;7:689–700.
58 Edwards JP, Ho AL, Tee MC, et al: Wound protectors reduce surgical site infection: a meta-analysis of randomized controlled trials. Ann Surg 2012; 256:53–59.
59 Simi M, Leardi S, Minervini S, et al: Early complications after surgery for Crohn's disease. Neth J Surg 1990;42: 105–109.
60 Hennessey DB, Burke JP, Ni-Dhonochu T, et al: Preoperative hypoalbuminemia is an independent risk factor for the development of surgical site infection following gastrointestinal surgery: a multi-institutional study. Ann Surg 2010;252: 325–329.
61 Ho VP, Stein SL, Trencheva K, et al: Differing risk factors for incisional and organ/space surgical site infections following abdominal colorectal surgery. Dis Colon Rectum 2011;54:818–825.
62 Fry DE: Preventive systemic antibiotics in colorectal surgery. Surg Infect (Larchmt) 2008;9:547–552.

Benjamin L. Cohen, MD, MAS
Dr. Henry D. Janowitz Division of Gastroenterology
Icahn School of Medicine at Mount Sinai, One Gustave L. Levy Place, Box 1069
10029-6574, New York, NY, USA
E-Mail benjamin.cohen@mssm.edu

Rogler G, Herfarth H, Hibi T, Nielsen OH (eds): Anti-Tumor Necrosis Factor Therapy in Inflammatory Bowel Disease.
Front Gastrointest Res. Basel, Karger, 2015, vol 34, pp 159–163 (DOI: 10.1159/000381597)

The 'Ideal' Anti-TNF Patient: Indications for Anti-TNF Therapy in Crohn's Disease

My-Linh Tran-Minh • Clotilde Baudry • Matthieu Allez

Service de Gastroentérologie, Hôpital Saint-Louis, APHP, INSERM U1160, Université Paris Diderot, Sorbonne Paris Cité, Paris, France

Abstract

The introduction of anti-TNF monoclonal antibodies to the therapeutic arsenal has represented a major advance in the management of Crohn's disease (CD). Anti-TNF agents are able to induce and maintain remission of the disease over time. These treatments also have the ability to close fistulae, heal mucosal lesions, and reduce rates of hospitalizations and surgeries. Such properties have been demonstrated in randomized clinical trials and have been confirmed in patient cohorts. Anti-TNF monoclonal antibodies represent the most effective agents currently available for the treatment of CD. Three anti-TNF monoclonal antibodies have demonstrated efficacies for the treatment of this disease: infliximab, adalimumab and certolizumab pegol. They are classically administered following a step-up approach to patients with refractory disease who are unresponsive to conventional therapies or are steroid-dependent. They may be used earlier in the disease course to treat patients presenting with aggressive disease or features predictive of poor prognosis. Indeed, several studies have suggested that early intervention with combination therapy may modify the long-term course of CD. The higher efficacies of these therapies compared to those of classical treatments have incited clinicians to have more ambitious objectives, such as endoscopic healing. In this chapter, we describe the major randomized controlled trials that have demonstrated the efficacies of infliximab, adalimumab and certolizumab pegol in the treatment of luminal CD, and that, together with data on safety, have defined their drug labeling. We also summarize the current international guidelines and discuss their usage in clinical practice.

Introduction

The therapeutic objectives for the management of Crohn's disease (CD) have considerably evolved over the last decade, from the control of symptoms to more ambitious objectives, including the complete control of inflammation, as assessed by biological markers such as CRP, endoscopy or imaging. It is now documented that the complete control of inflammation is correlated with a better outcome. The armamentarium for the management of CD includes steroids, immunomodulators (thiopurines and methotrexate), and anti-TNF agents. More recently, a new class of treatment has been introduced, targeting the migration of immune cells to the inflamed tissue. Anti-TNF agents are still the most efficient treatment available for CD. However, it appears unreasonable to give this treatment to all CD patients. Thus, the appropriate candidates have to be selected to receive it. As discussed in this chapter, some patients with an aggressive disease at presentation or with predictors of poor outcome are good candidates to receive anti-TNF therapy early in the course of their disease. For those who are not a candidate for the early introduction of an anti-TNF agent, this therapy may be introduced later if the disease is still active despite receiving classical treatments or if these treatments are not tolerated. In this chapter, we review data on the efficacy and tolerance of anti-TNF agents in luminal CD, review international guidelines, and discuss their use in clinical practice.

Main Points

The efficacy of anti-TNF therapy in luminal CD has been demonstrated in several randomized clinical trials and has also been evaluated in retrospective studies. Its efficacy as induction therapy and maintenance therapy for fistulizing CD and for treating extra-intestinal manifestations are described in two other chapters of this book.

Efficacy as Induction Therapy for Luminal Crohn's Disease

A multi-center, double-blind study of 108 patients [1] with moderate to severe CD refractory to 5-aminosalicylic acid, corticosteroids and/or immunomodulators demonstrated an 81% clinical response rate at 4 weeks after treatment with 5 mg/kg infliximab compared with 17% in placebo-treated patients ($p < 0.001$). These impressive results have been confirmed in a large cohort from the University of Leuven, reporting a clinical response rate of 89% after induction therapy with infliximab [2]. A single randomized controlled trial (the SONIC study [3]) has performed a head-to-head comparison of infliximab and azathioprine for the induction of remission in patients with moderately severe CD who were naïve to both agents. Treatment with 5 mg/kg infliximab at 0–2 and 6 weeks and every 8 weeks was found to be superior to that with azathioprine alone (2.5 mg/kg) for the induction of steroid-free remission after 26 weeks (45 vs. 30%, $p < 0.01$). In the CLASSIC I trial [4], 299 anti-TNF-naïve patients with active CD were treated with adalimumab. An induction dose of 160 mg followed by a dose of 80 mg at 2 weeks were needed to achieve remission in 36% of the patients at 4 weeks compared to 12% of those receiving placebo ($p < 0.05$).

In the PRECISE-1 trial [5], 662 patients with moderately to severely active CD were randomized to receive 400 mg certolizumab pegol or placebo at weeks 0, 2 and 4 and then every 4 weeks until week 24. The clinical response at week 6 was 37% for certolizumab pegol and 26% for placebo ($p < 0.05$). At both weeks 6 and 26 (the co-primary endpoints), the corresponding clinical response rates were 22 and 12%, respectively ($p = 0.05$). At weeks 6 and 26, the rates of remission in the two groups did not differ significantly ($p = 0.17$).

Efficacy as Maintenance Therapy for Medically Induced Remission of Luminal Crohn's Disease

The pivotal maintenance trial of infliximab was ACCENT-1 [6]. This trial studied patients with moderate to severe luminal CD refractory to conventional treatment. All 573 patients received 5 mg/kg infliximab at week 0. Responders at week 2 were randomized to receive placebo or 5 or 10 mg/kg infliximab at weeks 2 and 6 and every 8 weeks. The median time to loss of response was longer in the patients who continued receiving infliximab (19 weeks on placebo, 38 weeks at 5 mg/kg, and >54 weeks at 10 mg/kg; $p = 0.0002$). Maintenance therapy with infliximab was superior to placebo at week 54 (remission rates of 14% on placebo, 28% at 5 mg/kg, and 38% at 10 mg/kg; $p < 0.05$). Patients on scheduled therapy had more mucosal healing, required fewer hospitalizations and surgery, and had a better quality of life.

In the CHARM trial [7], patients with moderate to severe CD refractory to conventional therapy or infliximab received 40 mg adalimumab every other week, adalimumab every week or placebo for remission maintenance. The remission rates were 43% on adalimumab vs. 17% on placebo ($p < 0.0001$) at week 26 and 38 vs. 12%, respectively ($p < 0.0001$), at week 56. The patients on adalimumab had fewer hospitalizations and surgery.

The PRECISE-2 trial [8] studied remission maintenance of patients with moderate to severe CD who responded to 400 mg open-label certolizumab pegol at 0, 2 and 4 weeks. The responders were randomized to continue 400 mg certolizumab pegol every 4 weeks or to receive a placebo. At week 26, the response rates were 63 and 36% for the patients on certolizumab pegol and placebo, respectively ($p < 0.001$).

Pediatric Crohn's Disease

Infliximab

The REACH trial [9] explored the efficacy and safety of infliximab in pediatric patients from 6 to 17 years of age with moderate to severe CD refractory to immunosuppressive therapy (n = 112). At week 10, the clinical response and clinical remission rates were 90 and 60%, respectively. These impressive results were maintained at week 54 at 64 and 56%, respectively.

Adalimumab

The IMAGINE trial [10] was a double-blind randomized evaluation of adalimumab administered to 192 children aged 6–17 years with moderate to severe CD despite concurrent treatment with oral corticosteroids and/or immunomodulator therapy. At week 26, 33.5% of the patients were in clinical remission.

Drug Labeling of Anti-TNF Agents in Crohn's Disease

In the European Union, infliximab and adalimumab are approved by the European Medicines Agency for the treatment of moderately to severely active CD in adults who have not responded to a full and adequate course of therapy with corticosteroids and/or immunomodulators or who are intolerant to or have medical contraindications for such therapies. In Europe, certolizumab pegol is only approved in Switzerland.

The US Food and Drug Administration (FDA)-approved indications for infliximab and adalimumab are the same as those approved by the European Medicines Agency. In the US, certolizumab pegol has also been approved and licensed by the FDA for moderate to severe CD maintenance therapy but not for the induction of remission.

Indications for Anti-TNF Therapy According to Guidelines

The European and American guidelines on the use of anti-TNF therapy have recently been updated. This therapy can be used both for the induction of remission and maintenance therapy after remission. We describe the indications of anti-TNF therapy for luminal disease.

The European Crohn's and Colitis Organization recommends the use of anti-TNF therapy to induce remission in patients with moderate or severe localized ileocecal involvement who have previously been refractory, dependent, or intolerant to steroids (statement 5B), although the use of azathioprine or methotrexate in combination with corticosteroids can be an option for patients with moderately active disease. Anti-TNF therapy is also an appropriate option for patients with ileocecal or colonic disease who are initially treated with systemic corticosteroids and relapse if there is evidence of active disease (statement 5C, 5D) [11].

For patients with extensive bowel disease, anti-TNF therapy should be used for those who have relapsed after treatment with corticosteroids and immunomodulators (statement 5E). According to the new guidelines presented in 2014, the early introduction of anti-TNF therapy should also be considered, especially in patients with clinical indicators of poor prognosis. This therapy is also an alternative for severe and refractory (to the use of proton pump inhibitors with corticosteroids and immunomodulators) esophageal and gastroduodenal disease (statement 5F).

If remission has been achieved with an anti-TNF agent, the European Crohn's and Colitis Organization recommends maintenance with regular anti-TNF therapy. However, there is no recommendation about the duration of treatment (statement 6F). Anti-TNF therapy could also be considered for patients receiving thiopurines who have experienced a relapse after checking adherence to therapy and the effective dose (statement 6E). There is no recommendation about choosing between infliximab and adalimumab (statement 5I).

There are special guidelines for pediatric CD [12]. Anti-TNF therapy is recommended for inducing and maintaining remission in children with chronically active luminal CD despite prior optimized immunomodulator therapy. This therapy is also recommended for inducing remission in children with active steroid-refractory disease. Regularly scheduled and not episodic treatment should be administered to maintain remission in patients responding to induction therapy with anti-TNF agents.

The American Gastroenterology Association (AGA) recommends using anti-TNF therapy to induce remission in patients with moderately severe CD refractory to standard therapies, including mesalamine, antibiotics, corticosteroids and immunomodulators. Infliximab and adalimumab are approved by the US FDA for this indication, unlike certolizumab pegol. For the maintenance of remission, the AGA recommends using anti-TNF drugs to maintain corticosteroid- or anti-TNF-induced remission, with or without thiopurines [13].

The guidelines of the Japanese Society of Gastroenterology regarding anti-TNF therapy are consistent with these guidelines [14].

From Theoretical Indications to Clinical Practice
Anti-TNF therapy for induction of remission should be started in patients with objective signs of inflammation. Analysis performed in the SONIC trial demonstrated a higher efficacy of infliximab only in CD patients with evidence of active disease, as defined by a CRP level of >5 mg/l or endoscopic lesions. Thus, it is recommended in clinical practice to demonstrate disease activity based on biological markers such as CRP, the blood cell count or fecal calprotectin or on endoscopic and imaging findings.

According to guidelines, anti-TNF therapy should be used for moderately to severely active CD. Clinical disease activity is classically categorized as mild, moderate, or severe, depending on clinical parameters, systemic manifestations and the global impact of the disease on the individual's quality of life. In clinical trials, moderate disease is defined by a CD activity index of >220 and severe disease by a CD activity index of >300.

Risk factors for poor prognosis have been identified that contribute to determining disease severity. These factors concern the localization and behavior of the disease (extensive bowel disease, upper gastrointestinal lesion, perianal disease, fistulizing or stricturing disease, or severe endoscopic lesion as defined by the presence of deep and extensive ulcers) or are related to the patient (young age at diagnosis or tobacco use) [15]. Patients with severe disease could probably benefit the most from early anti-TNF therapy.

Conclusions and Future Directions

In conclusion, anti-TNF agents are able to induce and maintain remission of CD over time, to heal mucosal lesions and to reduce rates of hospitalizations and surgeries. They represent the most effective agents currently available to treat CD, and their usage is classically recommended in patients who are unresponsive to conventional therapies. However, they may be used earlier in patients with aggressive disease or features predictive of poor prognosis. The predictors are, however, still mainly clinically based, and better predictors must be identified. Additionally, despite the optimal usage of these treatments, a significant fraction of patients still do not obtain good results [16]. These failures are not fully understood and are only partly explained by the immunogenicity of these agents [17]. A better understanding of these anti-TNF failures could help to identify predictors of nonresponse to a specific agent or class to provide better tools to clinicians who need to make therapeutic decisions.

References

1 Targan SR, Hanauer SB, van Deventer SJ, Mayer L, Present DH, Braakman T, et al: A short-term study of chimeric monoclonal antibody cA2 to tumor necrosis factor alpha for Crohn's disease. Crohn's Disease cA2 Study Group. N Engl J Med 1997;337:1029–1035.

2 Schnitzler F, Fidder H, Ferrante M, Noman M, Arijs I, Van Assche G, et al: Long-term outcome of treatment with infliximab in 614 patients with Crohn's disease: results from a single-centre cohort. Gut 2009;58:492–500.

3 Colombel JF, Sandborn WJ, Reinisch W, Mantzaris GJ, Kornbluth A, Rachmilewitz D, et al: Infliximab, azathioprine, or combination therapy for Crohn's disease. N Engl J Med 2010;362:1383–1395.

4 Hanauer SB, Sandborn WJ, Rutgeerts P, Fedorak RN, Lukas M, MacIntosh D, et al: Human anti-tumor necrosis factor monoclonal antibody (adalimumab) in Crohn's disease: the CLASSIC-I trial. Gastroenterology 2006;130:323–333; quiz 591.

5 Sandborn WJ, Feagan BG, Stoinov S, Honiball PJ, Rutgeerts P, Mason D, et al: Certolizumab pegol for the treatment of Crohn's disease. N Engl J Med 2007;357:228–238.

6 Hanauer SB, Feagan BG, Lichtenstein GR, Mayer LF, Schreiber S, Colombel JF, et al: Maintenance infliximab for Crohn's disease: the ACCENT I randomised trial. Lancet 2002;359:1541–1549.

7 Colombel J-F, Sandborn WJ, Rutgeerts P, Enns R, Hanauer SB, Panaccione R, et al: Adalimumab for maintenance of clinical response and remission in patients with Crohn's disease: the CHARM trial. Gastroenterology 2007;132:52–65.

8 Schreiber S, Khaliq-Kareemi M, Lawrance IC, Thomsen OØ, Hanauer SB, McColm J, et al: Maintenance therapy with certolizumab pegol for Crohn's disease. N Engl J Med 2007;357:239–250.

9 Hyams J, Crandall W, Kugathasan S, Griffiths A, Olson A, Johanns J, et al: Induction and maintenance infliximab therapy for the treatment of moderate-to-severe Crohn's disease in children. Gastroenterology 2007;132:863–873; quiz 1165–1166.

10 Hyams JS, Griffiths A, Markowitz J, Baldassano RN, Faubion WA, Colletti RB, et al: Safety and efficacy of adalimumab for moderate to severe Crohn's disease in children. Gastroenterology 2012;143:365–374.e2.

11 Dignass A, Van Assche G, Lindsay JO, Lémann M, Söderholm J, Colombel JF, et al: The second European evidence-based Consensus on the diagnosis and management of Crohn's disease: current management. J Crohns Colitis 2010;4:28–62.

12 Ruemmele FM, Veres G, Kolho KL, Griffiths A, Levine A, Escher JC, et al: Consensus guidelines of ECCO/ESPGHAN on the medical management of pediatric Crohn's disease. J Crohns Colitis 2014;8:1179–1207.

13 Terdiman JP, Gruss CB, Heidelbaugh JJ, Sultan S, Falck-Ytter YT: American Gastroenterological Association Institute guideline on the use of thiopurines, methotrexate, and anti-TNF-α biologic drugs for the induction and maintenance of remission in inflammatory Crohn's disease. Gastroenterology 2013;145:1459–1463.

14 Ueno F, Matsui T, Matsumoto T, Matsuoka K, Watanabe M, Hibi T: Evidence-based clinical practice guidelines for Crohn's disease, integrated with formal consensus of experts in Japan. J Gastroenterol 2013;48:31–72.

15 Zallot C, Peyrin-Biroulet L: Clinical risk factors for complicated disease: how reliable are they? Dig Dis Basel Switz 2012;30(suppl 3):67–72.

16 Allez M, Karmiris K, Louis E, Van Assche G, Ben-Horin S, Klein A, et al: Report of the ECCO pathogenesis workshop on anti-TNF therapy failures in inflammatory bowel diseases: definitions, frequency and pharmacological aspects. J Crohns Colitis 2010;4:355–366.

17 Chowers Y, Sturm A, Sans M, Papadakis K, Gazouli M, Harbord M, et al: Report of the ECCO workshop on anti-TNF therapy failures in inflammatory bowel diseases: biological roles and effects of TNF and TNF antagonists. J Crohns Colitis 2010;4:367–376.

Prof. Matthieu Allez
Service de Gastroentérologie, Hôpital Saint-Louis
1, avenue Claude Vellefaux
FR–75010 Paris (France)
E-Mail matthieu.allez@aphp.fr

Rogler G, Herfarth H, Hibi T, Nielsen OH (eds): Anti-Tumor Necrosis Factor Therapy in Inflammatory Bowel Disease.
Front Gastrointest Res. Basel, Karger, 2015, vol 34, pp 164–168 (DOI: 10.1159/000381598)

Predictor of Treatment Response

Hiroki Tanaka · Satoshi Motoya

IBD Center, Sapporo Kosei General Hospital, Sapporo, Hokkaido, Japan

Abstract

Anti-tumor necrosis factor (anti-TNF) therapies, including infliximab, adalimumab, and certolizumab pegol, are effective for the induction and maintenance of clinical remission in patients with moderate to severe Crohn's disease (CD). Although anti-TNF-based therapies have markedly revolutionized the treatment of CD, these drugs are very expensive and are associated with increased risks of melanoma, opportunistic infections, and lymphoma. In this review, we discuss the clinical predictors of the anti-TNF treatment response in CD patients. Current data suggest that a shorter disease duration, an inflammatory disease phenotype, and an increased C-reactive peptide level are associated with a good response to an anti-TNF agent. Nevertheless, the identification of additional predictors of this response in CD patients might be beneficial for patient safety and cost reduction and allow for the individualized treatment of CD patients in the future.

Introduction

Crohn's disease (CD), a chronic inflammatory disorder of the gastrointestinal tract, generally follows a relapsing and remitting course [1]. Anti-tumor necrosis factor (anti-TNF) therapies, including infliximab, adalimumab, and certolizumab pegol, are effective for the induction and maintenance of clinical remission in patients with moderate to severe CD [2–11]. Anti-TNF-based therapies have markedly revolutionized the treatment of CD; however, these drugs are very expensive and are associated with increased risks of melanoma [12], opportunistic infections [13], and lymphoma [14]. It is believed that few patients with CD require anti-TNF therapy. CD patients with factors associated with poor prognosis, such as presentation at young age, stricturing disease, requirement for initial treatment with steroids, and perianal disease at diagnosis, are recommended to undergo early induction with anti-TNF agents [15]. Placebo-controlled clinical trials have revealed that approximately 50–65% of CD patients do not respond to induction therapy with anti-TNF agents [2, 4–6, 8]. Furthermore, 18.2–37% of patients who initially respond to anti-TNF treatment lose responsiveness over time [16, 17]. Because of the high cost of these drugs and the potential risks involved, determining the predictors of anti-TNF treatment response is economically and clinically important. Unfortunately, the studies assessing the factors that predict patient response to anti-TNF treatments are mostly post hoc analyses of randomized controlled trials (RCT) or observational studies, and few reports have provided important evidence. In this review, we summarize recent findings on the predictors of anti-TNF treatment response in CD patients.

Disease-Related Predictors

A longer disease duration is a predictive factor associated with a lower rate of anti-TNF response in CD patients. Lofberg et al. have reported that a longer disease duration is associated with a lower rate of clinical remission on week 4 of adalimumab treatment [18]. In addition, Peters et al. have shown that a longer disease duration before the start of adalimumab treatment increases the risk of failed induction therapy after 3 months of the treatment [19]. Furthermore, subgroup analyses in the Crohn's Trial of the Fully Human Antibody Adalimumab for Remission Maintenance (CHARM)/Additional Long-Term Dosing With HUMIRA to Evaluate Sustained Remission and Efficacy in CD (ADHERE) trial of adalimumab have revealed that a shorter disease duration improves the clinical remission rate at week 56. In particular, the long-term remission rates were consistently high in the <2-year disease duration subgroup from week 56 in the CHARM trial and week 108 in the ADHERE trial [20]. A longer disease duration is also a poor prognostic factor in patients treated with certolizumab pegol. The Pegylated Antibody Fragment Evaluation in CD: Safety and Efficacy 2 (PRECiSE 2) trial showed the achievement of a response to certolizumab pegol treatment at week 26 in 89.5% of patients with a diagnosis of <1 year compared with 57.3% of those with a diagnosis of ≥5 years ($p < 0.05$) [21].

When the CD phenotype is considered, patients with a stricturing or penetrating disease phenotype are less likely to respond to anti-TNF therapy than those with an inflammatory disease phenotype. Laharie et al. have demonstrated that the response to infliximab at week 2 is higher in patients with an inflammatory disease phenotype than in those with a stricturing disease phenotype [22]. In addition, intestinal strictures are associated with an increased risk of failed induction therapy [19]. Furthermore, patients with an inflammatory disease phenotype may show a sustained clinical benefit compared with those with stricturing and penetrating disease phenotypes [23]. The rates of steroid-free remission in patients treated with infliximab or adalimumab are also similar [24]. In fistulizing CD, a concomitant rectovaginal fistula is a poor prognostic indicator of successful infliximab therapy [25].

Patients with isolated colonic disease are reportedly more likely to respond to anti-TNF treatment. For CD patients treated with infliximab, the short-term treatment response at weeks 4–24 is better in those with isolated colonic disease [22, 26–28]. In contrast, Cohen et al. have reported that isolated colonic disease is highly associated with an earlier time-dose escalation in patients treated with adalimumab [29].

Patient-Related Predictors

Studies reporting patient characteristic-related prognostic factors vary, although several studies have assessed smoking habits. Smokers treated with infliximab are less likely to exhibit a short-term treatment response than nonsmokers [27, 30]. Smoking is also highly associated with an earlier time-dose escalation in patients treated with adalimumab [29].

For adalimumab treatment, male sex [29], a family history of inflammatory bowel disease [29], a higher body mass index [31], and a greater CD activity index at baseline [31, 32] are important predictors of the dose escalation requirement. Loftus et al. have reported that patients in the western and southern regions of the USA have markedly lower rates of weekly dosing with adalimumab than those in the northeast [33]. Furthermore, Chaparro et al. have reported that the presence of extraintestinal manifestations is associated with a higher risk of loss of adalimumab efficacy [34].

In addition, younger age has been reported to be a good predictor of a short-term clinical response to infliximab treatment [26, 28].

A Serological Marker: C-Reactive Protein

Some reports have suggested that an elevated C-reactive protein (CRP) level at baseline is a prognostic factor for disease remission. In the Clinical Assessment of Adalimumab Safety and Efficacy Studied as Induction Therapy in CD (CLASSIC I) trial, the difference in the rate of remission between adalimumab- and placebo-treated patients was greater in the subgroup of patients with week 0 CRP concentrations of ≥1.0 mg/dl than in those with concentrations of <1.0 mg/dl [5]. In a phase II study of certrizumab pegol, patients with baseline CRP concentrations of ≥1.0 mg/dl showed clearer separation between the active treatment and placebo [4]. For infliximab, the Study of Biologic and Immunomodulator Naïve Patients in Crohn's Disease (SONIC) trial revealed that the rate of corticosteroid-free clinical remission at week 26 in both combination-therapy and infliximab groups was higher in subgroups of patients with higher baseline CRP concentrations (≥0.8 mg/dl) compared with an azathioprine group [35]. In addition, Peters et al. have reported that patients with higher CRP concentrations (>0.5 mg/dl) are more likely to respond to induction therapy after 3 months [19]. However, Baert et al. have shown that an abnormally high CRP concentration at the start of treatment is a predictor of adalimumab dose escalation [36].

Prior Use of Anti-TNF Agents

The primary response to adalimumab is reportedly higher in anti-TNF-naïve patients than in those that have received prior anti-TNF treatment [36]. Several additional studies have shown that prior anti-TNF agent use is a predictor of loss of responsiveness or adalimumab dose escalation [19, 31].

Concomitant Immunomodulators

RCT data have demonstrated that the combination therapy of infliximab and azathioprine is more effective than infliximab monotherapy for achieving a clinical response and mucosal healing in CD (SONIC study) [35] but that the use of methotrexate as the concomitant immunosuppressive agent is not superior to infliximab monotherapy [37]. The effectiveness of anti-TNF monotherapy versus combination therapy has been evaluated in several observational studies, but the results are conflicting [38].

Conclusions and Future Directions

Various predictors of anti-TNF treatment response in CD have been reported. However, these predictors should not be used until further validation has been obtained. For example, the RCT SONIC trial has suggested that combined treatment with infliximab and azathioprine is a predictor of anti-TNF treatment response in CD patients [35]. However, additional studies assessing combination therapy with infliximab and azathioprine are required because some large-scale cohort studies have reported conflicting results [39, 40]. Most of the aforementioned predictors of anti-TNF treatment response have been obtained by post hoc analyses of RCTs or observational studies; thus, further data obtained using larger-scale cohorts and meta-analyses or prospective studies are required. Reports demonstrating the loss of efficacy of anti-TNF treatment in patients with a longer disease duration and a stricturing disease phenotype or improved efficacy with increased CRP concentrations may provide important information for selecting CD patients who are suitable for anti-TNF therapy during the initial disease stages. Nevertheless, additional studies investigating predictors of the response to anti-TNF treatment in CD patients will be beneficial for patient safety and cost reduction. In addition, the identification of additional predictors might allow for individualized therapy for CD patients in the future. We hope that more important predictors of anti-TNF treatment response in CD patients will be identified with the accumulation of additional information in the future.

References

1 Cosnes J, Cattan S, Blain A: Long-term evolution of disease behavior of Crohn's disease. Inflamm Bowel Dis 2002;8:244–250.

2 Targan SR, Hanauer SB, van Deventer SJ: A short-term study of chimeric monoclonal antibody cA2 to tumor necrosis factor alpha for Crohn's disease. Crohn's Disease cA2 Study Group. N Engl J Med 1997;337:1029–1035.

3 Hanauer SB, Feagan BG, Lichtenstein GR: Maintenance infliximab for Crohn's disease: the ACCENT I randomised trial. Lancet 2002;359:1541–1549.

4 Schreiber S, Rutgeerts P, Fedorak RN: A randomized, placebo-controlled trial of certolizumab pegol (CDP870) for treatment of Crohn's disease. Gastroenterology 2005;129:807–818.

5 Hanauer SB, Sandborn WJ, Rutgeerts P: Human anti-tumor necrosis factor monoclonal antibody (adalimumab) in Crohn's disease: the CLASSIC I trial. Gastroenterology 2006;130:323–333.

6 Sandborn WJ, Feagan BG, Stoinov S: Certolizumab pegol for the treatment of Crohn's disease. N Engl J Med 2007;357:228–238.

7 Sandborn WJ, Hanauer SB, Rutgeerts P: Adalimumab for maintenance treatment of Crohn's disease: results of the CLASSIC II trial. Gut 2007;56:1232–1239.

8 Sandborn WJ, Rutgeerts P, Enns R: Adalimumab induction therapy for Crohn disease previously treated with infliximab: a randomized trial. Ann Intern Med 2007;146:829–838.

9 Schreiber S, Khaliq-Kareemi M, Lawrance IC: Maintenance therapy with certolizumab pegol for Crohn's disease. N Engl J Med 2007;357:239–250.

10 Colombel J-F, Sandborn WJ, Rutgeerts P: Adalimumab for maintenance of clinical response and remission in patients with Crohn's disease: the CHARM trial. Gastroenterology 2007;132:52–65.

11 Sandborn WJ, Schreiber S, Feagan BG: Certolizumab pegol for active Crohn's disease: a placebo-controlled, randomized trial. Clin Gastroenterol Hepatol 2011;9:670–678.e3.

12 Singh S, Nagpal SJ, Murad MH: Inflammatory bowel disease is associated with an increased risk of melanoma: a systematic review and meta-analysis. Clin Gastroenterol Hepatol 2014;12:210–218.

13 Targownik LE, Bernstein CN: Infectious and malignant complications of TNF inhibitor therapy in IBD. Am J Gastroenterol 2013;108:1835–1842.

14 Siegel CA, Marden SM, Persing SM: Risk of lymphoma associated with combination anti-tumor necrosis factor and immunomodulator therapy for the treatment of Crohn's disease: a meta-analysis. Clin Gastroenterol Hepatol 2009;7:874–881.

15 D'Haens GR, Panaccione R, Higgins PD: The London position statement of the World Congress of Gastroenterology on biological therapy for IBD with the European Crohn's and Colitis Organization: when to start, when to stop, which drug to choose, and how to predict response? Am J Gastroenterol 2011;106:199–212.

16 Gisbert JP, Panés J: Loss of response and requirement of infliximab dose intensification in Crohn's disease: a review. Am J Gastroenterol 2009;104:760–767.

17 Billioud V, Sandborn WJ, Peyrin-Biroulet L: Loss of response and need for adalimumab dose intensification in Crohn's disease: a systematic review. Am J Gastroenterol 2011;106:674–684.

18 Löfberg R, Louis EV, Reinisch W: Adalimumab produces clinical remission and reduces extraintestinal manifestations in Crohn's disease: results from CARE. Inflamm Bowel Dis 2012;18:1–9.

19 Peters CP, Eshuis EJ, Toxopeüs FM: Adalimumab for Crohn's disease: long-term sustained benefit in a population-based cohort of 438 patients. J Crohns Colitis 2014;8:866–875.

20 Schreiber S, Reinisch W, Colombel JF: Subgroup analysis of the placebo-controlled CHARM trial: increased remission rates through 3 years for adalimumab-treated patients with early Crohn's disease. J Crohns Colitis 2013;7:213–221.

21 Schreiber S, Colombel JF, Bloomfield R: Increased response and remission rates in short-duration Crohn's disease with subcutaneous certolizumab pegol: an analysis of PRECiSE 2 randomized maintenance trial data. Am J Gastroenterol 2010;105:1574–1582.

22 Laharie D, Salzmann M, Boubekeur H: Predictors of response to infliximab in luminal Crohn's disease. Gastroenterol Clin Biol 2005;29:145–149.

23 Sprakes MB, Ford AC, Warren L: Efficacy, tolerability, and predictors of response to infliximab therapy for Crohn's disease: a large single centre experience. J Crohns Colitis 2012;6:143–153.

24 Zorzi F, Zuzzi S, Onali S: Efficacy and safety of infliximab and adalimumab in Crohn's disease: a single centre study. Aliment Pharmacol Ther 2012;35:1397–1407.

25 Topstad DR, Panaccione R, Heine JA: Combined seton placement, infliximab infusion, and maintenance immunosuppressives improve healing rate in fistulizing anorectal Crohn's disease. Dis Colon Rectum 2003;46:577–583.

26 Vermeire S, Louis E, Carbonez A: Demographic and clinical parameters influencing the short-term outcome of anti-tumor necrosis factor (infliximab) treatment in Crohn's disease. Am J Gastroenterol 2002;97:2357–2363.

27 Arnott ID, McNeill G, Satsangi J: An analysis of factors influencing short-term and sustained response to infliximab treatment for Crohn's disease. Aliment Pharmacol Ther 2003;17:1451–1457.
28 Lémann M, Mary JY, Duclos B: Infliximab plus azathioprine for steroid-dependent Crohn's disease patients: a randomized placebo-controlled trial. Gastroenterology 2006;130:1054–1061.
29 Cohen RD, Lewis JR, Turner H: Predictors of adalimumab dose escalation in patients with Crohn's disease at a tertiary referral center. Inflamm Bowel Dis 2012;18:10–16.
30 Parsi MA, Achkar JP, Richardson S: Predictors of response to infliximab in patients with Crohn's disease. Gastroenterology 2002;123:707–713.
31 Bultman E, de Haar C, van Liere-Baron A: Predictors of dose escalation of adalimumab in a prospective cohort of Crohn's disease patients. Aliment Pharmacol Ther 2012;35:335–341.
32 Sandborn WJ, Colombel JF, Schreiber S: Dosage adjustment during long-term adalimumab treatment for Crohn's disease: clinical efficacy and pharmacoeconomics. Inflamm Bowel Dis 2011;17:141–151.
33 Loftus EV Jr, Pan X, Zurawski P: Adalimumab real-world dosage pattern and predictors of weekly dosing: patients with Crohn's disease in the United States. J Crohns Colitis 2011;5:550–554.
34 Chaparro M, Panes J, García V: Long-term durability of infliximab treatment in Crohn's disease and efficacy of dose 'escalation' in patients losing response. J Clin Gastroenterol 2011;45:113–118.
35 Colombel JF, Sandborn WJ, Reinisch W: Infliximab, azathioprine, or combination therapy for Crohn's disease. N Engl J Med 2010;362:1383–1395.
36 Baert F, Glorieus E, Reenaers C: Adalimumab dose escalation and dose de-escalation success rate and predictors in a large national cohort of Crohn's patients. J Crohns Colitis 2013;7:154–160.
37 Feagan BG, McDonald JW, Panaccione R: Methotrexate in combination with infliximab is no more effective than infliximab alone in patients with Crohn's disease. Gastroenterology 2014;146:681–688.e1.
38 Dulai PS, Siegel CA, Colombel JF: Systematic review: monotherapy with antitumour necrosis factor α agents versus combination therapy with an immunosuppressive for IBD. Gut 2014;63:1843–1853.
39 Jurgens M, Mahachie John JM, Cleynen I: Levels of C-reactive protein are associated with response to infliximab therapy in patients with Crohn's disease. Clin Gastroenterol Hepatol 2011;9:421–427.e1.
40 Schnitzler F, Fidder H, Ferrante M: Long-term outcome of treatment with infliximab in 614 patients with Crohn's disease: results from a single-centre cohort. Gut 2009;58:492–500.

Hiroki Tanaka
IBD Center, Sapporo Kosei General Hospital
Kita-3, Higashi-8, Chuo-ku
Sapporo, Hokkaido 060–0033 (Japan)
E-Mail hirokit@mtc.biglobe.ne.jp

Rogler G, Herfarth H, Hibi T, Nielsen OH (eds): Anti-Tumor Necrosis Factor Therapy in Inflammatory Bowel Disease.
Front Gastrointest Res. Basel, Karger, 2015, vol 34, pp 169–177 (DOI: 10.1159/000381600)

Step-Up or Top-Down, Combination with Immunosuppression or Not?

Christiane Barthel · Eduard F. Stange

Department Internal Medicine I, Robert-Bosch-Krankenhaus, Stuttgart, Germany

Abstract

In Crohn's disease and ulcerative colitis, there are different philosophies regarding the principal therapeutic approach. In this review, we discuss the pros and cons of an initial aggressive top-down strategy using a combination of anti-TNF agents and an immunomodulator (commonly a thiopurine) versus a more gradual step-up from steroids to an immunomodulator to anti-TNF therapy as required by the response to therapy. Further, despite extensive positive evidence, thiopurines have come under attack following new negative studies, requiring a balanced view. Finally, the indications for a combination of thiopurines with an anti-TNF agent are considered in detail.

Introduction

In Crohn's disease (CD) and ulcerative colitis, the current therapeutic algorithms are complex (fig. 1, 2), and the current treatment strategies include 5-aminosalicylates, corticosteroids, immunomodulators and biologicals, particularly anti-TNF antibodies and anti-integrins. Individualized treatment regimens are mandatory, especially for patients with unusual courses of the disease. In this brief and noncomprehensive article, we cover some of the relevant literature and give recommendations based on our personal opinion.

Step-Up or Top-Down

Up to now, two different treatment approaches have been discussed for the therapy of inflammatory bowel disease (IBD): the principles of 'step-up' or 'top-down' therapy. The principle of 'step-up' therapy is characterized by a step-by-step escalation as required by the therapeutic response. The 'top-down' therapy comprises an aggressive therapy with both a biological and an immunomodulator at the earliest time point of the disease course.

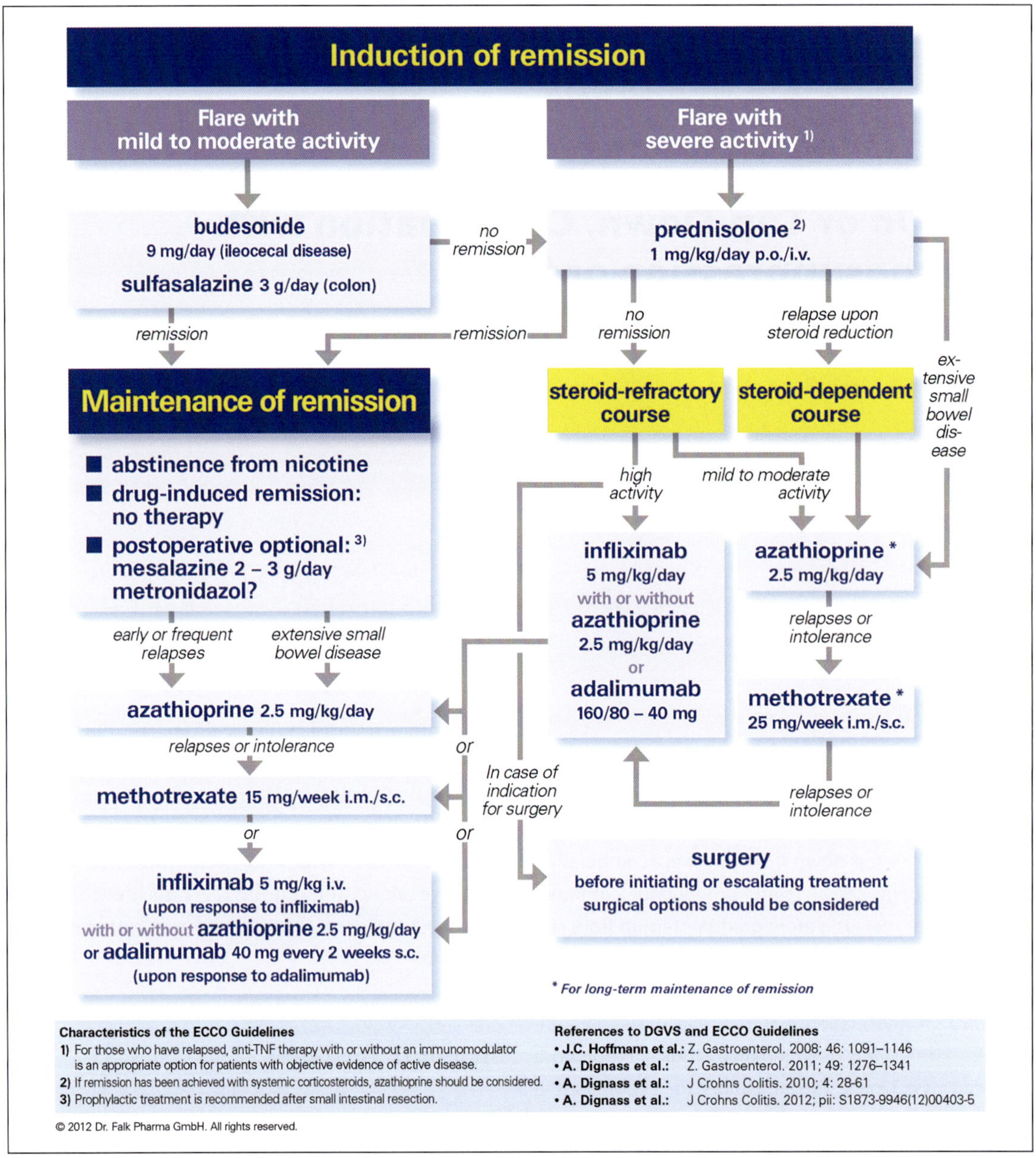

Fig. 1. Therapeutic algorithm for Crohn's disease. Mit freundlicher Genehmigung der Dr. Falk Pharma GmbH.

In the current literature, there is one fully published study that compared 'step-up' with 'top-down' therapy in patients with active CD [1]. In this study, the effectiveness of early use of combined immunomodulators (infliximab in combination with azathioprine or 6-mercaptopurine) was compared with conventional management (CM) (induction with corticosteroids) in patients with active CD who had not previously received glucocorticoids, antimetabolites

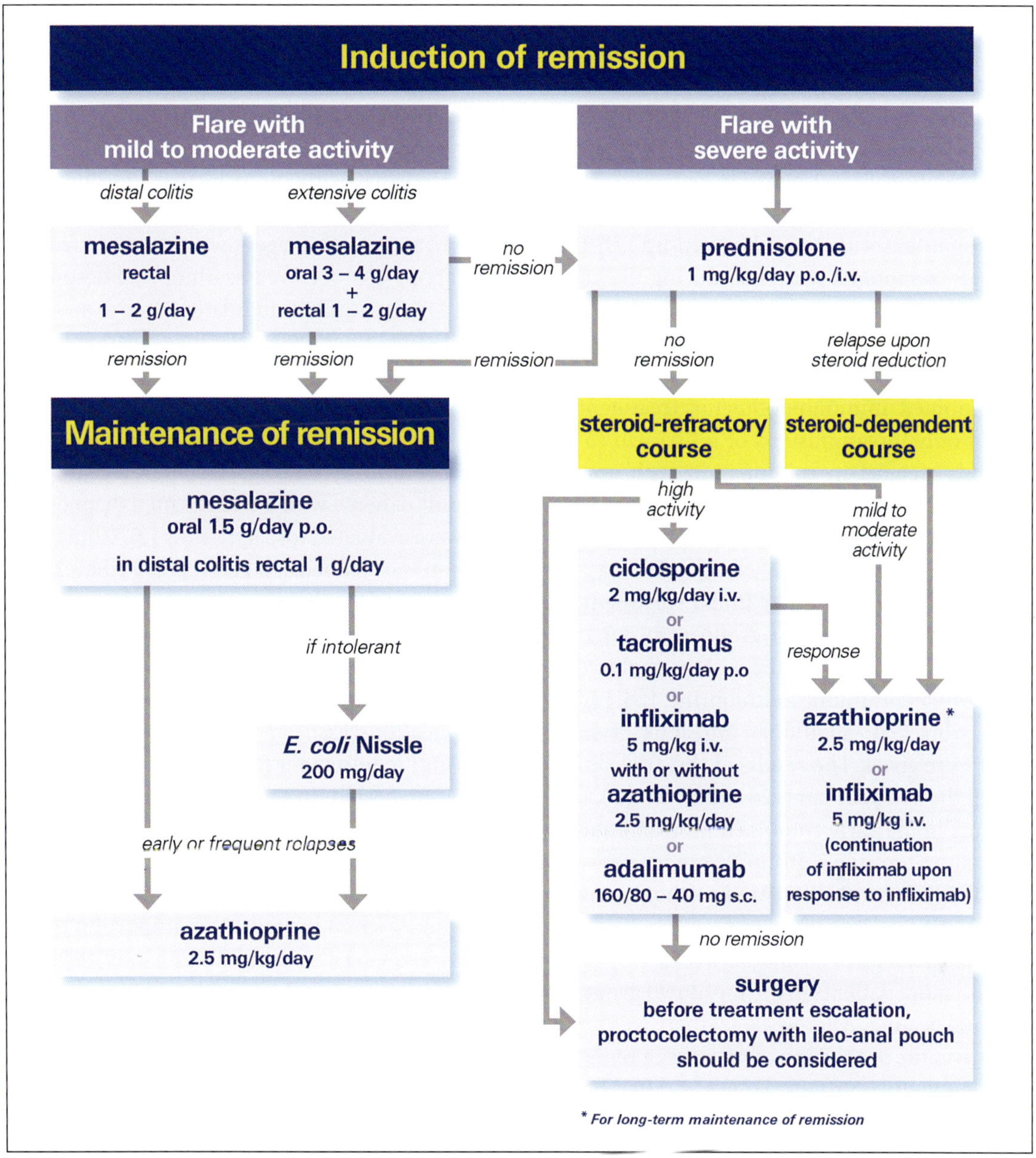

Fig. 2. Therapeutic algorithm for ulcerative colitis. Mit freundlicher Genehmigung der Dr. Falk Pharma GmbH.

or infliximab. Active CD was defined as a CD activity index (CDAI) score of greater than 200 points for a minimum of 2 weeks before randomization. Patients between 16–75 years old who had been diagnosed with CD within the past 4 years were included in the study. Patients with an immediate need for surgery, symptomatic stenosis or ileal or colonic strictures with pre-stenotic dilatation were excluded. Furthermore, patients with a positive tuberculin test, a positive stool culture for pathogens or pregnancy were excluded. Clinical remission/response was defined according to the CDAI score. In total, 133 patients were randomly assigned to receive either early combined immunomodulator (67 patients) or conventional treatment (66 patients). In the CM group, the patients received escalating therapy beginning with steroids ('step-up'). If these patients' symptoms worsened during the course of corticosteroid treatment, therapy with azathioprine was added (2–2.5 mg/kg body weight). In the reference group, the patients allocated to early combined immunomodulator treatment received only three infusions of infliximab (5 mg/kg body weight) in combination with azathioprine (2–2.5 mg/kg body weight) during weeks 0, 2 and 6. If the patients responded to and tolerated azathioprine, therapy with azathioprine was continued ('top-down'). After initial treatment, the patients in the top-down group with persisting symptoms were also treated with methylprednisolone while continuing azathioprine. If the symptoms worsened, additional infusions of infliximab were given. The results of this trial showed that in the first year (after 26 and 52 weeks), more patients in the early combined immunomodulator group ('top-down group') were in corticosteroid-free remission compared to the patients in the CM group ('step-up group') (60 vs. 35.9% and 61.5 vs. 42.2% after 26 and 52 weeks, respectively), and more patients in the top-down group had mucosal healing. After week 52, there was no difference in the proportion of patients in remission between the two groups. However, after 2 years of follow-up, significantly more patients in the top-down group showed mucosal healing than those in the step-up group (75 vs. 21%). The study design had several limitations that have to be addressed. First, it was a randomized but unblinded study, which was associated with all known limitations of physician and patient bias. Furthermore, remission was defined as 'corticosteroid-free clinical remission', which leads to a further a priori bias against the 'corticosteroid arm'. Since many step-up patients also received azathioprine after the failure of corticosteroid reduction, differences in the treatment response between these similarly treated groups are unlikely. Most importantly, the final analysis demonstrated that with the principal top-down approach, about 80% of the patients who did not require an anti-TNF agent were over-treated and that about 40% received azathioprine despite no need for an immunomodulator.

Recently, the OP004 trial investigating the effectiveness of early combined immunomodulator with adalimumab (ECI) in comparison to CM was presented. Following a cluster randomization of 39 community-based gastroenterology practices, adult patients with a documented diagnosis of CD were evaluated for 24 months [2]. Clinical remission was defined as a Harvey-Bradshaw Index score ≤4 in the absence of corticosteroids. The primary outcome was defined as the proportion of patients in remission after 12 months, and the secondary endpoints were defined as the rates of complications associated with CD, hospitalization, and requirement for surgery over the entire follow-up period. In total, 15.1% of the 1,084 patients in the ECI group and 6.5% of the 898 patients in the CM group received a combination of antimetabolite/adalimumab treatment after 12 months. After 24 months, the proportion of patients receiving this combination was 19.7% in the ECI group and 9.6% in the CM group. It is noteworthy that 66% of those in the ECI- and 62% of those in the CM group were in clinical remission after 12 months, which became 73 and 65%, respectively, after 24 months. However, highly significant and clinically important differences in the rates of complications, hospitalization and surgery over 24 months were observed in favor of the patients in the ECI group compared to those in the CM group. The authors of this trail concluded that early combined immunomodulator treatment was more effective in preventing CD-related complications compared to CM. However, again, the trial was open, and the combination of an immunomodulator and adalimumab had not been validated in prior trials. Detailed analysis of the study requires the fully published paper. Taken together, both top-down and conventional treatment are compatible with the superiority of the top-down arm with respect to mucosal healing and complications, but the aspired long term-effect of these treatments on clinical remission is lacking.

Thiopurines in Accelerated Step-Up

As an alternative to 'top-down' therapy, the early use of thiopurines (azathioprine, 6-mercaptopurine) has been suggested ('accelerated step-up'), as these compounds have been a mainstay of drug therapy for decades in CD and, although less evidence-based, in ulcerative colitis. Thiopurines are characterized by their slow onset of action. The effect of thiopurines has been described to occur approximately 12 weeks after the initiation of therapy, and therefore, thiopurines are commonly used for the maintenance of IBD (especially for patients with steroid dependence) but are less commonly used for the induction of remission [3]. This is based on extensive meta-analytic evidence that emphasizes the effectiveness and the importance of thiopurines in IBD [4–10]. A Cochrane meta-analysis concluded that thiopurines (azathioprine or 6-mercaptopurine) effectively maintained remission in CD patients with an odds ratio between 2 and 3 compared to placebo [4, 8] but induction therapy provided no benefit [5]. The meta-analysis by Gordon et al. [6] evaluated the efficacy and safety of purine analogs for the maintenance of surgically-induced remission in CD and showed that thiopurines were superior to placebo for the maintenance of surgically-induced remission in patients with CD. Finally, in another Cochrane meta-analysis, azathioprine therapy appeared to be more effective than placebo for the maintenance of remission in ulcerative colitis [7]. The evidence for methotrexate is much more limited and essentially involves a single large randomized trial in CD [11]. Unfortunately, in the absence of industry support, further trials with this drug are unlikely to be performed.

Despite this extensive evidence base, the use of thiopurines has recently been described to be controversial based on two new studies. Cosnes et al. performed an open-label trial of adults diagnosed with CD for less than 6 months and compared the efficacy of early treatment with azathioprine with CM in patients who were at high risk for disabling disease during a 3-year follow-up period [12]. The primary endpoint was defined as corticosteroid and anti-TNF therapy-free remission during the first 3 years after study inclusion. The authors showed that administration of azathioprine within 6 months of CD diagnosis was not more effective than CM regarding the extension of clinical remission. However, 60% of the patients in the control group also received azathioprine in the second or third year (similar to the study by D'Haens). This similarity of the treatment strategies between the two study groups makes an interpretation of the results difficult and only shows the frequent need of immunosuppressive therapy in this patient cohort.

Panés et al. performed a smaller placebo-controlled trial in which the efficacy of mercaptopurine therapy for 'all' patients newly diagnosed with CD was investigated [13]. The patients were randomly assigned to receive azathioprine or placebo. Only corticosteroids, but no other concomitant medication, were allowed for the control of disease activity. The primary endpoint was defined as corticosteroid therapy-free remission. In this study, early azathioprine therapy was not more effective than placebo for achieving sustained corticosteroid therapy-free remission. The patients in the azathioprine arm had more adverse events (20.6 vs. 11.1%), but severe relapses were significantly less frequent in the azathioprine arm than in the placebo arm (11.8 vs. 30.2%). One of the limitations of this trial was that half of the patients in both groups prematurely discontinued the study. In addition, the study apparently entered many patients into the trial that simply did not require immunosuppression and therefore had no benefit. As discussed previously [14], it is not surprising that treatment with azathioprine was not generally superior to placebo under these trial conditions [14].

Additionally, the phenotype classification of CD has an important role in patient management and may help to define and even predict the clinical course of patients with CD [15]. The disease phenotype can be determined according to the Montreal classification [16]: age of onset, location and behavior. Initially, it is usually characterized by a nonstenosing nonpenetrating behavior but with progression over time due to cumulative structural damage to a fibro-stenosing and/or penetrating phenotype. The recent study by Magro et al. investigated the long-term evolution of disease behavior of CD and tried to identify parameters that predicted phenotypic progression [15]. In this trial, 368 male and 368 female were followed for 12.3 years; 87% of the patients had a nonstenosing nonpenetrating behavior phenotype at diagnosis, and 28.5% and 23.5% of these patients progressed to the fibrostenosing and penetrating phenotypes, respectively. Half of the patients started azathioprine treatment and 13.9% received treatment with anti-TNF-α prior to a change in the phenotype. This study showed that monotherapy with azathioprine as well as combination therapy with azathioprine/anti-TNFα before a phenotypic change delayed disease progression compared to not receiving either treatment. This trial also demonstrated that upper gastrointestinal tract involvement, male gender, and use of steroids with or without steroid dependence were associated with a higher risk for disease progression. At any rate, this study provides additional evidence that patients selected based on their need for immunomodulator treatment benefit from this treatment with respect to disease activity and phenotypic progression.

Combination with Immunosuppression

There is good evidence that azathioprine works best in combination with an effective agent for remission induction, e.g. a steroid or infliximab [14]. A randomized, double-blind study (Study of Biologic and Immunomodulator Naive Patients in CD (SONIC)) evaluated the efficacy of infliximab monotherapy (5 mg/kg body weight), azathioprine monotherapy (2.5 mg/kg body weight), and the two drugs combined in 508 adults with moderate to severe CD who had not undergone previous immunosuppressive or biologic therapy. Infusions were applied at weeks 0, 2, 6 and every 8 weeks thereafter [17]. The eligible patients had early CD for at least 6 weeks and had a CDAI score of 220–450. Patients were included who were corticosteroid-dependent, under consideration for a second course of systemic corticosteroids within 12 months or who had not responded to treatment with either mesalazine (≥2.4 g/day) or budesonide (≥6 mg/day). Patients with short bowel syndrome, an abscess or a symptomatic stricture, a history of abdominal surgery, a history of tuberculosis, an opportunistic infection or an active infection with hepatitis B or C or HIV were excluded. Clinical remission was defined as an absolute CDAI score of less than 150 points, and corticosteroid-free clinical remission was defined as clinical remission in patients who had not received budesonide at a daily dose of more than 6 mg or systemic corticosteroids for at least 3 weeks. The primary efficacy endpoint was the rate of corticosteroid-free clinical remission at week 25. The secondary efficacy endpoints were the rates of corticosteroid-free clinical remission at all other time points. Of the 508 patients who underwent randomization, 170 patients received azathioprine monotherapy, 169 patients received infliximab monotherapy and 169 patients received a combination therapy of azathioprine and infliximab. At week 26, patients with moderate to severe CD treated with infliximab and azathioprine (56.8%) or infliximab monotherapy (44.4%)

were more likely to have corticosteroid-free clinical remission than those treated with azathioprine monotherapy (30.0%). The combination therapy was the most effective treatment. This trial had several limitations, especially regarding the inclusion criteria, since only corticosteroid-dependent patients or nonresponders to budesonide and mesalazine with active CD were included in the study. Particularly, treatment with mesalazine is not an effective treatment option in patients with active CD, implying that a proportion of patients did not receive appropriate treatment prior to study inclusion. This study showed that the use of azathioprine in combination with infliximab in early stages of the disease is more effective than the typical sequential treatment algorithm, but it remains unclear when to use anti-TNF: immediately or only upon a nonresponse to steroids, 6-MP, azathioprine or methotrexate. A similar study has been performed in ulcerative colitis, in which with respect to remission, azathioprine and infliximab were comparable, but the combination of these drugs was superior to either drug alone [18].

The combined treatment with an immunosuppressant and infliximab confers the advantage of additive efficacy as well as less anti-chimeric antibody formation induced by the hybrid antibody and, as a consequence, enhanced infliximab levels [19]. Although methotrexate was recently described to similarly reduce antibody formation, somewhat surprisingly, there was no clinical benefit to this drug [20]. It remains unclear whether the 'combo' benefit due to thiopurines applies to the other anti-TNF antibodies on the market.

Another important aspect is the 'treat-to-target' aim of mucosal healing. As mentioned above, this endpoint is reached more often during combo treatment than during monotherapy with either agent and is associated with a more benign prognosis. However, it remains unclear whether treatment escalation in patients in remission only based on suboptimal mucosal healing makes sense. Unfortunately, such a trial has not been performed, and large patient numbers would be required to evaluate the resulting safety issues.

The Markov model analysis by Scott et al. [21] demonstrated that the addition of an immunosuppressive drug to anti-TNF therapy increases treatment efficacy for infliximab in IBD, outweighing the additive risk. The use of combination therapy appears to add no significant risk for serious complications (e.g. lymphomas, lymphoma-related complications, infection and surgical complications) than the risk seen with anti-TNF or immunosuppressive monotherapy in patients aged from 35 to 65 years. In older patients (>65 years old), the risk of serious infections and non-Hodgkin's lymphomas were higher in combination therapy compared to anti-TNF monotherapy. Young males with limited disease also cause some additional concern due to the risk of hepatosplenic T-cell lymphoma. Decisions need to be made individually, but for most patients who clinically require a combination therapy, the benefits will probably outweigh the risks [21].

Finally, there is increasing evidence that if azathioprine is combined with an anti-TNF agent, about half of the patients remain in remission even if the anti-TNF agent is stopped [22]. Importantly, even in those that relapse, the reintroduction of the antibody works in most patients, suggesting that after achieving remission with the combination, a reduction to thiopurine monotherapy should be attempted. An extensive discussion of the potential induction of adverse events during combination therapy may be found in Dulai et al. [19].

Conclusions and Recommendations

Based on this state of evidence, we recommend the following:

1. Thiopurines should be used liberally for maintenance treatment in those patients with IBD who turn out to be steroid-dependent and may also be used postoperatively in CD patients.

2. Thiopurines should not be instituted to rapidly induce remission because of their known delayed effect.

3. The combination of a thiopurine with an anti-TNF agent should be instituted in those who require enhanced therapy because it is effective and relatively safe (except in those >65 years old), and the anti-TNF agent may be discontinued after therapeutic success in about half of the patients.

4. It is not evidence-based to escalate therapy in a patient in clinical remission simply to achieve mucosal healing.

References

1 D'Haens G, Baert F, v Assche G, Caenepeel P, Vergauwe P, Tuynman H, De Vos M: Early combined immunosuppression or conventional management in patients with newly diagnosed Crohn's disease: an open randomised trial. Lancet 2008;371:660–667.

2 Khanna R, Levesque BG, Bressler B, Zou G, Stitt L, Greenberg GR, Panaccione R, Bitton A, Pare P, Vermeire D, D'Haens G, MacIntosh D, Sandborn WJ, Vandervoort MK, Morris JC, Feagan BG: OP004. Early combined immunosuppression for the management of Crohn's disease: a community-based cluster randomized trial. JCC 2014;8:S2–S3.

3 Konidari A, El Matary W: Use of thiopurines in inflammatory bowel disease: safety issues. World J Gastrointest Pharmacol Ther 2014;5:63–76.

4 Prefontaine E, Sutherland LR, Mac Donald JK, Cepoiu M: Azathioprine or 6-mercaptopurine for maintenance of remission in Crohn's disease. Cochrane Database Syst Rev 2009; 1:CD000067.

5 Chande N, Tsoulis DJ, MacDonald JK: Azathioprine or 6-mercaptopurine for induction of remission in Crohn's disease. Cochrane Database Syst Rev 2013; 4:CD000545.

6 Gordon M, Taylor K, Akoberg AK, Thomas AG: Azathioprine and 6-mercaptopurine for maintenance of surgically-induced remission in Crohn's disease. Cochrane Database Syst Rev 2014; 8:CD010233.

7 Timmer A, McDonald JW, Tsoulis DJ, MacDonald JK: Azathioprine and 6-mercaptopurine for maintenance of remission in ulcerative colitis. Cochrane Database Syst Rev 2012; 9:CD000478.

8 Louis E, Irving P, Beaugerie L: Use of azathioprine in IBD: modern aspects of an old drug. Gut 2014;63:1695–1699.

9 Louis E, Mary JY, Vernier-Massouille G, Grimaud JC, Bouhnik Y, Laharie D, Dupas JL, Pillant H, Picon L, Veyrac M, Flamant M, Savoye G, Jian R, Devos M, Porcher R, Paintaud G, Piver E, Colombel JF, Lemann M; Groupe D'etudes Thérapeutiques Des Affections Inflammatoires Digestives: Maintenance of remission among patients with Crohn's disease on antimetabolite therapy after infliximab therapy is stopped. Gastroenterology 2012;142:63–70.

10 Reinisch W, Angelberger S, Petritsch W, Shonova O, Lukas M, Bar-Meir S, Teml A, Schaeffler E, Schwab M, Dilger K, Greinwald R, Mueller R, Stange EF, Herrlinger KR; International AZT-2 Study Group: Azathioprine versus mesalazine for prevention of postoperative clinical recurrence in patients with Crohn's disease with endoscopic recurrence: efficacy and safety results of a randomized, double-blind, double-dummy, multicenter trial. Gut 2010;59:752–759.

11 McDonald JW, Wang Y, Tsoulis DJ, MacDonald JK, Feagan BG: Methotrexate for induction of remission in refractory Crohn's disease. Cochrane Database Syst Rev 2014;8:CD003459.

12 Cosnes J, Bourrier A, Laharie D, Nahon S, Bouhnik Y, Carbonnel F, Dupas JL, Reimund JM, Savoye G, Jouet P, Moreau J, Mary JY, Colombel JF; Groupe d'Étude Thérapeutiques des Affections Inflammatoires du Tube Digestif: Early combination of azathioprine vs conventional management of Crohn's disease: a randomized controlled trial. Gastroenterology 2013;145:758–765.

13 Panés J, Lopéz-Sanromán A, Bermejo F, Garcia-Sánchez V, Esteve M, Torres Y, Domènch E, Piqueras M, Gomez-Garcia M, Gutiérrez A, Taxonera C, Sans M; AZTEC Study Group: Early azathioprine therapy is no more effective than placebo for newly diagnosed Crohn's disease. Gastroenterology 2013;145:766–774.

14 Herrlinger K, Stange EF: The debated role for thiopurines in Crohn's disease. JCC 2013;8:172–174.

15 Magro F, Rodrigues-Pinto E, Coelho R, Andrade A, Santos-Antunes J, Lopes S, Camila-Dias C, Macedo G: Is it possible to change phenotype progression in Crohn's disease in the era of immunomodulaters? Predictive factors of phenotype progression. Am J Gastroenterol 2014;109:1026–1036.

16 Silverberg MS, Satsangi J, Ahmad T, Arnott ID, Bernstein CN, Brant SR, Caprilli R, Colombel JF, Gasche C, Geboes K, Jewell DP, Karban A, Loftus EV, Peña AS, Riddell RH, Sachar DB, Schreiber S, Steinhart AH, Targan SR, Vermeire S, Warren BF: Toward an integrated clinical, molecular and serological classification of inflammatory bowel disease: report of a Working Party of the 2005 Montreal World Congress of Gastroenterology. Can J Gastroenterol 2005;19(suppl A):5A–36A.

17 Colombel JF, Sandborn W, Reinisch W, Mantzaris G, Kornbluth A, Rachmilewitz D, Lichtiger S, D'Haens G, Diamond RH, Broussard DL, Tang KL, Janneke van der Woude C, Rutgeerts P: Infliximab, azathioprine, or combination therapy for Crohn's disease. N Engl J Med 2010;362:1383–1395.

18 Panaccione R, Ghosh S, Middleton S, Márquez JR, Scott BB, Flint L, van Hoogstraten HJ, Chen AC, Zheng H, Danese S, Rutgeerts P: Combination therapy with infliximab and azathioprine is superior to monotherapy with either agent in ulcerative colitis. Gastroenterology 2014;146:392–400.

19 Dulai PS, Siegel CA, Colombel JF, Sandborn WJ, Peyrin-Biroulet L: Systematic review: monotherapy with antitumour necrosis factor α agents versus combination therapy with an immunosuppressive for IBD. Gut 2014;63:1843–1853.

20 Feagan BG, McDonald JW, Panaccione R, Enns RA, Bernstein CN, Ponich TP, Bourdages R, Macintosh DG, Dallaire C, Cohen A, Fedorak RN, Paré P, Bitton A, Saibil F, Anderson F, Donner A, Wong CJ, Zou G, Vandervoort MK, Hopkins M, Greenberg GR: Methotrexate in combination with infliximab is no more effective than infliximab alone in patients with Crohn's disease. Gastroenterology 2014;146:681–688.

21 Scott FI, Vajravelu R, Bewtra M, Mantani R, Lee D, Goldberg D, Lewis JL: The benefit to risk balance of combining infliximab with azathioprine varies with age: a Markov model. Gastroenterology 2015;13:302–309.e11.

22 Papamichael K, Casteele NV, Gils A, Tops S, Hauenstein S, Singh S, Princen F, Van Assche G, Rutgeerts P, Vermeire S, Ferrante M: Long-term outcome of patients with Crohn's disease who discontinued infliximab therapy upon clinical remission. Clin Gastroenterol Hepatol 2015, DOI: 10.1016/j.cgh.2014.11.026.

Eduard F. Stange
Department Internal Medicine I, Robert-Bosch-Krankenhaus
Auerbachstrasse 110
DE–70376 Stuttgart (Germany)
E-Mail eduard.stange@rbk.de

Rogler G, Herfarth H, Hibi T, Nielsen OH (eds): Anti-Tumor Necrosis Factor Therapy in Inflammatory Bowel Disease.
Front Gastrointest Res. Basel, Karger, 2015, vol 34, pp 178–184 (DOI: 10.1159/000381601)

The 'Ideal' Anti-TNF Patient: Indications for Anti-TNF Therapy in Ulcerative Colitis

Tadakazu Hisamatsu

Division of Gastroenterology and Hepatology, The Third Department of Internal Medicine, Kyorin University School of Medicine, Tokyo, Japan

Abstract

Recently, the efficacy of anti-TNF agents in refractory UC patients has been reported. Promising results of large scale clinical trials encourage us. while we also have unsolved issues in daily practice such as how to evaluate mucosal healing, long-term prognosis of patients treated with anti-TNF agents, and possibility of cessation of anti-TNF agents in well controlled patients.

Introduction

Ulcerative colitis (UC) is a chronic inflammatory disease causing chronic inflammation of the colonic mucosa. UC is characterized by a relapsing and remitting course; therefore, both inducing and maintaining remission are important in the treatment of UC. Anti-TNF agents show efficacy as both an induction and a maintenance therapy. Recently, the concept that UC should be considered as a progressive disease that causes disability of the colon has been proposed [1, 2], and it has been expected that anti-TNF therapy can change the natural history of UC [3]. On the other hand, we have several issues to resolve concerning the use of anti-TNF agents in UC: the indication of anti-TNF therapy in UC, the long-term prognosis of patients treated with anti-TNF agents, the concomitant use of immunomodulators, the possibility of stopping anti-TNF therapy in well-controlled patients, and so on. In this chapter, the efficacy of anti-TNF agents in UC is reviewed, and the 'ideal' patient with UC indicated for anti-TNF therapy is discussed.

Efficacy of Anti-TNF Therapy in Ulcerative Colitis

Previously, several large scale, double-blind, placebo-controlled studies of anti-TNF therapy for UC were performed (table 1). In the Active UC Trial (ACT)1 study (infliximab; IFX), the

Table 1. Efficacy of anti-TNF agents for the treatment of UC

Study	Anti-TNF agent	Enrolled patients	Primary endpoint (week)	Clinical response (vs. placebo)	Clinical remission (vs. placebo)	Ref.
ACT1	IFX	moderate to severe active UC despite treatment with concurrent medications (corticosteroid alone or in combination with AZA/6MP)	Clinical response at 8 W (decrease from baseline in Mayo score ≥30% and ≥3 points, rectal bleeding subscore 0 or 1 or decrease from baseline ≥1)	5 mg/kg: 69.4% (vs. 37.2%) at 8 W 45.5% (vs. 19.8%) at 54 W	5 mg/kg: 38.3% (vs. 14.9%) at 8 W 34.7% (vs. 16.5%) at 54 W	[4]
ACT2	IFX	moderate to severe active UC despite treatment with concurrent medications (as in ACT1 +/– 5-ASA)	Same as ACT1	5 mg/kg: 64.5% (vs. 29.3%) at 8 W 47.1% (vs. 26.0%) at 30 W	5 mg/kg: 33.9% (vs. 5.7%) at 8 W 25.6% (vs. 10.6%) at 30 W	[4]
ULTRA-1	ADA	Mayo score of ≥6 points and endoscopic subscore of ≥2 points despite treatment with corticosteroids and/or immunosuppressants	Clinical remission at 8 W (Mayo score ≤2 with no individual subscore >1)	160/80 mg: 54.6% (vs. 44.6%) at 8 W	160/80 mg: 18.5% (vs. 10%) at 8 W	[5]
ULTRA-2	ADA	moderate to severe UC receiving concurrent treatment with oral corticosteroids or immunosuppressants	(1) Clinical remission at 8 W (2) Clinical remission at 52 W (Mayo score ≤2 with no individual subscore >1)	50.4% (vs. 34.6%) at 8 W 30.2% (vs. 18.3%) at 52 W	16.5% (vs. 9.3%) at 8 W 17.3% (vs. 8.5%) at 52 W	[6]
PURSUIT-SC (Phase 3)	GLM	Mayo score: 6–12; endoscopic subscore ≥2	Clinical response at 6 W (decrease in Mayo score from baseline ≥30% and ≥3 points, rectal bleeding subscore 0 or 1 or decrease from baseline ≥1)	200/100 mg: 51.0% (vs. 30.3%) at 6 W 400/200 mg: 54.9% (vs. 30.3%) at 6 W	200/100 mg: 17.8% (vs. 6.4%) at 6 W 400/200 mg: 17.9% (vs. 6.4%) at 6 W	[7]
PURSUIT-M	GLM	Patients who responded to induction therapy with golimumab (50 or 100 mg every 4 W)	Maintenance of clinical response through 54 W among responders to GLM induction therapy (decrease in Mayo score from baseline ≥30% and ≥3 points, rectal bleeding subscore 0 or 1 or decrease from baseline ≥1)	50 mg every 4 W: 47% (vs. 31.2%) at 54 W 100 mg every 4 W: 49.7% (vs. 31.2%) at 54 W	100 mg every 4 W: 27.8% (vs. 15.6%) at both 30 and 54 W	[8]

W = Weeks.

treatment response and remission rates were 69.4 and 38.8% at week 8 and were 45.5 and 34.7% at week 54, respectively. In the ACT2 study (IFX), the treatment response and remission rates were 64.5 and 33.9% at week 8 and were 47.1 and 25.6% at week 30, respectively. The patients enrolled in the ACT1 study had moderate to severe active UC despite treatment with concurrent medications (corticosteroid alone or in combination with azathioprine (AZA)/mercaptopurine), while aminosalicylate-resistant patients were additionally enrolled in ACT2 [4]. In both the Ultrarunners Longitudinal Tracking (ULTRA)-1 and ULTRA-2 studies (adalimumab; ADA), the primary endpoint was clinical remission, which was different from other clinical trials such as the ACT and Program of UC Research Studies Utilizing an Investigational Treatment (PURSUIT) studies. The clinical remission rates were 18.5% at week 8 for the ULTRA-1 study and 16.5% at week 8 and 17.3% at week 52 for the ULTRA-2 study [5, 6]. In the PURSUIT-Subcutaneous (PURSUIT-SC) study, the clinical response rates of golimumab (GLM) were 51.0% in the 200/100 mg group and 54.9% in the 400/200 mg group at week 6 [7]. In the PURSUIT-Maintenance (PURSUIT-M) study, the clinical response rates to maintenance therapy were 47% in the 50 mg every 4 weeks group and 49.7% in the 100 mg every 4 weeks group [8]. As shown in table 1, the patients enrolled in these studies were mainly moderate to severe UC patients who were resistant to concurrent medications. Therefore, these patients are considered as appropriate candidates for anti-TNF therapy. In many studies, except for ULTRA-1 and ULTRA-2, the clinical response rate was defined as the primary endpoint. The clinical response rates were 50–70%. However the results were obtained from only very short-term observation (at week 6–8). In addition, about 30% of the clinical response rates were observed in placebo groups. These issues may emphasize the importance of clinical remission rates and mucosal healing rates as more objective primary endpoints.

Since there are no head-to-head comparative clinical trials among anti-TNF agents in UC, we cannot provide a conclusion regarding a definition of the superiority or the equivalence of anti-TNF agents. Several systematic reviews reported that the trends favored IFX over both ADA and GLM, although there was no statistically significant difference [9, 10]. However, this issue is inconclusive because of the lack of accumulated evidence. The choice of an anti-TNF agent should be decided based on not only the power of its efficacy but also its safety and cost, as well as the patient's adherence to the treatment.

Anti-TNF Agents as a Rescue Therapy for Severe Refractory Ulcerative Colitis

Anti-TNF agents have been used as a rescue therapy for severe refractory UC cases. An open-label, randomized controlled trial compared the efficacy of IFX with that of cyclosporine A (CsA) in acute severe UC patients who had been refractory to intravenous (IV) steroid therapy. In this clinical trial, 58 patients were treated with CsA, and 57 patients were treated with IFX. There were no significant differences between the IFX and CsA groups regarding the clinical response at day 7 (CsA 86% vs. IFX 84%), the treatment failure rate at day 98 (CsA 60% vs. IFX 54%), the colectomy-free survival rate at day 98, or severe adverse effects (CsA 16% vs. IFX 25%) [11].

The long-term efficacy in preventing colectomy (median follow-up duration, 37 months) was not significantly different between the IFX and CsA strategies in severe UC patients refractory to IV steroids [12]. Although serious adverse effects such as infection occurred in severe UC patients who were refractory to IV steroid therapy, rescue therapy with IFX or CsA in patients refractory to IV steroids was not associated with an increased risk for postoperative complications compared with IV steroids alone [13]. In addition to the clinical benefit and the risk of adverse effects, the medical cost of rescue therapy is an important issue for refractory UC patients. A study in the Netherlands demonstrated that the mean in-hospital costs were significantly higher in the CsA group, while the total costs up to 3 months after the initiation of rescue therapy were significantly higher in the IFX group [14]. Of course, medical costs should be assessed and discussed in each country.

The efficacy of oral tacrolimus (TAC), which is another calcineurin inhibitor, has been reported [15, 16], and TAC was approved as a treatment for refractory UC patients in Japan in 2009. To define the comparative efficacy of oral TAC and IFX in refractory UC patients, an open-label, randomized study has been conducted in Japan.

Table 2. Clinical remission and mucosal healing in UC patients with anti-TNF agents

Study	Anti-TNF agent	Definition of mucosal healing	Mucosal healing (vs. placebo)	Clinical remission (vs. placebo)	Ref.
ACT1	IFX	Mayo subscore of 0 or 1	5 mg/kg: 62.0% (vs. 33.9%) at 8 W 45.5% (vs. 18.2%) at 54 W	5 mg/kg: 38.3% (vs. 14.9%) at 8 W 34.7% (vs. 16.5%) at 54 W	[4]
ACT2	IFX	Mayo subscore of 0 or 1	5 mg/kg: 60.3% (vs. 30.9%) at 8 W 47.1% (vs. 46.31%) at 30 W	5 mg/kg: 33.9% (vs. 5.7%) at 8 W 25.6% (vs. 10.6%) at 30 W	[4]
ULTRA-1	ADA	Mayo subscore of 0 or 1	160/80 mg: 46.9% (vs. 41.5%) at 8 W 80/40 mg: 37.7% (vs. 41.5%) at 8 W	160/80 mg: 18.5% (vs. 10%) at 8 W	[5]
ULTRA-2	ADA	Mayo subscore of 0 or 1	50.4% (vs. 34.6%) at 8 W 30.2% (vs. 18.3%) at 52 W	16.5% (vs. 9.3%) at 8 W 17.3% (vs. 8.5%) at 52 W	[6]
PURSUIT-SC (Phase 3)	GLM	Mayo subscore of 0 or 1	200/100 mg: 42.3% (vs. 28.7%) at 6 W 400/200 mg: 45.1% (vs. 28.7%) at 6 W	200/100 mg: 17.8% (vs. 6.4%) at 6 W 400/200 mg: 17.9% (vs. 6.4%) at 6 W	[7]
PURSUIT-M	GLM	Mayo subscore of 0 or 1	50 mg every 4 W: 41.7% (vs. 26.6%) at 54 W 100 mg every 4 W: 42.4% (vs. 26.6%) at 54 W	50 mg every 4 W: 23.2% (vs.15.6%) 100 mg every 4 W: 27.8% (vs. 15.6%) at both 30 and 54 W	[8]

W = Weeks.

Is Mucosal Healing an Objective Parameter?

As described, relatively higher clinical response rates (~30%) were observed in placebo groups in several large-scale clinical trials (table 1). Therefore, to evaluate the efficacy of treatment and to monitor disease activity, objective markers are necessary. Colonoscopy is useful to evaluate disease activity in UC more objectively than in Crohn's disease. In table 2, mucosal healing was defined as a Mayo subscore of 0 or 1 in major large-scale clinical trials. The mucosal healing rates varied among trials, but the results for the treatment groups were superior (by about 30%) to those for the placebo groups, except for the results of the ULTRA-1 study. Therefore, the mucosal healing rates could be considered as a more objective parameter than the clinical response rates. However, at the same time, we can see curious findings in those clinical trials. In almost all trials, the mucosal healing rates were superior to the clinical remission rates (table 2). For example, in the ACT1 study, the clinical remission rate at week 54 was 34.7%, while mucosal the healing rate at week 54 was 45.5%. We should carefully assess these results. In all of the clinical trials described here, mucosal healing was defined as a Mayo subscore of 0 or 1. Therefore, the patient population in which mucosal healing was judged could include many patients with a Mayo subscore of 1. This factor may have caused the curious observation that the mucosal healing rates were superior to the clinical remission rates in several clinical trials. 'Complete mucosal healing' should be defined as a Mayo subscore of 0, and it may be very important to discuss long-term prognosis and maybe anti-TNF therapy cessation.

Recently, mucosal healing has been confirmed as an independent predictor of the long-term outcome of anti-TNF therapy in patients with UC. Based on additional analysis of the patients enrolled in the ACT1 study, those with a lower week 8 endoscopy subscore were less likely to progress to colectomy through 54 weeks of follow-up. These data suggested that endoscopic findings at week 8 could be a predictive marker for long-term prognosis, including the risk of colectomy, in patients treated with IFX [17]. Based on a retrospective analysis of 285 patients with refractory UC treated with IFX, independent predictors of colectomy-free survival included short-term clinical response, the baseline CRP level, and mucosal healing [18]. Thus, there is no doubt that endoscopic findings are a good, objective marker for evaluating disease activity and the treatment response and for predicting the long-term prognosis of UC patients treated with anti-TNF agents. The definition of 'complete mucosal healing' and the possibility of interobserver bias should be discussed by expert panels.

Concomitant Use of Thiopurine with an Anti-TNF Agent for the Treatment of Ulcerative Colitis

A randomized, double-blind, controlled study demonstrated that UC patients receiving combination therapy (IFX + AZA) have a significant clinical benefit. The patients with moderate to severe UC (Mayo scores of 6–8 and 9–12, respectively) who were anti-TNF therapy-naïve and AZA-free (either AZA-naïve or AZA-free for at least 3 months before enrollment) were enrolled in the study. The corticosteroid-free remission rate at week 16 was 40% in the combination therapy group, compared with 22% in the IFX monotherapy group. The mucosal healing rate was 63% in the combination therapy group, 55% in the IFX monotherapy group and 37% in the AZA monotherapy group [19]. Thus, in the short term, especially in anti-TNF therapy-naïve and AZA-free patients, combination therapy will be promising. However, the long-term efficacy and the risk of adverse effects using this combination therapy should be investigated. In addition, in patients who have already been treated with an anti-TNF agent or AZA, the clinical benefit of adding the other drug has not been demonstrated. Regarding ADA and GLM, large-scale clinical trials have not been performed.

Anti-TNF Discontinuation in Ulcerative Colitis – Is it Possible or Not?

Successful withdrawal of anti-TNF therapy has been reported in rheumatoid arthritis patients with the concomitant use of methotrexate [20, 21]. In IBD, a few prospective studies in Crohn's disease patients with the concomitant use of thiopurine have been reported. In a prospective cohort study (infliximab discontinuation in Crohn's disease patients in stable remission on combined therapy with immunosuppressors; STORI), IFX discontinuation in 115 Crohn's disease patients with steroid-free remission for at least 6 months who were treated for at least 1 year with scheduled IFX and thiopurine showed an estimated relapse rate over 1 year and 2 years of 44 and 52%, respectively [22]. In the STORI study, higher CRP and calprotectin levels were identified as risk factors for relapse, while mucosal healing may be associated with reduced relapse risk. So far, no clinical trial of the withdrawal of anti-TNF agents in UC has been reported. UC patients with the concomitant use of thiopurine and with complete mucosal healing (e.g. Mayo subscore of 0) could be candidates for stopping anti-TNF therapy.

Conclusions

Moderate to severe refractory UC is an appropriate indication for the use of anti-TNF agents. Anti-TNF agents are effective for the induction of clinical remission and mucosal healing. Anti-TNF agents, especially IFX, could also be used as a rescue therapy in severe UC patients refractory to IV steroids. The long-term efficacy of anti-TNF agents for maintaining remission and a reduced risk of surgery has been expected; however, further prospective studies are necessary to draw such conclusions. Finally, we should rank anti-TNF therapy among the treatment options for steroid-dependent and steroid-resistant UC.

References

1 Torres J, Billioud V, Sachar DB, Peyrin-Biroulet L, Colombel JF: Ulcerative colitis as a progressive disease: the forgotten evidence. Inflamm Bowel Dis 2012;18: 1356–1363.

2 Ochsenkühn T, D'Haens G: Current misunderstandings in the management of ulcerative colitis. Gut 2011;60:1294–1299.

3 Billiet T, Rutgeerts P, Ferrante M, Van Assche G, Vermeire S: Targeting TNF-α for the treatment of inflammatory bowel disease. Expert Opin Biol Ther 2014;14: 75–101.

4 Rutgeerts P, Sandborn WJ, Feagan BG, Reinisch W, Olson A, Johanns J, Travers S, Rachmilewitz D, Hanauer SB, Lichtenstein GR, de Villiers WJ, Present D, Sands BE, Colombel JF: Infliximab for induction and maintenance therapy for ulcerative colitis. N Engl J Med 2005; 353:2462–2476.

5 Reinisch W, Sandborn WJ, Hommes DW, D'Haens G, Hanauer S, Schreiber S, Panaccione R, Fedorak RN, Tighe MB, Huang B, Kampman W, Lazar A, Thakkar R: Adalimumab for induction of clinical remission in moderately to severely active ulcerative colitis: results of a randomised controlled trial. Gut 2011; 60:780–787.

6 Sandborn WJ, van Assche G, Reinisch W, Colombel JF, D'Haens G, Wolf DC, Kron M, Tighe MB, Lazar A, Thakkar RB: Adalimumab induces and maintains clinical remission in patients with moderate-to-severe ulcerative colitis. Gastroenterology 2012;142:257–265.e1–e3.

7 Sandborn WJ, Feagan BG, Marano C, Zhang H, Strauss R, Johanns J, Adedokun OJ, Guzzo C, Colombel JF, Reinisch W, Gibson PR, Collins J, Järnerot G, Hibi T, Rutgeerts P; PURSUIT-SC Study Group: Subcutaneous golimumab induces clinical response and remission in patients with moderate-to-severe ulcerative colitis. Gastroenterology 2014;146: 85–95; quiz e14–e15.

8 Sandborn WJ, Feagan BG, Marano C, Zhang H, Strauss R, Johanns J, Adedokun OJ, Guzzo C, Colombel JF, Reinisch W, Gibson PR, Collins J, Järnerot G, Rutgeerts P; PURSUIT-Maintenance Study Group: Subcutaneous golimumab maintains clinical response in patients with moderate-to-severe ulcerative colitis. Gastroenterology 2014;146:96–109. e1.

9 Stidham RW, Lee TC, Higgins PD, Deshpande AR, Sussman DA, Singal AG, Elmunzer BJ, Saini SD, Vijan S, Waljee AK: Systematic review with network meta-analysis: the efficacy of anti-TNF agents for the treatment of Crohn's disease. Aliment Pharmacol Ther 2014;39: 1349–1362.

10 Thorlund K, Druyts E, Mills EJ, Fedorak RN, Marshall JK: Adalimumab versus infliximab for the treatment of moderate to severe ulcerative colitis in adult patients naïve to anti-TNF therapy: an indirect treatment comparison meta-analysis. J Crohns Colitis 2014;8:571–581.

11 Laharie D, Bourreille A, Branche J, Allez M, Bouhnik Y, Filippi J, Zerbib F, Savoye G, Nachury M, Moreau J, Delchier JC, Cosnes J, Ricart E, Dewit O, Lopez-Sanroman A, Dupas JL, Carbonnel F, Bommelaer G, Coffin B, Roblin X, Van Assche G, Esteve M, Färkkilä M, Gisbert JP, Marteau P, Nahon S, de Vos M, Franchimont D, Mary JY, Colombel JF, Lémann M; Groupe d'Etudes Thérapeutiques des Affections Inflammatoires Digestives: Ciclosporin versus infliximab in patients with severe ulcerative colitis refractory to intravenous steroids: a parallel, open-label randomised controlled trial. Lancet 2012;380:1909–1915.

12 Naves JE, Llaó J, Ruiz-Cerulla A, Romero C, Mañosa M, Lobatón T, Cabré E, Garcia-Planella E, Guardiola J, Domènech E: Long-term comparative efficacy of cyclosporine- or infliximab-based strategies for the management of steroid-refractory ulcerative colitis attacks. Inflamm Bowel Dis 2014;20: 1375–1381.

13 Nelson R, Liao C, Fichera A, Rubin DT, Pekow J: Rescue therapy with cyclosporine or infliximab is not associated with an increased risk for postoperative complications in patients hospitalized for severe steroid-refractory ulcerative colitis. Inflamm Bowel Dis 2014;20:14–20.

14 Löwenberg M, Duijvis NW, Ponsioen C, van den Brink GR, Fockens P, D'Haens GR: Length of hospital stay and associated hospital costs with infliximab versus cyclosporine in severe ulcerative colitis. Eur J Gastroenterol Hepatol 2014;26:1240–1246.

15 Ogata H, Matsui T, Nakamura M, Iida M, Takazoe M, Suzuki Y, Hibi T: A randomised dose finding study of oral tacrolimus (FK506) therapy in refractory ulcerative colitis. Gut 2006;55:1255–1262.

16 Ogata H, Kato J, Hirai F, Hida N, Matsui T, Matsumoto T, Koyanagi K, Hibi T: Double-blind, placebo-controlled trial of oral tacrolimus (FK506) in the management of hospitalized patients with steroid-refractory ulcerative colitis. Inflamm Bowel Dis 2012;18:803–808.

17 Colombel JF, Rutgeerts P, Reinisch W, Esser D, Wang Y, Lang Y, Marano CW, Strauss R, Oddens BJ, Feagan BG, Hanauer SB, Lichtenstein GR, Present D, Sands BE, Sandborn WJ: Early mucosal healing with infliximab is associated with improved long-term clinical outcomes in ulcerative colitis. Gastroenterology 2011;141:1194–1201.

18 Arias MT, Vande Casteele N, Vermeire S, de Buck van Overstraeten A, Billiet T, Baert F, Wolthuis A, Van Assche G, Noman M, Hoffman I, D'Hoore A, Gils A, Rutgeerts P, Ferrante M: A panel to predict long-term outcome of infliximab therapy for patients with ulcerative colitis. Clin Gastroenterol Hepatol 2015;13:531–538.

19 Panaccione R, Ghosh S, Middleton S, Márquez JR, Scott BB, Flint L, van Hoogstraten HJ, Chen AC, Zheng H, Danese S, Rutgeerts P: Combination therapy with infliximab and azathioprine is superior to monotherapy with either agent in ulcerative colitis. Gastroenterology 2014;146:392–400.e3.

20 Saleem B, Keen H, Goeb V, Parmar R, Nizam S, Hensor EM, Churchman SM, Quinn M, Wakefield R, Conaghan PG, Ponchel F, Emery P: Patients with RA in remission on TNF blockers: when and in whom can TNF blocker therapy be stopped? Ann Rheum Dis 2010;69:1636–1642.

21 van den Broek M, Klarenbeek NB, Dirven L, van Schaardenburg D, Hulsmans HM, Kerstens PJ, Huizinga TW, Dijkmans BA, Allaart CF: Discontinuation of infliximab and potential predictors of persistent low disease activity in patients with early rheumatoid arthritis and disease activity score-steered therapy: subanalysis of the BeSt study. Ann Rheum Dis 2011;70:1389–1394.

22 Louis E, Mary JY, Vernier-Massouille G, Grimaud JC, Bouhnik Y, Laharie D, Dupas JL, Pillant H, Picon L, Veyrac M, Flamant M, Savoye G, Jian R, Devos M, Porcher R, Paintaud G, Piver E, Colombel JF, Lemann M; Groupe D'etudes Thérapeutiques Des Affections Inflammatoires Digestives: Maintenance of remission among patients with Crohn's disease on antimetabolite therapy after infliximab therapy is stopped. Gastroenterology 2012;142:63–70.

Tadakazu Hisamatsu, MD, PhD
Division of Gastroenterology and Hepatology
The Third Department of Internal Medicine, Kyorin University School of Medicine
6-20-2 Shinkawa, Mitaka-shi, Tokyo 181-8611 (Japan)
E-Mail thisamatsu@ks.kyorin-u.ac.jp

Rogler G, Herfarth H, Hibi T, Nielsen OH (eds): Anti-Tumor Necrosis Factor Therapy in Inflammatory Bowel Disease.
Front Gastrointest Res. Basel, Karger, 2015, vol 34, pp 185–189 (DOI: 10.1159/000381602)

Predictors of the Treatment Response

Hyo Jong Kim

Division of Gastroenterology, Department of Internal Medicine, Kyung Hee University School of Medicine, Seoul, Republic of Korea

Abstract

Slowly but surely, in almost a decade, researchers have been provided with convincing evidence for the important role of anti-TNF therapy and a potential mechanism for the efficacy of anti-TNF therapy in the management of ulcerative colitis. Now, researchers are taking another big step forward to identify predictors of the treatment response to anti-TNF therapy in order to deliver personalized care. Identifying predictors involves a wide repertoire of genetic, epigenetic, and clinical events, as well as pharmacokinetics. Along with rapidly progressing experimental studies aiming to understand the molecular pathways of TNF-α, evidence gained from analyses of pivotal clinical trials and accumulating data from longer periods of patient exposure have opened up multiple avenues of investigation for the development of comprehensive composite predictors of the treatment response of ulcerative colitis patients to anti-TNF therapy.

Introduction

Anti-TNF therapy for ulcerative colitis (UC) is a success story. The total incidence rate of colectomy for medically refractory UC has declined substantially since 2005, paralleling the increased use of anti-TNF therapy in these patients [1]. However, work remains to be done since anti-TNF therapy is not effective for every patient with UC. One-third of patients are primary nonresponders to anti-TNF therapy [2]. Emerging therapeutic agents with different mechanisms of action [3, 4] could provide a realistic option for this subset of patients. Consequently, the identification of predictors of the treatment response to anti-TNF therapy would be of great importance to patients with UC and would help to reduce the burden of UC on society.

Limitations of Single Predictors

Several studies have reported on predictors of the treatment response to anti-TNF therapy, including clinical, laboratory, immunologic, and treatment-related markers [5, 6], although these findings have not been universally consistent and require validation in long-term studies of larger cohorts.

Benefits of Composite Predictors

A more comprehensive approach using composite predictors such as a panel of markers is required, as UC displays heterogeneity in terms of treatment response and pathogenesis and as no single marker has been associated with the treatment response [7]. Recently, Arias et al. [8] combined factors that were independently associated with either relapse- or colectomy-free survival to create a risk panel in 285 patients with refractory UC who were followed up for an average of over 5 years. The risk panel was composed of five predictors of the long-term outcome of anti-TNF therapy: absence of short-term complete clinical response, absence of short-term mucosal healing, presence of perinuclear antineutrophil cytoplasmic antibodies, baseline hypoalbuminemia and baseline CRP elevation. An increase in these risk factors from 0 or 1 to 4 or 5 within 60 months was associated with a 25.5-fold increase in the risk of colectomy. These results confirm those from earlier, independent studies that disease activity prior to the initiation of infliximab (IFX) therapy is an independent predictor of the treatment response to IFX [9].

Mechanisms Leading to Predictors

Disease Activity

Among the factors in the risk panel, elevated CRP levels and hypoalbuminemia may be surrogate markers for baseline disease activity that represent more severe inflammation and diffuse ulcerative disease. Although the mechanisms leading to baseline disease activity serving as an independent predictor of the treatment response to IFX are unknown, increasing evidence suggests that disease activity accelerates anti-TNF drug clearance. IFX clearance increased by 20% with an increase in the pre-infusion CRP concentration from 3 to 14 mg/l [10], and a low serum CRP level at a follow-up colonoscopy in patients treated with an anti-TNF agent was recently identified as a predictor of mucosal healing [11]. Patients with hypoalbuminemia have a lower remission rate after IFX treatment, and an association between the baseline serum albumin concentrations and the serum IFX concentrations has also been reported recently [12].

Disease Phenotype

In addition to disease severity, disease phenotype is implicated as a predictor of the treatment response to anti-TNF agents. Interestingly, the disease duration differentially affects the treatment response to anti-TNF therapy between UC and Crohn's disease (CD). A shorter duration of disease predicts a good response to anti-TNF therapy in CD, as demonstrated by post hoc analyses of the results from a large clinical trial [13]. This was also demonstrated in pediatric populations [14]. In contrast, a shorter disease duration is associated with a higher risk of colectomy in UC. A disease duration ≥2 years at the start of IFX treatment was a predictor of colectomy-free survival in adult UC patients [8]. In children with UC, a disease duration <20 months before IFX initiation increased the likelihood of a colectomy within 1 year [15]. Historically, 15% of patients with UC will develop a severe attack requiring intensive inpatient medical therapy. Among these patients, data have consistently shown that 30–40% of patients will require an urgent colectomy [16]. Hypothetically, these differences may be related to a higher inflammatory burden in patients with severe and extensive UC than in patients with CD due to a greater inflamed intestinal surface, resulting in higher production of TNF-α that must be neutralized and greater loss of the anti-TNF drug in the intestinal lumen, [17, 18]. Accordingly, in acute UC, high levels of fecal IFX and low levels of serum IFX are predictors of induction therapy failure and subsequent colectomy [19, 20].

Predictors and Pharmacokinetics

In patients with severe UC, disease activity and the disease phenotype affect IFX pharmacokinetics, leading to lower exposure to IFX in UC patients than in patients with CD. Due to this mechanism, most predictors representing the baseline disease severity of UC should be associated with long-term outcomes of IFX therapy. Therefore, despite the involvement of common TNF-mediated proinflammatory pathways, patients with UC and CD require individualized approaches for the prediction of their treatment response to IFX.

What Genetic Factors and the Gene Expression Signature Hold

Given these findings, composite predictors mainly based on clinical and laboratory markers may be incomplete to explicitly describe the complex relationship between these predictors and the treatment response to anti-TNF therapy due to the multifactorial and unclear mechanisms underlying a disease like UC. Thus, genetic and gene expression markers should be considered in addition to clinical and laboratory markers.

Limitations of Genetics

When considering genetic susceptibility as the cornerstone of UC etiology, genetic markers are more attractive candidates as predictors of the treatment response. The few candidate gene association studies of anti-TNF-α therapy that have been reported have not shown a consistent association [21, 22]. Based on the report of their association with the susceptibility to UC, *IL23R* SNPs have been examined, but the results were not practically applicable [23]. Most genetic association studies suggested that UC risk-associated genes could not fully predict the treatment response to anti-TNF therapy. Consistently, a recent study of 163 inflammatory bowel disease (IBD) risk loci showed that the genetic risk score was not associated with the disease phenotype in UC [24]. These findings raise the possibility that genetic markers provide limited clinical utility for predicting drug responses in UC. Nevertheless, there is plenty of room for optimism. Future studies of genetic variants and the influence of epigenetic changes may have sufficient predictive power to be useful clinically.

Benefits of a Gene Expression Signature

Another experimental approach to further define the influence of genetic variation on the treatment response to anti-TNF agents is to characterize the expression profile of proinflammatory cytokines in colonic biopsies from patients with UC. Many gene expression studies have been performed mainly based on the unrealistic assumption that the association between gene expression and the treatment response is direct and isolated [25]. Arijs et al. [26] performed a gene-array study using mRNA from pre-IFX treatment rectal mucosal biopsy samples from patients with active UC, in which a panel of the top five differentially expressed genes predicted the treatment response to IFX with 95% sensitivity and 85% specificity. Although further validation is required, the authors suggested that advanced studies of a gene expression signature may enable the identification of gene variants that could be utilized as valuable markers for the prediction of the treatment response and as useful targets for the development of new therapeutic strategies.

Comprehensive Composite Predictors

Eventually, biomarkers will probably need to be combined with genetic data and phenotype to identify the subgroups of patients that are most likely to respond to treatment. Such a comprehensive composite predictor combining phenotype, serological biomarkers, known IBD susceptibility-associated SNPs, and separate loci from a novel pharmacogenetic genome-wide association study have been proposed as a predictive model of primary nonresponse to IFX treatment among pediatric patients with IBD with good discriminatory value [27]. Although these findings require validation in a prospective, independent cohort, they suggest that comprehensive composite predictors can be valuable for the identification of patients who will not benefit from this class of therapy. Fortunately, new genes (e.g., IL-9 and PRKCDBP) that are highly expressed and correlated with disease activity are being identified [28, 29], and our knowledge of highly sensitive biologic markers (e.g., anti-OmpC antibodies) continues to expand [30].

Conclusions and Future Directions

There is optimism that accurate comprehensive composite predictors composed of combinations of clinical, laboratory, and serologic markers, environmental factors and genetic and gene expression markers will be proposed. This will allow us to be more refined in personalized care. However, a sense of urgency is needed because the advent of several new classes of biologics will further challenge the selection of the right patient for anti-TNF therapy in the treatment algorithm of UC. In this context, we need to develop better insight into the interrelationship between the various immunologic mechanisms involved in the TNF-α signaling pathways before proposing accurate predictors of the treatment response to anti-TNF therapy using comprehensive composite predictors.

References

1 Reich KM, Chang HJ, Rezaie A, Wang H, Goodman KJ, Kaplan GG, Svenson LW, Lees G, Fedorak RN, Kroeker KI: The incidence rate of colectomy for medically refractory ulcerative colitis has declined in parallel with increasing anti-TNF use: a time-trend study. Aliment Pharmacol Ther 2014;40:629–638.

2 Rutgeerts P, Sandborn WJ, Feagan BG, Reinisch W, Olson A, Johanns J, Travers S, Rachmilewitz D, Hanauer SB, Lichtenstein GR, de Villiers WJ, Present D, Sands BE, Colombel JF: Infliximab for induction and maintenance therapy for ulcerative colitis. N Engl J Med 2005;353:2462–2476.

3 Feagan BG, Rutgeerts P, Sands BE, Hanauer S, Colombel JF, Sandborn WJ, Van Assche G, Axler J, Kim HJ, Danese S, Fox I, Milch C, Sankoh S, Wyant T, Xu J, Parikh A; GEMINI 1 Study Group: Vedolizumab as induction and maintenance therapy for ulcerative colitis. N Engl J Med 2013;369:699–710.

4 Sandborn WJ, Ghosh S, Panes J, Vranic I, Su C, Rousell S, Niezychowski W: Study A3921063 Investigators: Tofacitinib, an oral Janus kinase inhibitor, in active ulcerative colitis. N Engl J Med 2012;367:616–624.

5 Oussalah A, Evesque L, Laharie D, Roblin X, Boschetti G, Nancey S, Filippi J, Flourié B, Hebuterne X, Bigard MA, Peyrin-Biroulet L: A multicenter experience with infliximab for ulcerative colitis: outcomes and predictors of response, optimization, colectomy, and hospitalization. Am J Gastroenterol 2010;105:2617–2625.

6 Lee KM, Jeen YT, Cho JY, Lee CK, Koo JS, Park DI, Im JP, Park SJ, Kim YS, Kim TO, Lee SH, Jang BI, Kim JW, Park YS, Kim ES, Choi CH, Kim HJ: Efficacy, safety, and predictors of response to infliximab therapy for ulcerative colitis: a Korean multicenter retrospective study. J Gastroenterol Hepatol 2013;28:1829–1833.

7 Gerich ME, McGovern DP: Towards personalized care in IBD. Nat Rev Gastroenterol Hepatol 2014;11:287–299.

8 Arias MT, Casteele NV, Vermeire S, de Buck van Overstraeten A, Billiet T, Baert F, Wolthuis A, Van Assche G, Noman M, Hoffman I, D'Hoore A, Gils A, Rutgeerts P, Ferrante MA: A panel to predict long-term outcome of infliximab therapy for patients with ulcerative colitis. Clin Gastroenterol Hepatol 2015;13:531–538.

9 Seow CH, Newman A, Irwin SP, Steinhart AH, Silverberg MS, Greenberg GR: Trough serum infliximab: a predictive factor of clinical outcome for infliximab treatment in acute ulcerative colitis. Gut 2010;59:49–54.

10 Ternant D, Ducourau E, Perdriger A, Corondan A, Le Goff B, Devauchelle-Pensec V, Solau-Gervais E, Watier H, Goupille P, Paintaud G, Mulleman D: Relationship between inflammation and infliximab pharmacokinetics in rheumatoid arthritis. Br J Clin Pharmacol 2014;78:118–128.

11 Beigel F, Deml M, Schnitzler F, Breiteneicher S, Göke B, Ochsenkühn T, Brand S: Rate and predictors of mucosal healing in patients with inflammatory bowel disease treated with anti-TNF-alpha antibodies. PLoS One 2014;9:e99293.

12 Fasanmade AA, Adedokun OJ, Olson A, Strauss R, Davis HM: Serum albumin concentration: a predictive factor of infliximab pharmacokinetics and clinical response in patients with ulcerative colitis. Int J Clin Pharmacol Ther 2010;48:297–308.

13 Schreiber S, Reinisch W, Colombel JF, Sandborn WJ, Hommes DW, Robinson AM, Huang B, Lomax KG, Pollack PF: Subgroup analysis of the placebo-controlled CHARM trial: increased remission rates through 3 years for adalimumab-treated patients with early Crohn's disease. J Crohns Colitis 2013;7:213–221.

14 Lionetti P, Bronzini F, Salvestrini C, Bascietto C, Canani RB, Dé Angelis GL, Guariso G, Martelossi S, Papadatou B, Barabino A: Response to infliximab is related to disease duration in paediatric Crohn's disease. Aliment Pharmacol Ther 2003;18:425–431.
15 Mir SA, Nagy-Szakal D, Smith EO, Gilger MA, Kellermayer R: Duration of disease may predict response to infliximab in pediatric ulcerative colitis. J Clin Gastroenterol 2014;48:248–252.
16 Ho GT, Mowat C, Goddard CJ, Fennell JM, Shah NB, Prescott RJ, Satsangi J: Predicting the outcome of severe ulcerative colitis: development of a novel risk score to aid early selection of patients for second-line medical therapy or surgery. Aliment Pharmacol Ther 2004;19: 1079–1087.
17 Ordás I, Mould DR, Feagan BG, Sandborn WJ: Anti-TNF monoclonal antibodies in inflammatory bowel disease: pharmacokinetics-based dosing paradigms. Clin Pharmacol Ther 2012;91: 635–646.
18 Lin K, Mahadevan U: Pharmacokinetics of biologics and the role of therapeutic monitoring. Gastroenterol Clin North Am 2014;43:565–579.
19 Brandse JF, van der Kleij D, Wolbink GJ, Rigter IM, Baars PA, Lowenberg M, Ponsioen C, Jansen JM, van den Brink GR, Mathôt RA, D'Haens GR: The pharmacokinetics of infliximab induction therapy in patients with moderate to severe ulcerative colitis. Gastroenterology 2014;146(suppl 1):S–134.
20 Murthy S, Kevans D, Seow CH, Newman A, Steinhart AH, Silverberg MS, Greenberg GR: Association of serum infliximab and antibodies to infliximab to long-term clinical outcome in acute ulcerative colitis. Gastroenterology 2012; 142(suppl 1):S–388.
21 Mascheretti S, Hampe J, Kühbacher T, Herfarth H, Krawczak M, Fölsch UR, Schreiber S: Pharmacogenetic investigation of the TNF/TNF-receptor system in patients with chronic active Crohn's disease treated with infliximab. Pharmacogenomics J 2002;2:127–136.
22 Pierik M, Vermeire S, Steen KV, Joossens S, Claessens G, Vlietinck R, Rutgeerts P: Tumour necrosis factor-alpha receptor 1 and 2 polymorphisms in inflammatory bowel disease and their association with response to infliximab. Aliment Pharmacol The 2004;20:303–310.
23 Jürgens M, Laubender RP, Hartl F, Weidinger M, Seiderer J, Wagner J, Wetzke M, Beigel F, Pfennig S, Stallhofer J, Schnitzler F, Tillack C, Lohse P, Göke B, Glas J, Ochsenkühn T, Brand S: Disease activity, ANCA, and *IL23R* genotype status determine early response to infliximab in patients with ulcerative colitis. Am J Gastroenterol 2010;105:1811–1819.
24 Ananthakrishnan AN, Huang H, Nguyen DD, Sauk J, Yajnik V, Xavier RJ: Differential effect of genetic burden on disease phenotypes in Crohn's disease and ulcerative colitis: analysis of a North American cohort. Am J Gastroenterol 2014;109:395–400.
25 Olsen T, Goll R, Cui, G, Christiansen I, Florholmen J: TNF-alpha gene expression in colorectal mucosa as a predictor of remission after induction therapy with infliximab in ulcerative colitis. Cytokine 2009;46:222–227.
26 Arijs I, Li K, Toedter G, Quintens R, Van Lommel L, Van Steen K, Leemans P, De Hertogh G, Lemaire K, Ferrante M, Schnitzler F, Thorrez L, Ma K, Song XY, Marano C, Van Assche G, Vermeire S, Geboes K, Schuit F, Baribaud F, Rutgeerts P: Mucosal gene signatures to predict response to infliximab in patients with ulcerative colitis. Gut 2009; 58:1612–1619.
27 Dubinsky MC, Mei L, Friedman M, Dhere T, Haritunians T, Hakonarson H, Kim C, Glessner J, Targan SR, McGovern DP, Taylor KD, Rotter JI: Genome wide association (GWA) predictors of anti-TNFalpha therapeutic responsiveness in pediatric inflammatory bowel disease. Inflamm Bowel Dis 2010;16: 1357–1366.
28 Gerlach K, Hwang Y, Nikolaev A, Atreya R, Dornhoff H, Steiner S, Lehr HA, Wirtz S, Vieth M, Waisman A, Rosenbauer F, McKenzie AN, Weigmann B, Neurath MF: TH9 cells that express the transcription factor PU.1 drive T cell-mediated colitis via IL-9 receptor signaling in intestinal epithelial cells. Nat Immunol 2014;15:676–686.
29 Kim JW, Kim HJ, Lee CK, Shim JJ, Jang JY, Dong SH, Kim BH, Chang YW, Chi SG: Elevation of PRKCDBP, a novel transcriptional target of TNF-α, and its downregulation by infliximab in patients with ulcerative colitis. Dig Dis Sci 2014;59:2947–2957.
30 Kevans D, Waterman M, Milgrom R, Xu W, Van Assche G, Silverberg M: Serological markers associated with disease behavior and response to anti-TNF therapy in ulcerative colitis. J Gastroenterol Hepatol 2015;30:64–70.

Hyo Jong Kim, MD, PhD
Division of Gastroenterology, Department of Internal Medicine
Kyung Hee University School of Medicine, 23 Kyungheedae-ro, Dongdaemun-gu
Seoul 130-872 (Republic of Korea)
E-Mail hjkim@khmc.or.kr

Rogler G, Herfarth H, Hibi T, Nielsen OH (eds): Anti-Tumor Necrosis Factor Therapy in Inflammatory Bowel Disease.
Front Gastrointest Res. Basel, Karger, 2015, vol 34, pp 190–194 (DOI: 10.1159/000381603)

What Is the Right Dosage?

Pierre Michetti

Gastroenterology La Source-Beaulieu and Division of Gastroenterology, CHUV, Lausanne, Switzerland

Abstract

The optimal dosage of each anti-TNF agent is influenced by drug-specific as well as by disease-specific parameters, which play various roles in the pharmacodynamics of these drugs. The available data on infliximab, adalimumab and golimumab dose responses strongly suggest that the optimal initial dosing of these drugs could still be improved to better take into account individual patient and disease characteristics.

Introduction

The search for the optimal dosages of anti-TNF agents to treat inflammatory bowel disease started with the observation that higher doses are needed during induction and maintenance therapy to treat Crohn's disease (CD) compared with rheumatoid arthritis [1]. After an initial study indicated a 1 mg/kg body weight dose induced a less durable response than 5 or 10 mg/kg [2], Targan et al. [3] compared 5, 10 and 20 mg/kg infliximab in a landmark study that demonstrated the efficacy of infliximab in treating CD, but no clear dose-response relationship was observed across these dosages. Later studies, which have been recently reviewed, have confirmed that 5 mg/kg is the optimal dose for treating CD, administered with a loading regimen at weeks 0, 2 and 6 [4]. Despite years of clinical experience using infliximab and other anti-TNF agents to treat these conditions, the search for the optimal dosing regimen with the best risk/benefit ratio is still ongoing [5, 6].

In ulcerative colitis (UC), the issue of initial dosing has been evident since the first small clinical series of the use of infliximab, summarized at the time by Rutgeerts [7]. This issue expanded when subcutaneous forms of anti-TNF antibodies were introduced (adalimumab and golimumab).

The right dosage may no longer be seen as fixed because various dose escalation schedules may improve or restore responses in CD as well as in UC patients. Therefore, in this chapter, the initial dosing issues for infliximab, adalimumab and golimumab for the treatment of UC will be discussed. The use of trough levels to assist with dosing adjustments is certainly part of current treatment strategies for anti-TNF agents. However, trough levels are thus far only useful after induction because results are typically not available rapidly enough for initial patient management. Therefore, trough level-based management will not be discussed here because it is the focus of another chapter of this book by N. Vande Casteele.

Infliximab

Infliximab was the first anti-TNF agent tested to treat UC. In the first small randomized trial performed on 43 patients with steroid-refractory UC, 5 mg/kg infliximab at weeks 0 and 2, followed by 10 mg/kg open-label infliximab at week 6, did not induce remission more often than placebo [8]. However, the efficacy of infliximab was then demonstrated in two large randomized placebo-controlled trials (named ACT-1 and ACT-2), reported together by Rutgeerts et al. [9], which included 364 patients each. In these ACT trials, no differences were observed between the doses of 5 and 10 mg/kg administered at weeks 0, 2, 6 and every 8 weeks through week 46 (ACT-1) or through week 22 (ACT-2). Safety evaluations showed no differences among the different dose regimens. In a follow-up study of this large patient cohort, the colectomy rate was found to be lower in patients treated with infliximab compared to placebo, but again, there was no advantage of the higher dosing regimen [10]. In a recently published analysis of the whole patient populations of ACT-1 and ACT-2, a relationship between the serum concentration of infliximab and efficacy was observed in patients with moderate to severe UC [11]. More patients achieved higher quartiles of serum infliximab concentrations in the 10 mg/kg group compared to the 5 mg/kg group, but the efficacy did not appear to depend directly on the dose administered. The same relationship between serum concentration and efficacy has been confirmed in children [12].

These data suggest that the serum concentration of infliximab depends on factors other than the dose administered. In a prospective trial conducted in Sweden comparing the effects of 1 infusion of 5 mg/kg infliximab versus placebo on patients with acute severe colitis as well as in a cohort study of patients from Canada with moderate to severe UC treated with the standard infliximab regimen, greater efficacies were obtained in the less severely affected patients [13, 14], suggesting that disease burden may affect the response. Another factor influencing the serum concentration of infliximab may be a low serum albumin concentration, which affects FcRn-mediated antibody recycling, and thus, infliximab half-life [11, 15]. The serum infliximab concentration may, in turn, also depend on disease extension and/or severity. Finally, this concentration [16] and treatment outcome [17, 18] have been shown to be improved by the concomitant use of an immunosuppressant, but to date, there are no data suggesting that the initial or later dosing of infliximab may be altered in patients on combination therapy [17].

However, other studies have found a direct dose-response relationship for infliximab in UC. In a retrospective study performed to assess 41 patients with a secondary loss of response, dose intensification by doubling the injection dose to 10 mg/kg or reducing the dosing interval to 4–6 weeks restored response and remission in 90 and 46% of the patients, respectively [19].

Adalimumab

The use of adalimumab to treat UC was first limited to a small clinical series of patients who had lost response to infliximab or failed to tolerate this agent. The results were encouraging but suggested that a substantial minority of patients needed dose escalation [20, 21]. In the first large multicenter placebo-controlled clinical trial testing adalimumab safety and efficacy for treating UC, 390 patients were equally randomized to induction therapy at weeks 0 and 2 with 160/80 mg adalimumab, 80/40 mg adalimumab, or placebo [22]. At week 8, remission was obtained in 18.5% of the patients in the 160/80 mg group and in 10.0% of those in the 80/40 mg group compared with 9.2% of those in the placebo group. The difference was statistically significant versus placebo only for the higher induction dose regimen. The incidence rates of serious adverse events did not differ among the 3 groups. These results suggest that even higher doses of adalimumab are needed to achieve remission. Other aspects of the results seem to confirm this observation, such as the fact that efficacy was better in patients weighing less than 70 kg. Furthermore, the results were better in patients with less extensive disease and less inflammatory burden, also suggesting the presence of a better drug-to-target ratio in these patients [23]. In a second large randomized controlled trial, the efficacy of 160/80 mg adalimumab compared with placebo was confirmed in 494 patients with moderate to severe UC, but the 80/40 mg dose regimen was not included [24]. Overall, the results obtained using adalimumab to treat UC appear less impressive than those achieved with infliximab. Although a direct comparison of trials should not be considered conclusive, there are several reasons for the possible differences among the results reported for these two agents. The most obvious explanation involves the total TNF binding activity during the induction phase. Assuming that these two highly similar IgG1 antibodies have similar molecular weights, the difference between them would represent 730 mg for a 70 kg patient, which is more than twice the total amount of adalimumab administered during a 6-week induction period at the highest dose tested (320 mg). This low loading dose of adalimumab may play a more important role in UC than in CD because of the potential difference in the inflammatory burden in extensive colitis, in which a large mucosal surface may be inflamed. This difference may explain the higher rate of dose escalation observed in ULTRA-2 in patients who did not respond by week 8 to standard dosing compared to week 8 responders [25]. Other differences may affect the pharmacokinetics of these two drugs, but the magnitudes of these effects are likely to be much more limited in the average patient, especially during the induction phase, when anti-drug antibody development is still limited. These factors may play more prominent roles during maintenance therapy, when disease activity is less intense, explaining the good long-term results of adalimumab in patients who initially responded well to the medication [26, 27].

Golimumab

In contrast to infliximab and adalimumab, golimumab has been tested in UC without prior studies in CD. Thus, different dosing regimens have been directly assessed in this condition. Indeed, the first large randomized trial integrated double-blind phase 2 dose-finding and phase 3 dose-confirmation trials of a total of 1064 adults with UC (including 774 patients in the phase 3 trial) [28]. Patients were randomly assigned to groups and were given either placebo or golimumab doses of 100/50 mg (phase 2 only), 200/100 mg, or 400/200 mg, each 2 weeks apart. During the phase 2 part of the study, the median changes from baseline in the Mayo score were –1.0, –3.0, –2.0, and –3.0, respectively. During phase 3, the clinical response rates at week 6 were 51.0 and 54.9% among the patients given 200/100 mg and 400/200 mg golimumab, respectively, versus 30.3% for those given placebo (both $p \leq 0.0001$). The rates of serious adverse events and infections were low and were similar across all study groups. Golimumab (50 or 100 mg) maintained a clinical response through week 54 in the 464 patients who responded to induction therapy, but only patients who received 100 mg golimumab had clinical remission and mucosal healing at weeks 30 and 54 [29]. In a recent network meta-analysis, golimumab induction therapy was shown to be as efficacious as infliximab [30], further supporting the

Table 1. Characteristics and dosages of anti-TNF antibodies in ulcerative colitis

	Infliximab	Adalimumab	Golimumab
Brand name	Remicade	Humira	Simponi
Structure	Chimeric IgG1 kappa	Human IgG1 kappa	Human IgG1 kappa
Dosage in UC	5 mg/kg	160, 80 and 40 mg	200, 100 and 50 mg
Dosing schedule (weeks)	0, 2, 6 and every 8 weeks	0, 2 and every 2 weeks	0, 2, 4 and monthly
Dose escalation	10 mg/kg or every 4 weeks	40 mg weekly	100 mg monthly

argument that the initial binding activity should be regarded as an important parameter for the induction of a response to anti-TNF therapy in UC.

Conclusion

The right dosage of anti-TNF antibody for the treatment of UC depends on several factors, among which patient body weight, nutritional status and the burden of inflammation (disease extension and severity) play the most important roles. These parameters show more variability in UC than in CD, potentially explaining the less convincing data observed in the former condition. The initial dosing of adalimumab may in particular explain the suboptimal results observed with this drug in UC. Current recommendations for initial therapy and proposals for rescue dose escalation are presented in table 1. In the absence of convincing trough level management information during the induction phase of therapy, the highest evidence-based effective dose of each anti-TNF agent should be preferred.

References

1 Maini RN, Breedveld FC, Kalden JR, Smolen JS, Davis D, Macfarlane JD, Antoni C, Leeb B, Elliott MJ, Woody JN, Schaible TF, Feldmann M: Therapeutic efficacy of multiple intravenous infusions of anti-tumor necrosis factor alpha monoclonal antibody combined with low-dose weekly methotrexate in rheumatoid arthritis. Arthritis Rheum 1998;41:1552–1563.

2 McCabe RP, Woody J, vanDeventer S, Targan SR, Mayer L, vanHogezand R, Rutgeerts P, Hanauer SB, Podolsky D, Elson CO: A multicenter trial of cA2 anti-TNF chimeric monoclonal antibody in patients with active Crohn's disease. Gastroenterology 1996;110:A962.

3 Targan SR, Hanauer SB, van Deventer SJ, Mayer L, Present DH, Braakman T, DeWoody KL, Schaible TF, Rutgeerts PJ: A short-term study of chimeric monoclonal antibody cA2 to tumor necrosis factor alpha for Crohn's disease. Crohn's Disease cA2 Study Group. N Engl J Med 1997;337:1029–1035.

4 Kawalec P, Mikrut A, Wisniewska N, Pilc A: Tumor necrosis factor-alpha antibodies (infliximab, adalimumab and certolizumab) in Crohn's disease: systematic review and meta-analysis. Arch Med Sci 2013;9:765–779.

5 Armuzzi A, Lionetti P, Blandizzi C, Caporali R, Chimenti S, Cimino L, Gionchetti P, Girolomoni G, Lapadula G, Marchesoni A, Marcellusi A, Mennini FS, Salvarani C, Cimaz R: anti-TNF agents as therapeutic choice in immune-mediated inflammatory diseases: focus on adalimumab. Int J Immunopathol Pharmacol 2014;27:11–32.

6 Alten R, van den Bosch F: Dose optimization of infliximab in patients with rheumatoid arthritis. Int J Rheum Dis 2014;17:5–18.

7 Rutgeerts P: Infliximab for ulcerative colitis: the need for adequately powered placebo-controlled trials. Am J Gastroenterol 2002;97:2488–2489.

8 Probert CS, Hearing SD, Schreiber S, Kuhbacher T, Ghosh S, Arnott ID, Forbes A: Infliximab in moderately severe glucocorticoid resistant ulcerative colitis: a randomised controlled trial. Gut 2003;52:998–1002.

9 Rutgeerts P, Sandborn WJ, Feagan BG, Reinisch W, Olson A, Johanns J, Travers S, Rachmilewitz D, Hanauer SB, Lichtenstein GR, de Villiers WJ, Present D, Sands BE, Colombel JF: Infliximab for induction and maintenance therapy for ulcerative colitis. N Engl J Med 2005;353:2462–2476.

10 Sandborn WJ, Rutgeerts P, Feagan BG, Reinisch W, Olson A, Johanns J, Lu J, Horgan K, Rachmilewitz D, Hanauer SB, Lichtenstein GR, de Villiers WJ, Present D, Sands BE, Colombel JF: Colectomy rate comparison after treatment of ulcerative colitis with placebo or infliximab. Gastroenterology 2009;137:1250–1260; quiz 1520.

11 Adedokun OJ, Sandborn WJ, Feagan BG, Rutgeerts P, Xu Z, Marano CW, Johanns J, Zhou H, Davis HM, Cornillie F, Reinisch W: Association between serum concentration of infliximab and efficacy in adult patients with ulcerative colitis. Gastroenterology 2014;147:1296–1307.e5.

12 Adedokun OJ, Xu Z, Padgett L, Blank M, Johanns J, Griffiths A, Ford J, Zhou H, Guzzo C, Davis HM, Hyams J: Pharmacokinetics of infliximab in children with moderate-to-severe ulcerative colitis: results from a randomized, multicenter, open-label, phase 3 study. Inflamm Bowel Dis 2013;19:2753–2762.

13 Jarnerot G, Hertervig E, Friis-Liby I, Blomquist L, Karlen P, Granno C, Vilien M, Strom M, Danielsson A, Verbaan H, Hellstrom PM, Magnuson A, Curman B: Infliximab as rescue therapy in severe to moderately severe ulcerative colitis: a randomized, placebo-controlled study. Gastroenterology 2005;128:1805–1811.

14 Seow CH, Newman A, Irwin SP, Steinhart AH, Silverberg MS, Greenberg GR: Trough serum infliximab: a predictive factor of clinical outcome for infliximab treatment in acute ulcerative colitis. Gut 2010;59:49–54.

15 Fasanmade AA, Adedokun OJ, Olson A, Strauss R, Davis HM: Serum albumin concentration: a predictive factor of infliximab pharmacokinetics and clinical response in patients with ulcerative colitis. Int J Clin Pharmacol Ther 2010;48: 297–308.

16 Hayes MJ, Stein AC, Sakuraba A: Comparison of efficacy, pharmacokinetics, and immunogenicity between infliximab mono- versus combination therapy in ulcerative colitis. J Gastroenterol Hepatol 2014;29:1177–1185.

17 Panaccione R, Ghosh S, Middleton S, Marquez JR, Scott BB, Flint L, van Hoogstraten HJ, Chen AC, Zheng H, Danese S, Rutgeerts P: Combination therapy with infliximab and azathioprine is superior to monotherapy with either agent in ulcerative colitis. Gastroenterology 2014;146:392–400.e3.

18 Armuzzi A, Pugliese D, Danese S, Rizzo G, Felice C, Marzo M, Andrisani G, Fiorino G, Nardone OM, De Vitis I, Papa A, Rapaccini GL, Guidi L: Long-term combination therapy with infliximab plus azathioprine predicts sustained steroid-free clinical benefit in steroid-dependent ulcerative colitis. Inflamm Bowel Dis 2014;20:1368–1374.

19 Cesarini M, Katsanos K, Papamichael K, Ellul P, Lakatos PL, Caprioli F, Kopylov U, Tsianos E, Mantzaris GJ, Ben-Horin S, Danese S, Fiorino G: Dose optimization is effective in ulcerative colitis patients losing response to infliximab: a collaborative multicentre retrospective study. Dig Liver Dis 2014;46:135–139.

20 Afif W, Leighton JA, Hanauer SB, Loftus EV Jr, Faubion WA, Pardi DS, Tremaine WJ, Kane SV, Bruining DH, Cohen RD, Rubin DT, Hanson KA, Sandborn WJ: Open-label study of adalimumab in patients with ulcerative colitis including those with prior loss of response or intolerance to infliximab. Inflamm Bowel Dis 2009;15:1302–1307.

21 Peyrin-Biroulet L, Laclotte C, Roblin X, Bigard MA: Adalimumab induction therapy for ulcerative colitis with intolerance or lost response to infliximab: an open-label study. World J Gastroenterol 2007;13:2328–2332.

22 Reinisch W, Sandborn WJ, Hommes DW, D'Haens G, Hanauer S, Schreiber S, Panaccione R, Fedorak RN, Tighe MB, Huang B, Kampman W, Lazar A, Thakkar R: Adalimumab for induction of clinical remission in moderately to severely active ulcerative colitis: results of a randomised controlled trial. Gut 2011; 60:780–787.

23 Travis S. Does it all ADA up? Adalimumab for ulcerative colitis. Gut 2011;60: 741–742.

24 Sandborn WJ, van Assche G, Reinisch W, Colombel JF, D'Haens G, Wolf DC, Kron M, Tighe MB, Lazar A, Thakkar RB: Adalimumab induces and maintains clinical remission in patients with moderate-to-severe ulcerative colitis. Gastroenterology 2012;142:257–265.e1–e3.

25 Wolf D, D'Haens G, Sandborn WJ, Colombel JF, Van Assche G, Robinson AM, Lazar A, Zhou Q, Petersson J, Thakkar RB: Escalation to weekly dosing recaptures response in adalimumab-treated patients with moderately to severely active ulcerative colitis. Aliment Pharmacol Ther 2014;40:486–497.

26 Colombel JF, Sandborn WJ, Ghosh S, Wolf DC, Panaccione R, Feagan B, Reinisch W, Robinson AM, Lazar A, Kron M, Huang B, Skup M, Thakkar RB: Four-year maintenance treatment with adalimumab in patients with moderately to severely active ulcerative colitis: Data from ULTRA 1, 2, and 3. Am J Gastroenterol 2014;109:1771–1780.

27 Thorlund K, Druyts E, Mills EJ, Fedorak RN, Marshall JK: Adalimumab versus infliximab for the treatment of moderate to severe ulcerative colitis in adult patients naive to anti-TNF therapy: an indirect treatment comparison meta-analysis. J Crohns Colitis 2014;8:571–581.

28 Sandborn WJ, Feagan BG, Marano C, Zhang H, Strauss R, Johanns J, Adedokun OJ, Guzzo C, Colombel JF, Reinisch W, Gibson PR, Collins J, Jarnerot G, Hibi T, Rutgeerts P, Group P-SS. Subcutaneous golimumab induces clinical response and remission in patients with moderate-to-severe ulcerative colitis. Gastroenterology 2014;146:85–95; quiz e14–e15.

29 Sandborn WJ, Feagan BG, Marano C, Zhang H, Strauss R, Johanns J, Adedokun OJ, Guzzo C, Colombel JF, Reinisch W, Gibson PR, Collins J, Jarnerot G, Rutgeerts P, Group PU-MS. Subcutaneous golimumab maintains clinical response in patients with moderate-to-severe ulcerative colitis. Gastroenterology 2014;146:96–109.e1.

30 Danese S, Fiorino G, Peyrin-Biroulet L, Lucenteforte E, Virgili G, Moja L, Bonovas S: Biological agents for moderately to severely active ulcerative colitis: a systematic review and network meta-analysis. Ann Intern Med 2014;160: 704–711.

Pierre Michetti, MD
Gastro-entérologie La Source-Beaulieu
Avenue Jomini 8
CH–1004 Lausanne (Switzerland)
E-Mail pmichetti@gesb.ch

Rogler G, Herfarth H, Hibi T, Nielsen OH (eds): Anti-Tumor Necrosis Factor Therapy in Inflammatory Bowel Disease.
Front Gastrointest Res. Basel, Karger, 2015, vol 34, pp 195–200 (DOI: 10.1159/000381604)

Fistulizing and Stricturing Crohn's Disease

Alain M. Schoepfer

Division of Gastroenterology and Hepatology, Centre Hospitalier Universitaire Vaudois/CHUV, Lausanne, Switzerland

Abstract

Most Crohn's disease (CD) patients will develop a complicated disease characterized by the occurrence of intestinal strictures and/or internal and/or perianal fistulas during their lifetime. Such complicated disease may be associated with considerable morbidity and professional and personal disabilities. Options for treating fibrostenotic CD include endoscopic balloon dilation, strictureplasty, and surgery. Anti-TNF therapy can influence concomitantly present acute inflammatory changes but does not correct underlying fibrotic processes. Treatment of perianal fistulizing disease is based on antibiotics, immunomodulators and anti-TNF drugs. Surgical measures to treat perianal fistulas include drainage by means of setons, temporary ileostomy, or proctectomy. The presence of internal fistulas often necessitates surgical measures. A close collaboration between a gastroenterologist and surgeon is mandatory to solve these interdisciplinary challenges. This article discusses general treatment principles for stricturing and fistulizing CD, with a special focus on anti-TNF therapy.

Introduction

Crohn's disease (CD) can phenotypically present as either an inflammatory, a stricturing, or a penetrating form [1, 2]. At diagnosis, most CD patients have an inflammatory phenotype, with stenosing and fistulizing phenotypes developing over time [1, 2]. About 20–30% of CD patients present with perianal lesions at diagnosis. A study from the Mayo Clinic reported a fistula occurrence rate of 35% over time in these patients [3]. Of these fistulas, 54% were perianal, 24% were enteroenteric, 9% were rectovaginal, and 13% involved other locations (enterocutaneous, enterovesicular, and Intraabdominal fistulas). The authors found a cumulative fistula prevalence of 33% at 10 years and a prevalence of 50% at 20 years after CD diagnosis [3]. Perianal fistulas can manifest with persistent anal pain, purulent discharge, and painful stool expulsion. These symptoms may also represent the initial manifestations of CD [4]. Most commonly, fistulous openings are located in the perianal skin, but they can also be identified in the scrotum, vulva, or groin.

Perianal fistulas are classified as either simple or complex based on their anatomic extensions. Simple fistulas are located in the dentate line, have a single external opening, and are not painful, and they are not accompanied by a rectovaginal fistula or an anorectal stricture. In contrast, complex fistulas are located above the dentate line, may have multiple openings, and can be associated with an abscess, pain, the presence of a

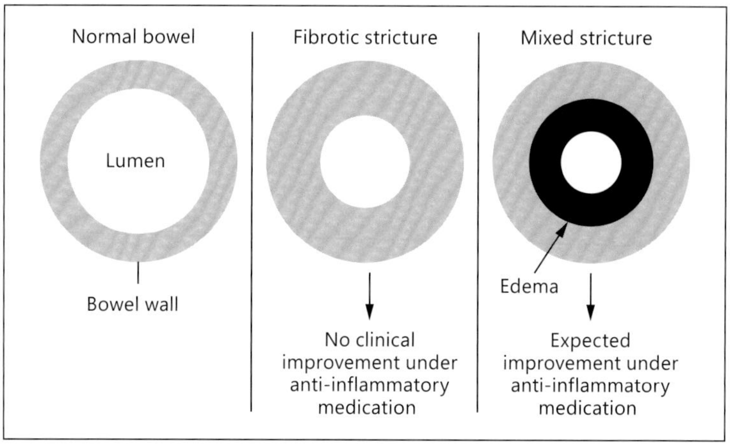

Fig. 1. The response of subocclusive symptoms to anti-inflammatory drugs depends on the stricture configuration. In the case of fibrotic strictures, no clinical improvement can be expected with anti-inflammatory medication, whereas improvement can be expected in the case of mixed strictures that share both inflammatory and fibrotic alterations.

rectovaginal fistula or an anorectal stricture or active rectal disease at endoscopy [5]. The risk of fistula development is higher in patients with colonic CD, particularly those with rectal involvement, compared with CD patients with isolated ileal disease [2]. Perianal fistulas are diagnosed by clinical examination and imaging (pelvic magnetic resonance imaging [MRI] is typically used) [6]. The activity of a perianal fistula can be measured using the perianal disease activity index, which evaluates five categories (discharge, pain, restriction of sexual activity, type of perianal disease, and degree of induration) [7]. Alternatively, the activity of a perianal fistula can be assessed by the finger compression technique (with the investigator using gentle finger compression), which detects a reduction of 50% in the number of draining fistulas observed at two or more consecutive visits [8]. Of note, the definition of 'response to therapy' for perianal CD fistula treatment varies from study to study. Thus, the particular methods to assess perianal disease activity should be taken into account when comparing different study results.

Nonperianal fistulas (such as enteroenteric, enterovesicular, and enterocutaneous fistulas) are diagnosed clinically and also using imaging techniques such as bowel MRI [6]. Randomized controlled data regarding the treatment of nonperianal fistulas are lacking. Fibrostenotic CD usually presents with symptoms of bowel obstruction (nausea, vomiting, and abdominal pain). CD-related strictures are mostly located in the ileocecal region [1, 2]. Active inflammation with edema accompanying a stricture may aggravate stricture-related symptoms. This review focuses on treatment strategies for fibrostenotic and fistulizing CD with particular emphasis on anti-TNF therapy.

Therapy of Stricturing Crohn's Disease

Options for treating stricturing (fibrostenotic) CD include anti-inflammatory medication, endoscopic balloon dilation and surgery.

Anti-Inflammatory Medication

CD patients with obstructive symptoms may improve following treatment with intravenous steroids for a short duration (3–4 days) [9]. The persistence of obstructive symptoms despite steroid use indicates the presence of fibrotic strictures without any relevant edema due to acute inflammation (fig. 1). Historically, bowel strictures have been considered to represent a contra-indication for treatment with anti-TNF drugs. However, patients with strictures composed of inflammatory and fibrotic features may benefit from infliximab (IFX) therapy (fig. 2) [10, 11]. Holtmann et al.

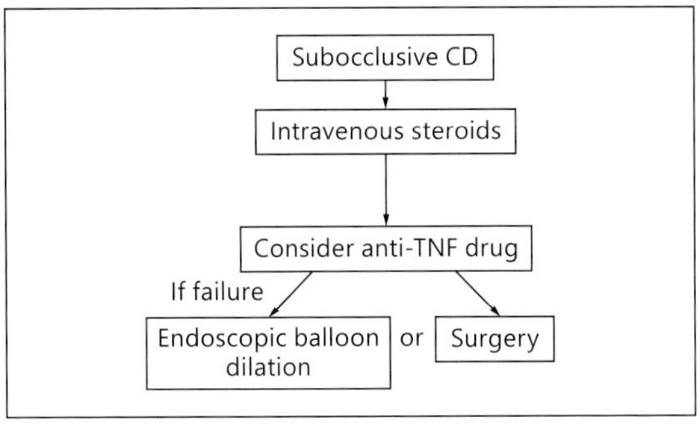

Fig. 2. Algorithm for the therapy of stricturing Crohn's disease. A clinical response to a short-duration therapy with intravenous steroids supports the presence of a mixed stricture with fibrotic and inflammatory features. These patients may profit from prolonged therapy with an anti-TNF drug. Only the use of infliximab for this particular indication has been reported.

retrospectively evaluated 21 CD patients treated with IFX, of whom 11 had inflammatory stenosis [12]. Nine of these patients responded well to IFX and became asymptomatic for a considerable period of time. Similarly, Pelletier et al. reported on a retrospective series of 14 CD patients with symptomatic strictures who were treated with IFX [13]. Of them, 8 patients were on maintenance IFX treatment at a median follow-up time of 18 months. The authors concluded that IFX therapy may be effective in patients with symptomatic strictures and should therefore be tested before considering surgery. Gasparetto et al. reported on IFX treatment in 7 pediatric CD patients with luminal strictures [14]. In 6 of these patients, the disappearance of inflammatory strictures was observed, whereas one child with ileal fibrotic stenosis required surgery [14]. Multivariate analyses of the TREAT registry and ACCENT I trial demonstrated that IFX treatment did not increase the likelihood of stenosis [15]. The literature search did not reveal any studies/case series involving the use of adalimumab or certolizumab pegol for the treatment of symptomatic stricturing CD. A treatment algorithm for fibrostenotic CD is presented in figure 2.

Endoscopic Balloon Dilatation, Strictureplasty, and Resective Surgery

Because a detailed discussion of endoscopic balloon dilatation, strictureplasty and resective surgery is outside of the scope of this article, we would like to refer to only a few key studies. Endoscopic balloon dilatation of CD-related intestinal strictures represents a nonsurgical alternative with a relatively low complication rate. Meta-analysis including 13 studies with a total of 347 CD patients who underwent balloon dilatation for mostly post-surgical strictures found that dilatation was technically successful in 86% of the patients and that clinical efficacy was achieved in 58% of the patients at a mean follow-up time of 33 months, with a major complication rate of 2% [16]. Thus, endoscopic balloon dilatation can represent a valuable alternative to surgery for CD patients suffering from short strictures [16].

Strictureplasty is feasible for short stenoses and yields similar results as bowel resection with respect to improvements in obstructive symptoms, the reoperation rate and the time interval to symptom recurrence [17, 18]. The question of whether intestinal resection is associated with longer recurrence-free survival compared to strictureplasty has not been clarified as of yet [19, 20].

Therapy of Perianal Fistulizing Crohn's Disease

Perianal fistulizing CD can be treated by different drugs and by surgical measures. No specific treatment may be required for asymptomatic simple perianal fistulas [5]. Therapy options for symptomatic simple perianal fistulas include noncutting seton or fistulotomy and antibiotics, such as metronidazole or ciprofloxacin [5]. Surgical treatment is generally recommended for complex perianal disease and includes abscess drainage and seton placement. Fistulectomy and fistulotomy should be used with caution given the risks of fecal incontinence [5]. Severe perianal disease refractory to any medical therapy may be treated using a diverting stoma or proctectomy.

The following drug categories are used for the treatment of complex perianal fistulas: antibiotics, immunomodulators (azathioprine/6-mercaptopurine and methotrexate), anti-TNF drugs (IFX, adalimumab, and certolizumab pegol), cyclosporine, and tacrolimus. This chapter will focus on anti-TNF drug treatment. Regarding the use of antibiotics, immunomodulators, and calcineurin inhibitors, we kindly refer to the guidelines of the European Crohn's and Colitis Organization [21].

Infliximab

Efficacy has been demonstrated with the use of IFX for the induction and maintenance of perianal fistula closure in randomized controlled trials. Treatment of simple and complex perianal fistulas with 5 mg/kg IFX at weeks 0, 2, and 6 induced complete fistula closure (defined as the cessation of all drainage observed at two visits 1 month apart) in 17/31 (55%) of patients [22]. In the ACCENT II trial, an initial response rate of 69% (195/306) was documented at week 14, and responders were randomized to receive 5 mg/kg every 8 weeks or placebo [23]. At week 54, 33/91 (36%) of patients on IFX experienced complete fistula closure compared to 19/98 (19%) of those on placebo ($p = 0.009$). Response, defined as >50% fistula closure on clinical assessment, was documented in 46% of patients on IFX compared to 23% of those on placebo ($p = 0.01$) [23]. Long-term efficacy data for the use of IFX to treat CD patients with perianal fistulas are limited. Bouguen et al. evaluated 156 CD patients who underwent IFX treatment for perianal fistulizing disease [24]. After a median follow-up time of 250 weeks, 108/156 (69%) of the patients had at least one fistula closure. The cumulative probabilities of first fistula closure were 40 and 65% at 1 and 5 years, respectively. Factors that predicted fistula closure were ileocolonic disease (hazard ratio [HR] = 1.88), concomitant immunosuppressant use (HR = 2.58), duration of seton drainage <34 weeks (HR = 2.31), and long duration of IFX treatment (HR = 1.76). Among the 108 patients with fistula closure, the cumulative probabilities of first fistula recurrence were 16.6 and 40.1% at 1 and 5 years, respectively [24].

Adalimumab

In the placebo-controlled CHARM trial, 117 of 778 CD patients had actively draining perianal fistulas [25, 26]. The patients were treated with 80 mg adalimumab at week 0 and 40 mg at week 2, and they were then randomized at week 4 to receive either 40 mg every 2 weeks, 40 mg weekly, or placebo. Patients with draining fistulas were evaluated for healing at weeks 26 and 56 as the secondary endpoint. Thirty percent (21/70) of all of the randomized patients on active adalimumab maintenance treatment had complete healing at both time points, compared with 13% (6/47) of those on placebo maintenance ($p < 0.04$). Of all the patients with healed fistulas at week 56, 90% (28/31) maintained fistula healing for 1 further year of open-label adalimumab therapy [27]. Dewint et al. performed a randomized, double-blind, placebo-controlled trial to evaluate the efficacy of adalimumab combined with ciprofloxacin (given twice daily at 500 mg for 12 weeks) versus adalimumab monotherapy for the treatment of fistulas in 76 CD patients with active perianal fistulizing disease [28]. The primary endpoint was clinical response, defined as a 50% reduction in fistulas from baseline to week 12. The secondary endpoint was remission, which was defined as the closure of all fistulas. Clinical response was observed in 71% of patients treated with adalimumab and ciprofloxacin compared to 47% of those treated with adalimumab and placebo ($p = 0.047$). Similarly, the remission rate at week 12 was significantly higher in the combination group compared to the adalimumab plus placebo group (65 vs. 33%, $p = 0.009$). Of note, there was no longer a difference in clinical response between the two treatment groups at week 24 ($p = 0.22$).

Certolizumab Pegol

Schreiber et al. evaluated patients from PRECiSE 2 (n = 108) with draining fistulas at baseline who received open-label induction with certolizumab pegol [29]. At week 6, responders (n = 58) were randomized to receive certolizumab or placebo every 4 weeks. A total of 55/58 patients suffered from perianal fistulas. At week 26, 36% of patients in the certolizumab pegol group had 100% fistula closure compared with 17% of those in the placebo group (p = 0.038). An open-label phase IV study of 60 CD patients demonstrated complete perianal fistula closure in 36% of the patients at week 6 and in 55% at week 26 [30].

Therapy of Nonperianal Fistulizing Crohn's Disease

The management of nonperianal fistulizing CD remains an interdisciplinary challenge. Of note, randomized trials studying treatment strategies for nonperianal fistulizing CD are lacking. Treatment options include medication (see above) and surgical procedures [5]. An in-depth review of nonperianal fistulizing CD is out of the focus of this review, and we therefore refer to comprehensive guidelines [5].

Conclusions and Future Directions

Most CD patients will experience a complication in the form of bowel strictures and/or fistulas (perianal or nonperianal) during their lifetime. In the case of sub-occlusive symptoms, a trial with intravenous steroids can be performed to find out if the patient has a mixed (fibrotic-inflammatory) stricture. Patients with a mixed stricture who respond to this trial may profit from anti-TNF therapy. Perianal fistulas should be drained by setons before anti-inflammatory drugs are started. IFX, adalimumab, and certolizumab pegol have demonstrated clinical efficacy in the treatment of perianal fistulizing CD. The treatment of internal fistulas represents an interdisciplinary challenge to gastroenterologists, radiologists, and surgeons.

References

1 Cosnes J, Cattan S, Blain A, Beaugerie L, Carbonnel F, Parc R, Gendre JP: Long-term evolution of disease behavior of Crohn's disease. Inflamm Bowel Dis 2002;8:244–250.

2 Cosnes J, Gower- Rousseau C, Seksik P, Cortot A: Epidemiology and natural history of inflammatory bowel diseases. Gastroenterology 2011;140:1785–1794.

3 Schwartz DA, Loftus EV Jr, Tremaine WJ, Panaccione R, Harmsen WS, Zinsmeister AR, Sandborn WJ: The natural history of fistulizing Crohn's disease in Olmsted County, Minnesota. Gastroenterology 2002;122:875–880.

4 Hellers G, Bergstrand O, Ewerth S, Holmström B: Occurrence and outcome after primary treatment of anal fistulae in Crohn's disease. Gut 1980;21:525–527.

5 Sandborn WJ, Fazio VW, Feagan BG, Hanauer SB: AGA technical review on perianal Crohn's disease. Gastroenterology 2003;125:1508–1530.

6 Van Assche G, Dignass A, Reinisch W, van der Woude CJ, Sturm A, De Vos A, Guslandi M, Oldenburg B, Dotan I, Marteau P, Ardizzone A, Baumgart DC, D'Haens G, Gionchetti P, Portela F, Vucelic B, Söderholm J, Escher J, Koletzko S, Kolho KL, Lukas M, Mottet C, Tilg H, Vermeire S, Carbonnel F, Cole A, Novacek G, Reinshagen M, Tsianos E, Herrlinger K, Oldenburg B, Bouhnik Y, Kiesslich R, Stange E, Travis S, Lindsay J; European Crohn's and Colitis Organisation (ECCO): The second European evidence-based consensus on the diagnosis and management of Crohn's disease: special situations. J Crohns Colitis 2010;4:63–101.

7 Irvine EJ: Usual therapy improves perianal Crohn's disease as measured by a new disease activity index. Mc Master IBD Study Group. J Clin Gastroenterol 1995;20:27–32.

8 Present DH, Rutgeerts P, Targan S, Hanauer SB, Mayer L, van Hogezand RA, Podolsky DK, Sands BE, Braakman T, DeWood KL, Schaibl TF, van Deventer SJ: Infliximab for the treatment of fistulas with Crohn's disease. N Engl J Med 1999;340:1398–1405.

9 Sandborn WJ, Feagan BG, Hanauer SB, Lochs H, Lofberg R, Modigliani R, Present DH, Rutgeerts P, Scholmerich J, Stange EF, Sutherland LR: A review of activity indices and efficacy endpoints for clinical trials of medical therapy in adults with Crohn's disease. Gastroenterology 2002;122:512–530.

10 Pelletier AL, Kalisazan B, Wienckiewicz J, Bouarioua N, Soulé JC: Infliximab treatment for symptomatic Crohn's disease strictures. Aliment Pharmacol Ther 2009;29:279–285.

11 Louis E, Boverie J, Dewit O, Baert F, De Vos M, D'Haens G; Belgian IBD Research Group: Treatment of small bowel subocclusive Crohn's disease with infliximab: an open pilot study. Acta Gastroenterol Belg 2007;70:15–19.

12 Holtmann M, Wanitschke R, Helisch A, Bartenstein P, Galle PR, Neurath M: Anti-TNF antibodies in the treatment of inflammatory intestinal stenoses in Crohn's disease. Z Gastroenterol 2003; 41:11–17.

13 Pelletier AL, Kalisazan B, Wienckiewicz J, Bouarioua N, Soulé JC: Infliximab treatment for symptomatic Crohn's disease strictures. Aliment Pharmacol Ther 2009;29:279–285.

14 Gasparetto M, Corradin S, Vallortigara F, Cananzi M, Guariso G: Infliximab and pediatric stricturing Crohn's disease: a possible alternative to surgery? Experience of seven cases. Acta Gastroenterolog Belg 2012;75:58–60.

15 Lichtenstein GR, Olson A, Travers S, Diamond RH, Chen DM, Pritchard ML, Feagan BG, Cohen RD, Salzberg BA, Hanauer SB, Sandborn WJ: Factors associated with the development of intestinal strictures or obstructions in patients with Crohn's disease. Am J Gastroenterol 2006;101:1030–1038.

16 Hassan C, Zullo A, De Francesco V, Ierardi E, Giustini M, Pitidis A, Taggi F, Winn S, Morini S: Systematic review: endoscopic dilatation in Crohn's disease. Aliment Pharmacol Ther 2007;26: 1457–1464.

17 Dietz DW, Laureti S, Strong SA, Hull TL, Church J, Remzi FJ, Lavery IC, Fazio VW: Safety and long-term efficacy of strictureplasty in 314 patients with obstruction small bowel Crohn's disease. J Am Coll Surg 2001;192:330–338.

18 Fearnhead NS, Chowdhury R, Box B, George BD, Jewell DP, Mortensen NJ: Long-term follow-up of strictureplasty for Crohn's disease. Br J Surg 2006;93: 475–482.

19 Yamamoto T, Fazio VW, Tekkis PP. Safety and efficacy of strictureplasty for Crohn's disease: a systematic review and meta-analysis. Dis Colon Rectum 2007; 50:1968–1986.

20 Fichera A, Lovadina S, Rubin M, Cimino F, Hurst RD, Michelassi F: Patterns and operative treatment of recurrent Crohn's disease: a prospective longitudinal study. Surgery 2006;140:649–654.

21 Dignass A, Van Assche G, Lindsay JO, Lémann M, Söderholm J, Colombel JF, Danese S, D'Hoore A, Gassull M, Gomollon F, Hommes DW, Michetti P, O'Morain C, Oresland T, Windsor A, Stange EF, Travis SPL; European Crohn's and Colitis Oreganisation (ECCO): The second European evidence-based consensus on the diagnosis and management of Crohn's disease: current management. J Crohns Colitis 2010;4:28–62.

22 Present DH, Rutgeerts P, Targan S, Hanauer SB, Mayer L, van Hogezand RA, Podolsky DK, Sands BE, Braakman T, DeWoody KL, Schaible TF, van Deventer SJ: Infliximab for the treatment of fistulas in patients with Crohn's disease. N Engl J Med 1999;340:1398–1405.

23 Sands BE, Anderson FH, Bernstein CN, Chey WY, Feagan BG, Fedorak RN, Kamm MA, Korzenik JR, Lashner BA, Wild G, Wolf DC, Marsters PA, Travers SB, Blank MA, van Deventer SJ: Infliximab maintenance therapy for fistulazing Crohn's disease. N Engl J Med 2004; 350:876–885.

24 Bouguen G, Siproudhis L, Gizard E, Wallenhorst T, Billioud V, Bretagne JF, Bigard MA, Peyrin-Biroulet L: Clin Gastroenterol Hepatol 2013;11:975–981.

25 Colombel JF, Sandborn WJ, Rutgeerts P, Enns R, Hanauer SB, Panaccione R, Schreiber S, Byczkowski D, Li J, Kent JD, Pollack PF: Adalimumab for maintenance of clinical response and remission in patients with Crohn's disease: the CHARM Trial. Gastroenterology 2007;132:52–65.

26 Colombel JF, Schwartz DA, Sandborn WJ, Kamm MA, D'Haens G, Rutgeerts P, Enns R, Panaccione R, Schreiber S, Li J, Kent JD, Lomax KG, Pollack PF: Adalimumab for the treatment of fistulas in patients with Crohn's disease. Gut 2009; 5:940–948.

27 Colombel JF, Schwartz DA, Sandborn WJ, Kamm MA, D'Haens G, Rutgeerts P, Enns R, Panaccione R, Schreiber S, Li J, Kent JD, Lomax KG, Pollack PF: Adalimumab for the treatment of fistulas in patients with Crohn's disease. Gut 2009;5:940–948.

28 Dewint P, Hansen BE, Verhey E, Oldenburg B, Hommes DW, Peirik M, Ponsioen CI, van Dullemen HM, Russel M, van Bodegraven AA, van der Woude CJ: Adalimumab combined with ciprofloxacin is superior to adalimumab monotherapy in perianal fistula closure in Crohn's disease: a randomized, double-blind, placebo controlled study (ADAFI). Gut 2014;63:292–299.

29 Schreiber S, Lawrance IC, Thomsen O, Hanauer SB, Bloomfield R, Sandborn WJ: Randomised clinical trial: certolizumab pegol for fistulas in Crohn's disease – subgroup results from a placebo-controlled study. Aliment Pharmacol Ther 2011;33:185–193.

30 Vavricka SR, Schoepfer AM, Bansky G, Binek J, Felley C, Geyer M, Manz M, Rogler G, de Saussure P, Sauter B, Scharl M, Seibold F, Straumann A, Michetti P; Swiss IBDnet: Efficacy and safety of certolizumab pegol in an unselected Crohn's disease population: 26-week data of the FACTS II survey. Inflamm Bowel Dis 2011;17:1530–1539.

Alain M. Schoepfer, MD
Division of Gastroenterology and Hepatology
Centre Hospitalier Universitaire Vaudois/CHUV, Rue de Bugnon 44, 07/2409
CH–1011 Lausanne (Switzerland)
E-Mail Alain.schoepfer@chuv.ch

Rogler G, Herfarth H, Hibi T, Nielsen OH (eds): Anti-Tumor Necrosis Factor Therapy in Inflammatory Bowel Disease.
Front Gastrointest Res. Basel, Karger, 2015, vol 34, pp 201–205 (DOI: 10.1159/000381606)

Postoperative Anti-TNF Therapy in the Management of Crohn's Disease

Arthur Barrie · Miguel Regueiro

Inflammatory Bowel Disease Center and Division of Gastroenterology, Hepatology and Nutrition, University of Pittsburgh Medical Center, Pittsburgh, Pa., USA

Abstract

The management of postoperative Crohn's disease has evolved over the years. Historically, treatment was initiated for recurrent symptoms, i.e. clinical recurrence. Later, it was determined that endoscopic Crohn's disease recurrence was quite common and clinically silent. An era of postoperative prevention trials followed, involving the evaluation of medications, such as 5-aminosalicylates, antibiotics, and thiopurine analogs. In the past decade, there have been a number of postoperative prevention studies investigating anti-tumor necrosis factor (TNF) drugs. The type of patient who would benefit from and the timing of postoperative anti-TNF therapy remain unclear. In this review, the evidenced-based data for postoperative anti-TNF treatment is summarized, and a suggested approach to postoperative patient management is provided.

The postoperative recurrence of Crohn's disease has historically been inevitable for the vast majority of patients. However, the introduction of prophylactic anti-tumor necrosis factor (TNF) therapy after surgery has been proven to be one of the most important advances in the care of Crohn's disease patients in the last 10 years. In the prebiologic era, natural history studies have found that 70–90% of Crohn's disease patients develop endoscopic evidence of recurrent disease within 1 year of surgery and that 30–60% become symptomatic within 3–5 years of surgery [1–3]. Consequently, 50% of these patients require repeat surgery within 5 years of their first surgery. Standard medical therapies, including antibiotics, aminosalicylates, and immunomodulators, have been shown to only modestly reduce the risk of clinical and endoscopic disease recurrence. In contrast, growing evidence demonstrates that anti-TNF therapy is effective for suppressing disease recurrence and may have the potential to change the natural course of the disease after surgery (table 1).

Sorrentino et al. first reported the successful use of prophylactic anti-TNF therapy with infliximab to treat a Crohn's colitis patient after partial colonic resection, who went on to have a disease-free course for at least 4 years after surgery [4]. The group went on to perform a prospective pilot study comparing infliximab (5 mg/kg every 8 weeks) plus methotrexate (10 mg/week by mouth) versus mesalamine (2.4 g/day) to prevent postoperative recurrent disease [5]. Their study population consisted mostly of patients with stricturing ileocolonic Crohn's disease undergoing

Table 1. Postoperative Crohn's disease prevention trials investigating the rate of endoscopic recurrence with anti-TNF therapy versus control

	anti-TNF, %	Control, %
Sorrentino et al. [5] (MTX/IFX vs. 5ASA 2 years)	0	100 (5ASA)
Regueiro et al. [6] (IFX vs. PBO RCT 1 year)	9	85 (PBO)
Yoshida et al. [7] (IFX vs. PBO open 1 year)	21	81 (5ASA)
Armuzzi et al. [8] (IFX vs. AZA open 1 year)	9	40 (AZA)
Fernandez-Blanco et al. [19] (ADA)	10	N/A
Papamichael et al. [9] (ADA 6 months)	0	N/A
Savarino et al. [10] (ADA 3 years)	0	N/A
Aguas et al. [7] (ADA 1 year)	21	N/A
De Cruz et al. [20] (ADA vs. AZA 6 months)	6	38 (AZA)
Savarino et al. [11] (ADA vs. AZA vs. 5ASA 2 years)	6	65 (AZA), 83 (5ASA)

5ASA = 5-aminosalicylic acid; AZA = azathioprine; IFX = infliximab; MTX = methotrexate; PBO = placebo; RCT = randomized controlled trial.

their first surgery who were at moderate risk of disease recurrence based on age, disease duration, penetrating complications, surgical history and cigarette smoking status. The investigators reported that none of the 7 patients treated with infliximab and methotrexate had clinical or endoscopic recurrent disease at 2 years after surgery compared to 75% of the patients (n = 16) treated with only mesalamine.

Regueiro et al. subsequently performed the first randomized placebo-controlled trial examining the ability of anti-TNF therapy using infliximab (5 mg/kg every 8 weeks) to prevent the endoscopic recurrence of Crohn's disease at 1 year after ileal resection [6]. In a relatively small study of patients with ileal or ileocolonic disease at moderate to high risk of disease recurrence, the rate of endoscopic recurrence, defined by a Rutgeerts postoperative score of i2 or higher, was significantly lower in infliximab-treated patients (9.1%, n = 11) compared to placebo-treated patients (84.6%, n = 13) (p = 0.0006). Several follow-up randomized studies have verified that infliximab prevents recurrent disease. A 3-year randomized open trial of moderate-risk patients conducted by Yoshida et al. revealed that 21.4% of patients (n = 14) treated with infliximab (5 mg/kg every 8 weeks) had endoscopic recurrent disease at 1 year after ileocolonic or ileal resection compared to 81.3% of patients (n = 16) on no treatment (p = 0.004) [7]. Armuzzi et al. compared infliximab and azathioprine in a 1-year randomized open-label trial of high-risk patients and found that 9% of infliximab-treated patients (n = 11) had endoscopic recurrence compared to 40% of azathioprine-treated patients (n = 10) (p = 0.14) [8].

The protective effect of infliximab appears to be a class effect of TNF inhibitors and not a drug-specific effect because adalimumab has also been proven to prevent postoperative recurrent disease. Papamichael et al. published an open-label, 2-year study in which eight Crohn's patients at moderate to high risk of disease recurrence were treated with adalimumab (40 mg sc qowk) after ileocolonic resection [9]. After 2 years of treatment, 75% of the treated patients (n = 8) were in complete or near complete endoscopic remission. Savarino et al. published a case series demonstrating that adalimumab (40 mg sc qowk) prevented recurrent disease in 6 patients at moderate risk of recurrence for up to 3 years after surgery [10]. They subsequently performed a randomized three-armed controlled study comparing the efficacies of adalimumab (40 mg sc qowk), azathioprine (2 mg/kg/day), and mesalamine (3 g/day) for the prevention of postoperative recurrence in Crohn's patients at moderate to high risk after ileocolonic resection [11]. They found that adalimumab significantly lowered the rate of endoscopic and clinical recurrence at 2 years after surgery compared to azathioprine and mesalamine. Only 1 of 15 (6.3%) adalimumab-treated patients developed endoscopic recurrent disease during the follow-up period compared with 64.7% of the azathioprine-treated patients (n = 17) and 83.3% of the mesalamine-treated patients (n = 18) (p = 0.0017). Similar rates of clinical recurrence and statistical significance were found among the groups.

The efficacy of prophylactic anti-TNF therapy for the prevention of postoperative Crohn's disease recurrence has been supported by the studies that have been conducted to date. Postoperative natural history studies have taught us that most *but not all* of these patients develop recurrent disease. Thus, initiating anti-TNF therapy in all postoperative Crohn's disease patients would certainly result in the over treatment of a subset. Relevant to this concern, it is not known whether prophylactic anti-TNF therapy is more effective than waiting to treat recurrent disease. Yamamoto et al. investigated the impact of infliximab therapy on Crohn's disease patients who were in clinical remission but had endoscopic recurrent disease at 6 months after ileocolonic resection despite prophylactic mesalamine therapy (3 g/day) [12]. Eight of these patients were started on infliximab (5 mg/kg every 8 weeks), another eight were started on azathioprine (50 mg/day), and the remainder was maintained only on mesalamine. This group found that infliximab induced complete endoscopic remission in 38% of the patients at 6 months after starting treatment compared to only 13% of the azathioprine-treated patients and 0% of the mesalamine-treated patients (p = 0.10). Sorrentino et al. found similar results following the treatment of patients with endoscopic disease at 6 months after surgery with either infliximab (5 mg/kg every 8 weeks) or mesalamine (2.4 g/day) [13]. Fifty-four percent of the infliximab-treated patients (n = 13) were in endoscopic remission at 1 year after starting treatment compared to 0% of the mesalamine-treated patients (n = 11) (p = 0.01). Adalimumab appears to be equally effective in treating early recurrent disease, as Papamichael et al. showed that adalimumab promoted endoscopic healing in 60% of treated patients (n = 15) who had endoscopic disease at 6 months after surgery [9]. Overall, these studies suggest that anti-TNF therapy may be effective for the treatment of early recurrent disease in certain patients.

The risks versus benefits of continuing prophylactic anti-TNF therapy for patients in long-term remission have also been called into question considering the cost of treatment and the potential for rare, but serious, side effects. Long-term safety data for the use of infliximab for the treatment of Crohn's disease demonstrate that infliximab therapy is associated with a moderate risk of infection but that it does not increase the risk of mortality or malignancy [14, 15]. The same study has found that severe Crohn's disease and prednisone and narcotic use are associated with a higher risk of infection than infliximab therapy; thus, one could argue that the benefits of infliximab in the prevention of severe recurrent disease outweigh the infection risk. In our postoperative infliximab study, we found no increased risk of adverse events in infliximab-treated patients compared to placebo-treated patients, including postoperative complications, up to 1 year after surgery [16]. Preventive anti-TNF therapy has been found to be relatively safe in other postoperative studies, including a study of adalimumab conducted by Savarino et al., who reported that adalimumab-treated patients had fewer adverse events than azathioprine- and mesalamine-treated patients over a 2-year follow-up period [11].

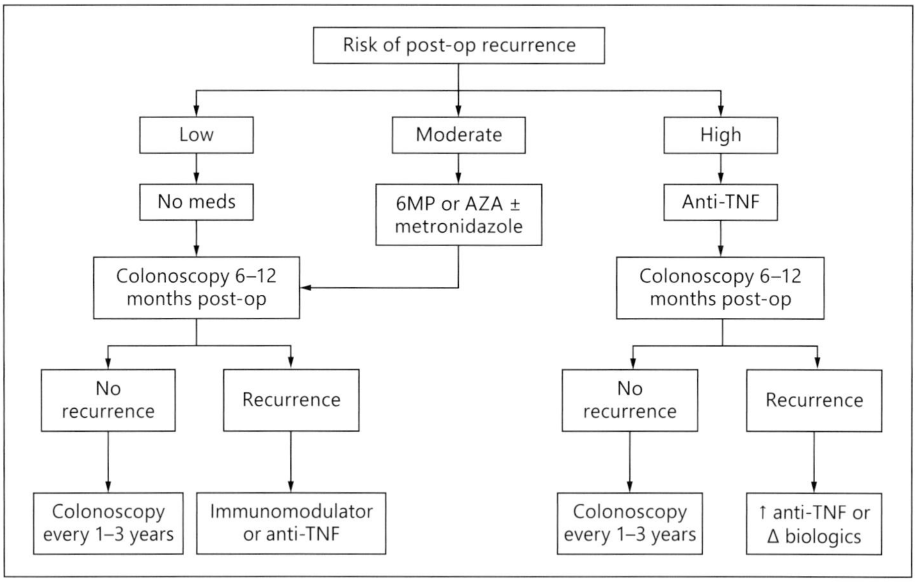

Fig. 1. Proposed treatment algorithm for the management of postoperative Crohn's disease. A low risk of postoperative recurrence was defined by longstanding Crohn's disease, 1st surgery, and short stricture. A moderate risk was defined by a less than 10-year history of Crohn's disease, long stricture and/or inflammatory disease. A high risk was defined by penetrating disease and/or 2 or more surgeries.

In contrast, the risks of stopping postoperative anti-TNF therapy appear to be higher than those of continuing treatment because we have found that patients in remission who stop infliximab are at a high risk of recurrent disease. After the completion of our 1-year study, we permitted patients to discontinue (or start) infliximab and followed them for an additional 5 years [17]. Eight of the original 11 infliximab-treated patients chose to stop therapy, and all 8 developed endoscopic recurrent disease, and 5 subsequently required repeat surgery. The 3 other original infliximab-treated patients continued their treatment, and none required repeat surgery during the study period. Twelve of the original 13 placebo patients had recurrence and chose to start infliximab, 7 of whom achieved endoscopic remission and required no repeat surgery during the study period. Overall, we found that patients who were treated with infliximab for at least 60% of the 5-year study period had a significantly lower risk of repeat surgery irrespective of their original treatment assignment (20.0 vs. 64.3%, p = 0.047). Sorrentino et al. found a similar high risk of recurrence, reporting that 83% of patients (n = 12), who were previously in remission for 3 years after surgery on infliximab developed endoscopic recurrent disease at 16 weeks after stopping treatment [18].

The following questions remain in the practical management of postoperative Crohn's disease: (1) which patients should receive immediate postoperative anti-TNF?; and (2) for which patients would it be reasonable to wait to treat endoscopic recurrence? In our practice, we target patients at high risk of postoperative recurrence for anti-TNF therapy (fig. 1). We start an anti-TNF agent within 4 weeks of surgery for patients with penetrating/fistulizing disease or those with 2 or more surgeries. We also consider patients who have progressed to surgery despite immunomodulator treatment as candidates for postoperative anti-TNF therapy. Waiting for endoscopic recurrence would be an alternative strategy for these patients, but more data are required. Ideally, we would like a noninvasive test that accurately identifies the earliest sign of postoperative Crohn's disease recurrence and a treatment that when started, completely heals the bowel. Until then, we recommend postoperative anti-TNF therapy for patients at high risk of recurrence.

Grant Support

None.

References

1 Rutgeerts P, Geboes K, Vantrappen G, et al: Predictability of the postoperative course of Crohn's disease. Gastroenterology 1990;99:956–963.
2 Olaison G, Smedh K, Sjodahl R: Natural course of Crohn's disease after ileocolic resection: endoscopically visualised ileal ulcers preceding symptoms. Gut 1992; 33:331–335.
3 Sachar DB: The problem of postoperative recurrence of Crohn's disease. Med Clin North Am 1990;74:183–188.
4 Sorrentino D, Terrosu G, Avellini C, et al: Prevention of postoperative recurrence of Crohn's disease by infliximab. Eur J Gastroenterol Hepatol 2006;18: 457–459.
5 Sorrentino D, Terrosu G, Avellini C, et al: Infliximab with low-dose methotrexate for prevention of postsurgical recurrence of ileocolonic Crohn disease. Arch Intern Med 2007;167:1804–1807.
6 Regueiro M, Schraut W, Baidoo L, et al: Infliximab prevents Crohn's disease recurrence after ileal resection. Gastroenterology 2009;136:441–450.e1; quiz 716.
7 Yoshida K, Fukunaga K, Ikeuchi H, et al: Scheduled infliximab monotherapy to prevent recurrence of Crohn's disease following ileocolic or ileal resection: a 3-year prospective randomized open trial. Inflamm Bowel Dis 2012;18:1617–1623.
8 Armuzzi A, Felice C, Papa A, et al: Prevention of postoperative recurrence with azathioprine or infliximab in patients with Crohn's disease: an open-label pilot study. J Crohns Colitis 2013;7:e623–e629.
9 Papamichael K, Archavlis E, Lariou C, et al: Adalimumab for the prevention and/ or treatment of post-operative recurrence of Crohn's disease: a prospective, two-year, single center, pilot study. J Crohns Colitis 2012;6:924–931.
10 Savarino E, Dulbecco P, Bodini G, et al: Prevention of postoperative recurrence of Crohn's disease by Adalimumab: a case series. Eur J Gastroenterol Hepatol 2012;24:468–470.
11 Savarino E, Dulbecco P, Bodini G, et al: Adalimumab is more effective than azathioprine and mesalamine at preventing postoperative recurrence of Crohn's disease: a randomized controlled trial. Am J Gastroenterol 2013;108:1731–1742.
12 Yamamoto T, Umegae S, Matsumoto K: Impact of infliximab therapy after early endoscopic recurrence following ileocolonic resection of Crohn's disease: a prospective pilot study. Inflamm Bowel Dis 2009;15:1460–1466.
13 Sorrentino D, Terrosu G, Paviotti A, et al: Early diagnosis and treatment of postoperative endoscopic recurrence of Crohn's disease: partial benefit by infliximab – a pilot study. Dig Dis Sci 2012; 57:1341–1348.
14 Lichtenstein GR, Feagan BG, Cohen RD, et al: Drug therapies and the risk of malignancy in Crohn's disease: results from the TREAT Registry. Am J Gastroenterol 2014;109:212–223.
15 Lichtenstein GR, Feagan BG, Cohen RD, et al: Serious infection and mortality in patients with Crohn's disease: more than 5 years of follow-up in the TREAT registry. Am J Gastroenterol 2012;107:1409–1422.
16 Regueiro M, El-Hachem S, Kip KE, et al: Postoperative infliximab is not associated with an increase in adverse events in Crohn's disease. Dig Dis Sci 2011;56: 3610–3615.
17 Regueiro M, Kip KE, Baidoo L, et al: Postoperative therapy with infliximab prevents long-term Crohn's disease recurrence. Clin Gastroenterol Hepatol 2014;12:1494–1502.e1.
18 Sorrentino D, Paviotti A, Terrosu G, et al: Low-dose maintenance therapy with infliximab prevents postsurgical recurrence of Crohn's disease. Clin Gastroenterol Hepatol 2010;8:591–599.e1; quiz e78–e79.
19 Fernández-Blanco I, Monturiol J, Martinez B, et al: Adalimumab in the prevention of postoperative recurrence of Crohn's disease. Gastroenterology 2010; 138:S692.
20 De Cruz P, Kamm MA, Hamilton AL, et al: Adalimumab prevents post-operative Crohn's disease recurrence, and is superior to thiopurines: early results from the POCER Study. Gastroenterology 2012;142:S212.

Miguel Regueiro, MD, Professor of Medicine
University of Pittsburgh School of Medicine, Co-Director, Inflammatory Bowel Disease Center
Division of Gastroenterology, Hepatology and Nutrition, University of Pittsburgh Medical Center
200 Lothrop Street, PUH-C Wing Mezzanine Level
Pittsburgh, PA 15213 (USA)
E-Mail mdr7@pitt.edu

Rogler G, Herfarth H, Hibi T, Nielsen OH (eds): Anti-Tumor Necrosis Factor Therapy in Inflammatory Bowel Disease.
Front Gastrointest Res. Basel, Karger, 2015, vol 34, pp 206–213 (DOI: 10.1159/000381607)

Anti-TNF-α Therapy for Extraintestinal Manifestations of Inflammatory Bowel Disease

Ole Haagen Nielsen[a] • Klaus Bendtzen[b] • Jannie Pedersen[a]

[a]Department of Gastroenterology, Medical Section, Herlev Hospital, Herlev, and [b]Institute for Inflammation Research, Rigshospitalet, University of Copenhagen, Copenhagen, Denmark

Abstract

The introduction of biological tumor necrosis factor (TNF)-α inhibitors has transformed the paradigm for the treatment of inflammatory bowel disease (IBD), i.e. Crohn's disease and ulcerative colitis. The specific TNF inhibitors currently approved for patients with IBD are infliximab, adalimumab and certolizumab pegol for Crohn's disease refractory to conventional treatment and infliximab, adalimumab, and golimumab for ulcerative colitis. Additionally, many patients with IBD have extraintestinal manifestations, and biological TNF inhibitors have also been shown to be of therapeutic benefit for these patients. The present chapter highlights these indications.

Introduction

Inflammatory bowel disease (IBD) encompasses multiple specific disorders, of which Crohn's disease (CD) and ulcerative colitis (UC) are the two prevailing entities [1, 2]. Included in the IBD disease spectrum are, however, various extraintestinal manifestations (EIMs) that vary from mild and transitory to severe and that are sometimes even more debilitating than the underlying intestinal disease itself [3]. Almost every organ system may be affected in IBD, including the musculoskeletal system, the skin, the eyes, the liver, the biliary tract, the lungs, the kidneys, and the hematologic and cardiovascular systems [3–8], suggesting that IBD may be a systemic disorder with predominantly bowel manifestations [9, 10]. EIMs are seen in up to 40% of patients with IBD depending on the study population and definitions used [11–15], and successful treatment of EIMs is therefore essential for improving the quality of life of many IBD patients [16].

Frequently occurring EIMs are immune mediated and are found in multiple organs like the spine (ankylosing spondylitis), the skin (erythema nodosum or pyoderma gangrenosum) and the eyes (uveitis or (epi)scleritis) (fig. 1). Others are associated with autoimmunity (e.g., primary sclerosing cholangitis) [3], whereas additional EIMs such as decreased mineral density, gallstones and kidney stones are considered to be driven by metabolic and nutritional consequences of malabsorption and/or chronic use of glucocorticoids [3]. Finally, EIMs may be a result of in-

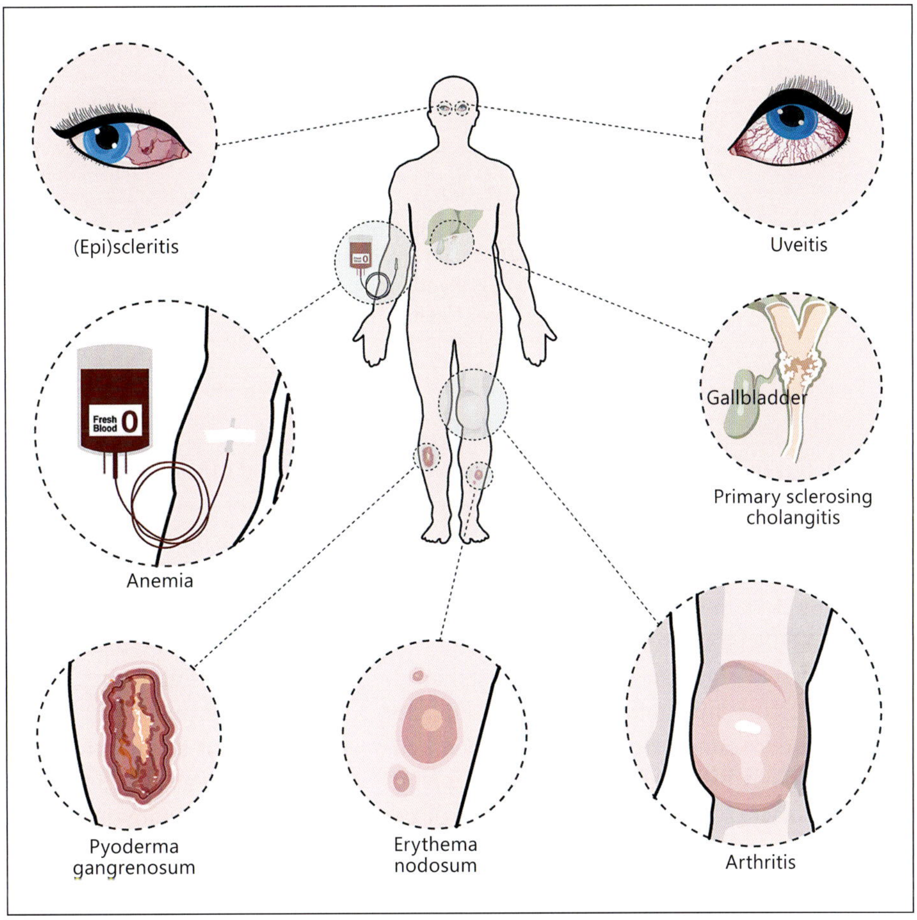

Fig. 1. Extraintestinal manifestations in inflammatory bowel disease that might be considered for treatment with biological TNF inhibitors.

testinal bacterial overgrowth and iatrogenic complications of therapy.

The resolution of EIMs most often parallels the course of IBD in terms of both timing and therapy required. These are therefore designated as 'inflammatory', although some EIMs, including axial arthritis, pyoderma gangrenosum, uveitis, and primary sclerosing cholangitis, seem to run a clinical course that is independent of IBD activity [6, 17]. The cumulative probability of developing EIMs increases with the duration of IBD [18], and in a large series of studies, the prevalence of EIMs is higher in CD than in UC [6, 19].

The introduction of biological tumor necrosis factor (TNF)-α inhibitors, including infliximab, adalimumab and certolizumab pegol in CD and infliximab, adalimumab and golimumab in UC, has proved to be one of the most significant advances in the care of IBD patients [20, 21]. The evidence in favor of TNF inhibitors for the treatment of IBD and their off-label use according to the approved indications for immune-mediated EIMs of IBD strongly support the use of biologics in the clinical setting and imply that the pathogenesis of intestinal and extraintestinal inflammation in IBD share common TNF-dependent mechanisms

Table 1. Extraintestinal manifestations (EIM) of IBD responding to biological TNF inhibitors categorized as associated with intestinal disease activity, independent of intestinal disease activity or 'paradoxical'

EIMs		
Associated with active IBD	Independent of IBD activity	TNF inhibitor-related (paradoxical)
Anemia	Axial arthropathy (i.e. sacroiliitis and ankylosing spondylitis)	Psoriasiform eczema
Peripheral arthropathy	Pyoderma gangrenosum	Eczema
Erythema nodosum	Uveitis	Xerosis cutis
(Epi)scleritis	Primary sclerosing cholangitis	Drug-induced lupus
		Arthralgia

(table 1). It is indeed likely that TNF is an essential proinflammatory mediator of an IBD-associated systemic immune response [22] and, therefore, that selective inhibition of this cytokine could at least partly explain the observed systemic benefits of anti-TNF therapies in these conditions.

Our current understanding suggests that although intestinal inflammation is a consequence of an abnormal immune response to environmental agents (likely bacterial) in genetically susceptible individuals [2, 23], further interaction of genetic predisposition with the response to luminal microbes might result in EIMs. It remains unclear, however, why the IBD phenotype includes so many EIMs, in what way disease pathogenesis is overlapping between IBD and EIM, and why certain patients develop a particular EIM whereas others do not.

Anemia is considered to be the most frequent EIM for both CD and UC (in up to 74% of patients with IBD) [24]. Arthritis is seen in 33 and 21% of CD and UC cases, respectively. The most common skin manifestations are erythema nodosum in 6 and 3% of CD and UC cases, respectively, pyoderma gangrenosum in 2% for both conditions, and psoriasis in 2 and 1% of CD and UC cases, respectively [6]. Risk factors include female gender and the severity of accompanying IBD.

Biological agents such as genetically engineered anti-TNF antibody constructs hold considerable promise for the management of IBD and several associated EIMs, and early administration of these agents is of great importance for preventing significant morbidity. However, EIMs occasionally occur as a result of biological therapy, i.e., paradoxical inflammation. For example, important drug-induced complications including lupus, psoriasis, and arthralgia may require discontinuation of the current therapy.

The aim of this article is to provide an update (July 2014) of the use of biological TNF inhibitors for EIMs accompanying IBD.

Extraintestinal Manifestations in Different Organs

Anemia

Anemia and iron deficiency are the most common EIMs of IBD at the time of both diagnosis and flares [24]. Anemia is more common in CD than in UC; women with CD are particularly at risk of anemia [25].

Iron deficiency without anemia is even more common than anemia and might subsequently lead to anemia [26]. The prevalence of iron deficiency without anemia in IBD patients ranges from 36 to 90% depending on the definition of iron deficiency and the type of study [27]. Notwithstanding, this condition may be considered as the rule rather than the exception in this setting, especially during disease flares.

Anemia in IBD is multifactorial and may occur as a result of blood loss from inflamed intestinal areas combined with impaired iron absorption and of the sequelae of inflammation, which hampers the availability of iron for erythropoiesis and erythroid progenitor cell proliferation [28–30]. In general, anemia found in patients with IBD is termed *'anemia of chronic disease'* and is more prevalent in subjects with complicated disease and in those insufficiently responding to therapy [30]. Interestingly, TNF may be directly involved in the pathophysiology of anemia of chronic disease, as it inhibits hepcidin, an important regulator of iron homeostasis [29]. Anemia in IBD may also be induced by drugs used to treat IBD, by vitamin deficiencies, or, more rarely, by various other factors such as renal insufficiency or hemolysis [31]. In general, treatment with TNF inhibitors might diminish the inflammatory burden [20] and lower the hepcidin levels, thereby normalizing the iron load and the hemoglobin levels, thus relieving anemia [32, 33].

Musculoskeletal Manifestations

IBD-associated or enteropathic arthropathy belongs to a group of seronegative inflammatory spondyloarthropathies, which include ankylosing spondylitis, reactive arthritis, psoriatic arthritis and undifferentiated spondyloarthropathy [34]. These conditions usually present as back pain due to sacroiliitis or ankylosing spondylitis. IBD patients are, however, also prone to the development of peripheral arthropathy. These musculoskeletal manifestations, which occur in up to 46% of IBD patients, may be accompanied by osteoporosis and widespread pain (fibromyalgia). They typically involve large joints in a pauci-articular, asymmetrical and migratory pattern and are often associated with relapses of IBD [34–36]. In contrast, the development and remission of axial arthropathy is frequently independent of the IBD state. IBD-related sacroiliitis is observed in 20–25% of patients, whereas HLA-B27-positive and -negative ankylosing spondylitis are each developed by 3–10% of IBD patients [35].

First-line drugs used for the treatment of mild to moderate inflammatory joint EIMs include acetaminophen, sulfasalazine and mesalazine [37]. Second-line agents include glucocorticoids, methotrexate and nonsteroidal anti-inflammatory drugs. Nevertheless, evidence has shown that treatment with biological TNF inhibitors is beneficial for relieving ankylosing spondylitis among patients with IBD [34, 38, 39].

Skin Manifestations

The reactive skin manifestations erythema nodosum and pyoderma gangrenosum are classically associated with IBD in 6 and 2% of patients, respectively [36, 40, 41]. Erythema nodosum often occurs with acute flares of IBD and is self-limiting or improves with treatment of the underlying IBD. Alternatively, pyoderma gangrenosum has a more severe and usually IBD-independent course.

These skin disorders usually respond to topical and systemic glucocorticoids, which are considered as the initial drugs of choice [37, 41]. However, in steroid-refractory cases and in cases with frequent relapses, biological TNF inhibitors have been administered with success [42, 43].

Ocular Manifestations

Ophthalmologic disorders develop in 2–6% of IBD patients; the most common of these EIMs are uveitis (often the anterior form) and (epi)scleritis [7, 36, 44]. Acute flares of IBD typically predispose patients to the development of (epi)scleritis, which usually responds to anti-inflammatory agents. Uveitis, on the other hand, is not always associated with active disease and usually requires more aggressive therapies.

First-line drugs used for these EIMs are anti-inflammatory agents. Glucocorticoids are especially important in uveitis, which may progress to blindness if not treated adequately. Recently, biological TNF inhibitors have also proved beneficial for the treatment of various ocular inflammatory conditions, including IBD-related EIMs such as uveitis and (epi)scleritis [45, 46]. Currently, the evidence is weaker for the latter condition, and most investigators consider anti-TNF biologicals as second-line therapies only [47].

Hepatobiliary Manifestations

Primary sclerosing cholangitis (PSC) is a condition causing damage to bile ducts in up to 3% in UC and 5% in CD patients, with a male predominance [4], and a significantly enhanced risk of developing local as well as colonic neoplastic complications is seen in up to 5% of patients [17]. The natural course of PSC appears to be independent of IBD, and the bile duct damage is usually irreversible and not responsive to medications. However, a recent report suggests benefits of treatment with TNF inhibitors [48]. This case report might be of importance, as the majority of patients with IBD and PSC ultimately require liver transplantation [17].

Hypersensitivity and Paradoxical Inflammation Induced by Biological TNF Inhibitors

Although side effects of TNF inhibitors occur, the clinical benefits remain undisputed in most of the cases mentioned above. Nevertheless, drug hypersensitivity to biologics occurs in approximately 12% of patients, requiring prompt drug withdrawal and, usually, an in-class switch to another agent [49].

Although biological TNF inhibitors have an overall favorable safety profile [20], quite unexpected manifestations in the skin, the joints, the brain and the peripheral nerves have been reported. Some of these manifestations are considered as paradoxical because TNF inhibitors by themselves should counteract these symptoms.

Skin

The cutaneous adverse manifestations associated with TNF inhibitors in the management of IBD include a wide range of dermatological manifestations (psoriasis-like, eczema-like and lichenoid eruptions, cutaneous lupus erythematosus, and nonmelanoma skin cancer). These disorders, including the paradoxical ones, should be promptly recognized and correctly diagnosed by gastroenterologists and dermatologists together to quickly establish an adequate treatment.

Psoriasis is more frequent in IBD than in the background population (11 vs. up to 2%) [10], and psoriasis is seen more often in patients with CD than in those with UC (11 and 6%, respectively) [50]. Although psoriasis is generally not considered as an EIM of IBD, the available data suggest this is a class-related side effect with a genetic linkage [51]. The overall frequency of new-onset psoriasiform skin lesions following TNF inhibitor treatment in a prospective study was 5%, with smoking as a major risk factor [51]. This complication does not relate to the age of the patients or to the duration of biological treatment [52–54]. Thus, psoriasiform eczema and eczema followed by xerosis cutis are the most commonly observed types of paradoxical skin inflammation associated with anti-TNF therapies [55]. These complications are generally attributed to a drug class effect that depends on TNF neutralization rather than a drug-specific adverse event, and they are usually reversible upon discontinuation or switching to another class of drugs [56]. Drug re-challenge with a second TNF inhibitor is, however, a possible option, although this option associated with a high recurrence rate of about half of these patients [51]. Stopping anti-TNF therapy is largely reserved for patients with severe psoriasis or for those who do not respond to topical therapies.

Drug-induced lupus occurs in approximately 1% of patients receiving anti-TNF biologics [57]. The symptoms disappear in nearly all cases upon discontinuation of the biologics. Challenging with another drug, including a second TNF inhibitor, is a potential option that results in a low recurrence of lupus [57].

Nonmelanoma skin cancer is reported to have a prevalence of 0.3–1.4% [57] in patients exposed to biological TNF inhibitors. All of these cases should immediately be referred to dermatologists for excision, and continued anti-TNF therapy should be considered on a case-by-case basis, as cessation of therapy with the TNF inhibitor is not routinely required.

Joint Manifestations
Some patients with IBD treated with biological TNF inhibitors (1–2%) complain of arthralgia, especially in the hands and the wrists, and morning stiffness, usually without signs of arthritis or synovitis [55]. Symptomatic treatment with acetaminophen should be considered as the first-line therapy, and only rarely is an in-class shift of drugs required.

Neurologic Adverse Reactions

Neurologic complications including peripheral neuropathy have rarely been associated with the use of biological TNF inhibitors. The exact prevalence of neurologic complications [20, 58] and the mechanism(s) underlying these phenomena are unknown [59]. In most cases, patients respond to withdrawal of the offending biologics, and additional immunosuppressive therapy has seldom been required [60–62]. Nerve conduction studies performed on patients with neuropathy in response to TNF inhibitors has, however, not revealed any common features [61].

Conclusions

During the last two decades, biological TNF inhibitors have revolutionized the treatment of IBD.

After the initial randomized controlled trials using protocols that were artificially designed because of regulatory requirements in registration studies, real-life clinical situations and subsequent clinical experience have taught clinicians to administer these drugs off-label according to their approved indications, including the management of some EIMs associated with IBD.

Thus, the success of treatment algorithms depends upon the optimization of each step of therapy and judgement about outcome, and the present algorithms for the treatment of EIMs of IBD are based upon therapeutic evidence, which is in constant flux. Future experience based on randomized, controlled trials may reveal some of the present areas of uncertainty and should provide further evidence for skillful tailored anti-TNF therapies to individual patients with IBD and EIMs. Furthermore, the armamentarium of biological drugs will be extended in the coming years, as the success of TNF inhibitors has become an inspirational model for other novel biological agents already marketed or in development, e.g., anti-α4/β7 monoclonal antibodies (which do not activate the JC virus), small molecules (e.g., Janus kinase inhibitors), and cytokine targets other than TNF [63–67]. Finally, stem cell therapies may become a future treatment option [68]. These new therapeutic principles will no doubt optimize the quality of life for future patients suffering from EIMs due to IBD.

References

1 Baumgart DC, Sandborn WJ: Crohn's disease. Lancet 2012;380:1590–1605.
2 Danese S, Fiocchi C: Ulcerative colitis. N Engl J Med 2011;365:1713–1725.
3 Larsen S, Bendtzen K, Nielsen OH: Extraintestinal manifestations of inflammatory bowel disease: epidemiology, diagnosis, and management. Ann Med 2010;42:97–114.
4 Gizard E, Ford AC, Bronowicki JP, et al: Systematic review: the epidemiology of the hepatobiliary manifestations in patients with inflammatory bowel disease. Aliment Pharmacol Ther 2014;40:3–15.

5 Kristensen SL, Lindhardsen J, Ahlehoff O, et al: Increased risk of atrial fibrillation and stroke during active stages of inflammatory bowel disease: a nationwide study. Europace 2014;16:477–484.
6 Vavricka SR, Brun L, Ballabeni P, et al: Frequency and risk factors for extraintestinal manifestations in the Swiss inflammatory bowel disease cohort. Am J Gastroenterol 2011;106:110–119.
7 Veloso FT, Carvalho J, Magro F: Immune-related systemic manifestations of inflammatory bowel disease. A prospective study of 792 patients. J Clin Gastroenterol 1996;23:29–34.
8 Williams H, Walker D, Orchard TR: Extraintestinal manifestations of inflammatory bowel disease. Curr Gastroenterol Rep 2008;10:597–605.
9 Ardizzone S, Puttini PS, Cassinotti A, et al: Extraintestinal manifestations of inflammatory bowel disease. Dig Liver Dis 2008;40 Suppl 2:S253–S259.
10 Danese S, Semeraro S, Papa A, et al: Extraintestinal manifestations in inflammatory bowel disease. World J Gastroenterol 2005;11:7227–7236.
11 Bernstein CN, Blanchard JF, Rawsthorne P, et al: The prevalence of extraintestinal diseases in inflammatory bowel disease: a population-based study. Am J Gastroenterol 2001;96:1116–1122.
12 Veloso FT: Extraintestinal manifestations of inflammatory bowel disease: do they influence treatment and outcome? World J Gastroenterol 2011;17:2702–2707.
13 Bernstein CN, Wajda A, Blanchard JF: The clustering of other chronic inflammatory diseases in inflammatory bowel disease: a population-based study. Gastroenterology 2005;129:827–836.
14 Ricart E, Panaccione R, Loftus EV Jr, et al: Autoimmune disorders and extraintestinal manifestations in first-degree familial and sporadic inflammatory bowel disease: a case-control study. Inflamm Bowel Dis 2004;10:207–214.
15 Huang BL, Chandra S, Shih DQ: Skin manifestations of inflammatory bowel disease. Front Physiol 2012;3:13.
16 Siebert U, Wurm J, Gothe RM, et al: Predictors of temporary and permanent work disability in patients with inflammatory bowel disease: results of the Swiss inflammatory bowel disease cohort study. Inflamm Bowel Dis 2013;19: 847–855.
17 Hirschfield GM, Karlsen TH, Lindor KD, et al: Primary sclerosing cholangitis. Lancet 2013;382:1587–1599.
18 Veloso FT, Ferreira JT, Barros L, et al: Clinical outcome of Crohn's disease: analysis according to the vienna classification and clinical activity. Inflamm Bowel Dis 2001;7:306–313.
19 Vind I, Riis L, Jess T, et al: Increasing incidences of inflammatory bowel disease and decreasing surgery rates in Copenhagen City and County, 2003–2005: a population-based study from the Danish Crohn colitis database. Am J Gastroenterol 2006;101: 1274–1282.
20 Nielsen OH, Ainsworth MA: Tumor necrosis factor inhibitors for inflammatory bowel disease. N Engl J Med 2013;369: 754–762.
21 Nielsen OH, Ainsworth MA: Which biological agents are most appropriate for ulcerative colitis? Ann Intern Med 2014; 160:733–734.
22 Winsauer C, Kruglov AA, Chashchina AA, et al: Cellular sources of pathogenic and protective TNF and experimental strategies based on utilization of TNF humanized mice. Cytokine Growth Factor Rev 2014;25:115–123.
23 Baumgart DC, Sandborn WJ: Inflammatory bowel disease: clinical aspects and established and evolving therapies. Lancet 2007;369:1641–1657.
24 Fiorino G, Allocca M, Danese S: Commentary: anaemia in inflammatory bowel disease–the most common and ignored extra intestinal manifestation. Aliment Pharmacol Ther 2014;39:227–228.
25 Hoivik ML, Reinisch W, Cvancarova M, et al: Anaemia in inflammatory bowel disease: a population-based 10-year follow-up. Aliment Pharmacol Ther 2014; 39:69–76.
26 Tussing-Humphreys L, Pusatcioglu C, Nemeth E, et al: Rethinking iron regulation and assessment in iron deficiency, anemia of chronic disease, and obesity: introducing hepcidin. J Acad Nutr Diet 2012;112:391–400.
27 Kulnigg S, Gasche C: Systematic review: managing anaemia in Crohn's disease. Aliment Pharmacol Ther 2006;24:1507–1523.
28 de Silva AD, Mylonaki M, Rampton DS: Oral iron therapy in inflammatory bowel disease: usage, tolerance, and efficacy. Inflamm Bowel Dis 2003;9: 316–320.
29 Semrin G, Fishman DS, Bousvaros A, et al: Impaired intestinal iron absorption in Crohn's disease correlates with disease activity and markers of inflammation. Inflamm Bowel Dis 2006;12:1101–1106.
30 Weiss G, Goodnough LT: Anemia of chronic disease. N Engl J Med 2005;352: 1011–1023.
31 Gasche C, Berstad A, Befrits R, et al: Guidelines on the diagnosis and management of iron deficiency and anemia in inflammatory bowel diseases. Inflamm Bowel Dis 2007;13:1545–1553.
32 Song SN, Iwahashi M, Tomosugi N, et al: Comparative evaluation of the effects of treatment with tocilizumab and TNF-alpha inhibitors on serum hepcidin, anemia response and disease activity in rheumatoid arthritis patients. Arthritis Res Ther 2013;15:R141.
33 Weiss G, Schett G: Anaemia in inflammatory rheumatic diseases. Nat Rev Rheumatol 2013;9:205–215.
34 Atzeni F, Defendenti C, Ditto MC, et al: Rheumatic manifestations in inflammatory bowel disease. Autoimmun Rev 2014;13:20–23.
35 De VM: Review article: joint involvement in inflammatory bowel disease. Aliment Pharmacol Ther 2004;20(suppl 4):36–42.
36 Su CG, Judge TA, Lichtenstein GR: Extraintestinal manifestations of inflammatory bowel disease. Gastroenterol Clin North Am 2002;31:307–327.
37 Van Bodegraven AA, Pena AS: Treatment of extraintestinal manifestations in inflammatory bowel disease. Curr Treat Options Gastroenterol 2003;6: 201–212.
38 Arvikar SL, Fisher MC: Inflammatory bowel disease associated arthropathy. Curr Rev Musculoskelet Med 2011;4: 123–131.
39 Jacques P, Van PL, Carron P, et al: Pathophysiology and role of the gastrointestinal system in spondyloarthritides. Rheum Dis Clin North Am 2012;38: 569–582.
40 Tavarela VF: Review article: skin complications associated with inflammatory bowel disease. Aliment Pharmacol Ther 2004;20(suppl 4):50–53.
41 Trost LB, McDonnell JK: Important cutaneous manifestations of inflammatory bowel disease. Postgrad Med J 2005;81: 580–585.

42 Ampuero J, Rojas-Feria M, Castro-Fernandez M, et al: Predictive factors for erythema nodosum and pyoderma gangrenosum in inflammatory bowel disease. J Gastroenterol Hepatol 2014;29: 291–295.
43 Marzano AV, Borghi A, Stadnicki A, et al: Cutaneous manifestations in patients with inflammatory bowel diseases: pathophysiology, clinical features, and therapy. Inflamm Bowel Dis 2014;20: 213–227.
44 Mintz R, Feller ER, Bahr RL, et al: Ocular manifestations of inflammatory bowel disease. Inflamm Bowel Dis 2004; 10:135–139.
45 Ally MR, Veerappan GR, Koff JM: Treatment of recurrent Crohn's uveitis with infliximab. Am J Gastroenterol 2008; 103:2150–2151.
46 Katsanos A, Asproudis I, Katsanos KH, et al: Orbital and optic nerve complications of inflammatory bowel disease. J Crohns Colitis 2013;7:683–693.
47 Levy-Clarke G, Jabs DA, Read RW, et al: Expert panel recommendations for the use of anti-tumor necrosis factor biologic agents in patients with ocular inflammatory disorders. Ophthalmology 2014; 121:785–796.
48 Duca I, Ramirez dlP, Estrada S, et al: Steroid-refractory ulcerative colitis and associated primary sclerosing cholangitis treated with infliximab. World J Gastroenterol 2013;19:590–593.
49 Nielsen OH, Seidelin JB, Munck LK, et al: Use of biological molecules in the treatment of inflammatory bowel disease. J Intern Med 2011;270:15–28.
50 Yates VM, Watkinson G, Kelman A: Further evidence for an association between psoriasis, Crohn's disease and ulcerative colitis. Br J Dermatol 1982; 106:323–330.
51 Tillack C, Ehmann LM, Friedrich M, et al: Anti-TNF antibody-induced psoriasiform skin lesions in patients with inflammatory bowel disease are characterised by interferon-gamma-expressing Th1 cells and IL-17A/IL-22-expressing Th17 cells and respond to anti-IL-12/IL-23 antibody treatment. Gut 2014;63: 567–577.
52 Fiorino G, Allez M, Malesci A, et al: Review article: anti TNF-alpha induced psoriasis in patients with inflammatory bowel disease. Aliment Pharmacol Ther 2009;29:921–927.
53 Guerra I, Algaba A, Perez-Calle JL, et al: Induction of psoriasis with anti-TNF agents in patients with inflammatory bowel disease: a report of 21 cases. J Crohns Colitis 2012;6:518–523.
54 Guerra I, Gisbert JP: Onset of psoriasis in patients with inflammatory bowel disease treated with anti-TNF agents. Expert Rev Gastroenterol Hepatol 2013; 7:41–48.
55 Cleynen I, Vermeire S: Paradoxical inflammation induced by anti-TNF agents in patients with IBD. Nat Rev Gastroenterol Hepatol 2012;9:496–503.
56 de Gannes GC, Ghoreishi M, Pope J, et al: Psoriasis and pustular dermatitis triggered by TNF-{alpha} inhibitors in patients with rheumatologic conditions. Arch Dermatol 2007;143:223–231.
57 Moran GW, Lim AW, Bailey JL, et al: Review article: dermatological complications of immunosuppressive and anti-TNF therapy in inflammatory bowel disease. Aliment Pharmacol Ther 2013; 38:1002–1024.
58 Benavente L, Moris G: Neurologic disorders associated with inflammatory bowel disease. Eur J Neurol 2011;18:138–143.
59 Stubgen JP: Tumor necrosis factor-alpha antagonists and neuropathy. Muscle Nerve 2008;37:281–292.
60 Alshekhlee A, Basiri K, Miles JD, et al: Chronic inflammatory demyelinating polyneuropathy associated with tumor necrosis factor-alpha antagonists. Muscle Nerve 2010;41:723–727.
61 Lozeron P, Denier C, Lacroix C, et al: Long-term course of demyelinating neuropathies occurring during tumor necrosis factor-alpha-blocker therapy. Arch Neurol 2009;66:490–497.
62 Richez C, Blanco P, Lagueny A, et al: Neuropathy resembling CIDP in patients receiving tumor necrosis factor-alpha blockers. Neurology 2005;64: 1468–1470.
63 Feagan BG, Rutgeerts P, Sands BE, et al: Vedolizumab as induction and maintenance therapy for ulcerative colitis. N Engl J Med 2013;369:699–710.
64 Neurath MF: Cytokines in inflammatory bowel disease. Nat Rev Immunol 2014; 14:329–342.
65 Sandborn WJ, Ghosh S, Panes J, et al: Tofacitinib, an oral Janus kinase inhibitor, in active ulcerative colitis. N Engl J Med 2012;367:616–624.
66 Sandborn WJ, Feagan BG, Rutgeerts P, et al: Vedolizumab as induction and maintenance therapy for Crohn's disease. N Engl J Med 2013;369:711–721.
67 Vermeire S, O'Byrne S, Keir M, et al: Etrolizumab as induction therapy for ulcerative colitis: a randomised, controlled, phase 2 trial. Lancet 2014;384: 309–318.
68 van Deen WK, Oikonomopoulos A, Hommes DW: Stem cell therapy in inflammatory bowel disease: which, when and how? Curr Opin Gastroenterol 2013; 29:384–390.

Ole Haagen Nielsen
Department of Gastroenterology, Medical Section, Herlev Hospital
University of Copenhagen, Herlev Ringvej 75
DK-2730 Herlev (Denmark)
E-Mail ohn@dadlnet.dk

Rogler G, Herfarth H, Hibi T, Nielsen OH (eds): Anti-Tumor Necrosis Factor Therapy in Inflammatory Bowel Disease.
Front Gastrointest Res. Basel, Karger, 2015, vol 34, pp 214–218 (DOI: 10.1159/000381608)

Anti-TNF Alpha Agents and Breastfeeding

Hythem Al-Sum • Cynthia V. Maxwell

Department of Obstetrics and Gynecology, Division of Maternal Fetal Medicine, Mount Sinai Hospital, University of Toronto, Toronto, Canada

Abstract

While anti-TNF alpha agents readily cross the placenta and enter the fetal circulation by the second trimester, comparatively miniscule amounts are secreted into human breast milk. Three agents, including infliximab, adalimumab, and certolizumab, have been shown to be expressed in breast milk at concentrations that are unlikely to impact neonatal health. Other agents, such as natalizumab and golimumab, require further investigation. At present, to avoid potential neonatal susceptibility to infection, live virus vaccines (such as rotavirus vaccine) are given after 6 months of life to ensure that antenatally acquired levels of the agents have left the neonate's system. Current knowledge does not suggest added risk from lactational exposure to these agents, so breast-feeding mothers should be encouraged to avoid discontinuation of the anti-TNF alpha agents needed to control their inflammatory bowel disease.

Introduction

Patients with inflammatory bowel disease (IBD) are advised to conceive during a quiescent stage of their disease. However, unplanned pregnancies are common, and women are often confronted with the need for medication therapy during pregnancy and the postpartum period. Pregnant women with IBD have a greater risk of adverse pregnancy outcomes when compared with the general population. However, if the disease is well controlled during pregnancy and postpartum, there may be a need to continue treatment, leading to neonatal exposure to medications during lactation. This chapter will review how breast milk is generated; how effectively the agents are secreted into the breast milk; and finally, the potential impact on the neonate.

Physiology of Human Lactation

Breast milk is secreted by specialized mammary epithelial cells that line a complex network of alveoli in order to provide nutrition for the newborn. The complex process of combining water, lipid, protein, carbohydrate and the breakdown products of items ingested by the mother (food, xenobiotics) has been reviewed in detail by McManaman and Neville [1]. Briefly, the main pathways used to secrete substances into breast milk include exocytosis (for protein secretion), transcytosis (for secretion of large proteins and macromolecules,

Table 1. Anti-TNF alpha agents typically in use to treat IBD (adapted from OH Nielson et al., 2014) [18]

Agent	Description
Infliximab	chimeric mouse/human monoclonal IgG1 antibody against TNF alpha
Adalimumab	fully human IgG1 antibody against TNF alpha
Certolizumab pegol	humanized monoclonal antibody Fab fragment linked to polyethylene glycol
Natalizumab	humanized monoclonal IgG4 antibody to alpha-4 integrin
Golimumab	complete IgG1 antibody against TNF alpha

including immunoglobulins and lipoprotein-bound drugs), membrane transport (such as ion, glucose and amino acid transport mechanisms) and occasionally paracellular mechanisms.

Breastfeeding during the first 6 months of neonatal life confers significant health benefits on the infant [2].

Physiology of Anti-TNF Alpha Agents and Their Passage into Breast Milk and the Neonate

TNF alpha and its receptors are found mainly in endometrial, decidual and placental tissues, and they work to protect embryos against stress [3]. Placental transfer of immunoglobulin G (IgG) by active transport mechanisms mediated by fetal Fc receptors has been documented, occurring in a progressive fashion with increasing gestational age [4].

Anti-TNF alpha immunoglobulins are mostly in the IgG1 class, with the exception of certolizumab (see table 1). While immunoglobulin A is the main immunoglobulin in human milk, anti-TNF alpha IgG has the potential to enter breast milk but is found in relatively minuscule amounts, given its large molecular size [5]. The impact on the nursing neonate is further diminished by the fact that such large proteins will be broken down by the neonate's digestive enzymes [6]. Certolizumab is a humanized monoclonal antibody Fab fragment linked to polyethylene glycol that, unlike immunoglobulins, does not cross into breast milk via active transport, but rather through passive diffusion [7].

There is evidence to suggest that the levels of some anti-TNF alpha agents (such as infliximab) persist longer in the neonatal system compared with the maternal system following transplacental transfer [8]. This is attributed to the substantially longer half-life in the relatively immature infant reticuloendothelial system [9]. However, as will be outlined, the vastly smaller amounts of these agents that pass into breast milk seem unlikely to impact neonatal health, despite this persistence.

Infliximab

Case reports suggest that infliximab has minimal passage into breast milk, such that levels are undetectable [8, 10, 11]. Subsequent studies analyzing breast milk samples showed either tiny amounts relative to the amount found in maternal sera [12] or undetectable levels in the breast milk as well as neonatal serum [13]. More recently, in a prospective series of 4 breast-fed infants whose mothers were treated with infliximab or adalimumab, both agents were detected in the breast milk using a sensitive immunoassay. However, the infliximab could not be detected in the infant's serum in one case, and a low level (1,700 ng/ml) was detected in another case. The authors note that this level is far below what is expected for transplacental transfer to the fetus and furthermore is below the therapeutic level [14].

Adalimumab
A recent short communication reporting an analysis of breast milk from a mother treated with adalimumab showed very low secretion levels, similar to infliximab [15]. Similarly, the drug was not detected in the serum of the nursing infant [16]. As of 2011, a consensus review committee noted that there was no commercially available test for adalimumab, thus making testing milk and serum more challenging [7].

Adalimumab was detected at very low concentrations in breast milk (2 cases) but not in the infant serum in one case in which infant testing was carried out [14].

Certolizumab
A study examining a small series of pregnant women treated with certolizumab found that sampling of breast milk at different stages revealed undetectable levels of the agent [17].

Natalizumab, Golimumab, and Other Anti-TNF Agents
No data were available on the presence of these agents in breast milk or infant serum at the time of preparation of this chapter.

Potential Effects of Anti-TNF Alpha Agents on Neonatal Health and Immune Function

While the overall suspected exposure of infants to anti-TNF alpha agents is minimal during breastfeeding, there are unanswered questions regarding the actual effects of the agents on neonatal and infant health. The higher transplacental levels of the agent infliximab do pose risks to the neonate, as these levels persist for months and can lead to severe infection, as described in the much-quoted report of an infant who succumbed to disseminated infection following live virus vaccination (Bacillus Calmette-Guerin) at 3 months of life [19]. While this vaccine is rarely given in North America compared with other parts of the world, it is common for infants to now receive the rotavirus vaccine prior to 6 months of life. As this and other future vaccinations may contain live viruses, careful assessment and follow-up of neonates born to mothers taking these agents during pregnancy is critical, with delay in their administration until after 6 months likely providing the solution. The role of *breast milk transfer* of these agents may provide minimal additional risk due to the low secretion rates but merits careful assessment. The evidence for infant health outcomes will be examined in the remainder of this section.

Infliximab
In a prospective assessment of two mothers who were treated during pregnancy and who breastfed at least part of the time while receiving infliximab, only one infant demonstrated measurable, albeit low, serum levels. However, at 18 and 22 months of follow-up, neither infant showed health or immune problems by the time of publication. The authors note that one of the infants born with low birth weight had caught up with expected growth percentiles by the age of 11 months [14]. Stengel and Arnold [11] reported on a breastfed infant whose mother maintained therapy during lactation; at 27 months, the infant showed no abnormalities.

Adalimumab
Two case reports give preliminary indication that the effect of adalimumab on the neonate is minimal, with no reported infectious or immune complications. In the first report, the newborn remained healthy at 6 months [20]. The second report detailed a mother with severe disease who continued to take regular doses of the agent during pregnancy and postpartum; her infant remained well at a 6-month follow-up, although details regarding breast milk and infant serum testing were not available [21].

A detailed prospective study of two infants exposed to adalimumab and followed until 14.5 or 15 months did not demonstrate significant drug effects or health issues (bearing in mind that only one infant had serum testing, and the drug was undetectable) [14]. One of these infants (the one who did not have the serum testing) did develop a common infantile disease, or acute laryngitis, at 10 months of age, and it was difficult to ascertain if the agent contributed to this condition.

The PIANO Study

The Pregnancy in Inflammatory Bowel Disease and Neonatal Outcomes (PIANO) Study is an ongoing, prospective cohort examining neonatal and infant outcomes in mothers with IBD [22, 23]. Results to date have been reported in abstract form and summarize the experience of 30 American IBD centers that have treated over 1,200 women to date, with a planned childhood follow-up period of 4 years. Mothers were divided into 4 groups: A – no treatment or unexposed; B – treatment with thiopurines; C – treatment with anti-TNF alpha agents, including infliximab, adalimumab, and certolizumab; and D – combination therapy with thiopurines and anti-TNF alpha agents. For the 1,052 women enrolled in the study as of 2012, 72% of their infants were breastfed. When mothers received single-agent treatment during lactation, infections were not increased in their infants relative to unexposed infants at a 12-month follow-up. However, for infants exposed to combination therapy via the lactating mother, there was a significant increase in infectious risks. There were no differences in growth or development among these cohorts. The conclusion of the authors was that as the infant approaches 12 months of age, possible defective immune system development might be related to exposure to a combination of immunomodulators and anti-TNF alpha agents.

Subsequent data from 2014, presented in abstract form, reported on 1,289 women enrolled to date. While this abstract did not report the details of breastfeeding rates or infectious morbidity in the infants, it did conclude that the achievement of developmental milestones was equivalent in exposed and nonexposed infants, and in some cases, those milestones were surpassed by the exposed individuals.

Summary

Caution must be exerted when recommending continuation of medications during breastfeeding. For many mothers with active IBD, discontinuation of medications such as anti-TNF alpha agents can have devastating effects and potentially reduce future treatment options. Evidence to date suggests that minimal exposure of the infant to the anti-TNF alpha agents infliximab, adalimumab and certolizumab during breastfeeding poses no significant health or immune risks. Areas that will require further detailed investigation include the infant health risks of exposure to combination IBD therapies through breast milk and the concentration and impact of newer agents, such as golimumab and natalizumab, in IBD therapy for lactating mothers.

References

1 McManaman JL, Neville MC: Mammary physiology and milk secretion. Adv Drug Deliv Rev 2003;55:629–641.

2 Gartner LM, Morton J, Lawrence RA, et al: Breastfeeding and the use of human milk. Pediatrics 2005;115:496–506.

3 Haider S, Knofler M: Human tumor necrosis factor: physiological and pathological roles in placenta and endometrium. Placenta 2009;30:111–123.

4 Kane SV, Acquah LA: Placental transport of immuonoglobulins: a clinical review for gastroenterologists who prescribe therapeutic monoclonal antibodies to women during conception and pregnancy. Am J Gastroenterol 2009; 104:228–233.

5 Arsenescu R, Arsenescu V, de Villiers WJ: TNF-alpha and the development of the neonatal immune system: implications for inhibitor use in pregnancy. Am J Gastroenterol 2011;106:559–562.
6 Moffatt DC, Bernstein CN: Drug therapy for inflammatory bowel disease in pregnancy and the puerperium. Best Pract Res Clin Gastroenterol 2007;21:835–847.
7 Mahadevan U, Cucchiara S, Hyams JS, et al: The London Position Statement of the World Congress of Gastroenterology on Biological Therapy for IBD With the European Crohn's and Colitis Organization: pregnancy and pediatrics. Am J Gastroenterol 2011;106:214–223.
8 Vasiliauskas EA, Church JA, Silverman N, et al: Case report: evidence for transplacnetal transfer of maternally administered infliximab to the newborn. Clin Gastro Hepatol 2006;4:1255–1258.
9 Steenholdt C, Al-Khalaf M, Ainsworth MA, et al: Therapeutic infliximab drug levels in a child born to a woman with ulcerative colitis treated until gestation week 31. J Crohns Colitis 2012;6:358–361.
10 Peltier M, James D, Ford J: Infliximab levels in breast-milk of a nursing Crohn's patient. Am J Gastroenterol 2001;96:P258.
11 Stengel JZ, Arnold HL: Is infliximab safe to use while breastfeeding? World J Gastroenterol 2008;14:3085–3087.
12 Ben-Horin S, Yavzori M, Kopylov U, et al: Detection of infliximab in breast milk of nursing mothers with inflammatory bowel disease. J Crohns Colitis 2011;5:555–558.
13 Kane S, Ford J, Cohen R, et al: Absence of infliximab in infants and breast milk from nursing mothers receiving therapy for Crohn's disease before and after delivery. J Clin Gastroenterol 2009;43:613–616.
14 Fritzche J, Pilch A, Mury D, et al: Infliximab and Adalimumab use during breastfeeding. J Clin Gastroenterol 2012;46:718–719.
15 Ben-Horin S, Yavzori M, Katz L, et al: Adalimumab level in breast milk of a nursing mother. Clin Gastroenterol Hepatol 2010;8:475–476.
16 Julsgaard M, BrownS, Gibson P, et al: Adalimumab levels in an infant. 2013;7:597–598.
17 Mahadevan U: Certolizumab use in pregnancy: low levels detected in cord blood. Gastroenterology 2009;136:A960.
18 Nielsen OH, Maxwell C, Hendel J: IBD medications during pregnancy and lactation. Nat Rev Gastroenterol Hepatol 2014;11:116–127.
19 Cheent K, Nolan J, Shariq S, et al: Case report: fatal case of disseminated BCG infection in an infant born to a mother taking infliximab for Crohn's disease. J Crohns Colitis 2010;4:603–605.
20 Mishkin DS, Van Diense W, Becker JM, et al: Successful use of Adalimumab (Humira) for Crohn's disease in pregnancy. Inflamm Bowel Dis 2006;12:827–828.
21 Vesga L, Terdiman JP, Mahadevan U: Adalimumab use in pregnancy. Gut 2005;54:890.
22 Mahadevan U, Martin CF, Sandler RS, et al: PIANO: a 1,000 patient prospective registry of pregnancy outcomes in women with IBD exposed to immunomodulators and biologic therapy. Gastroenterology 2012;142(suppl 1):S–149.
23 Mahadevan U, Martin CF, Chambers C, et al: Achievement of developmental milestones among offspring of women with inflammatory bowel disease: the PIANO registry. Gastroenterology 2014;146(suppl 1):S–1.

Dr. Cynthia V. Maxwell
Department of Obstetrics and Gynecology, Division of Maternal Fetal Medicine
Mount Sinai Hospital, University of Toronto
600 University Avenue, Toronto, Ontario M5G1X5 (Canada)
E-Mail CMaxwell@mtsinai.on.ca

Rogler G, Herfarth H, Hibi T, Nielsen OH (eds): Anti-Tumor Necrosis Factor Therapy in Inflammatory Bowel Disease.
Front Gastrointest Res. Basel, Karger, 2015, vol 34, pp 219–223 (DOI: 10.1159/000381609)

Anti-TNF Therapy before Surgery

Stephan R. Vavricka[a, b] · Michael Scharl[a] · Gerhard Rogler[a]

[a]Division of Gastroenterology and Hepatology, University Hospital Zurich, Zurich, and [b]Division of Gastroenterology and Hepatology, Triemlispital Zurich, Zurich, Switzerland

Abstract

Up to 80% of Crohn's disease (CD) patients and 10% of ulcerative colitis (UC) patients will require at least one bowel surgery during their lifetime. Other surgeries that are not related to inflammatory bowel disease may also be necessary for these patients. It is well known that the preoperative administration of steroids is associated with increased numbers of perioperative complications, anastomosis leaks and postoperative infections. For classical immunosuppressants, such as azathioprine and 6-mercaptopurine, significantly lower risks of the above-mentioned complications have been demonstrated. Thus, the careful consideration of preoperative therapy is crucial for the short-term and long-term outcomes of surgery in inflammatory bowel disease patients. The association of preoperative anti-TNF antibody therapy with a higher rate of postoperative complications has been debated in the literature. Two recent meta-analyses of CD patients have suggested that this therapy results in a slightly higher rate of postoperative infection complications in these patients, but its effects on UC patients are still unclear. This overview summarizes the current literature on the use of preoperative anti-TNF treatment and consecutive potential complications in CD and UC patients.

Introduction

Crohn's disease (CD) and ulcerative colitis (UC) comprise two chronic diseases in which affected patients present with inflammation along the gastrointestinal tract. Besides medical therapy, the operative management of inflammatory bowel disease (IBD) patients, especially CD patients, can be effective in managing disease complications and improving quality of life [1].

In CD patients, the frequency of surgery remains high [2, 3]. Some authors have reported that one-third of CD patients require intestinal resective surgery [4, 5]. Other publications have even reported that 75–80% of CD patients end up with at least one surgical resection during their lifetime [6–14]. In addition, 10% of UC patients undergo total proctocolectomy within a 5-year period following disease diagnosis [15, 16].

Unfortunately, many patients develop recurrence of CD even after surgery, requiring a second intervention [10, 17–19]. Thus, pre- and postoperative medical therapy may be crucial for the long-term outcomes of these patients.

Preoperative administration of more than 20 mg of systemic steroids (in contrast to topical steroids) has been associated with significantly increased risks of postoperative complications and infections. The impacts of azathioprine and 6-mercaptopurine on these risks are clearly lower. However, there is still a significantly increased risk of complications when immunosuppressives are administered at standard doses.

An especially high rate of postoperative complications has been seen in CD patients who have undergone abdominal surgery for penetrating disease [20–22]. Therefore, preoperative therapy for CD and UC patients needs careful consideration. The disease behavior, the intended surgery, and the risk of recurrence have to be taken into account. To estimate the benefit/risk ratio for an individual situation, it is necessary to know whether preoperative treatment with anti-TNF antibodies increases the risk of complications in IBD patients who have to undergo surgery.

Postoperative Complications in Patients on Preoperative Anti-TNF Therapy

The introduction of anti-TNF antibodies, such as infliximab, adalimumab, certolizumab pegol and golimumab, has resulted in the improved outcomes of CD and UC patients, but long-term data are still lacking [23, 24]. However, controversies exist regarding the potential adverse effects of these agents on surgery outcome. The immunosuppressive effects of biologics place patients at an increased risk of postoperative complications, including infectious complications. Appau et al. in 2008 and Kopylov et al. in 2012 have suggested that anti-TNF antibodies may be independently associated with septic complications and abscess formation during the postoperative period [25, 26]. Most studies focusing on CD patients have failed to demonstrate any impact of preoperative anti-TNF administration during the postoperative period [27–34]. Tay et al. have even suggested that patients receiving ant-TNF therapy before surgery have improved outcomes [35].

Most studies published so far, however, seem underpowered and probably do not allow for the reliable identification of potentially important clinical differences. Furthermore, most studies have been nonrandomized and unmatched. Two meta-analyses were performed that both showed increased infectious complication rates in IBD individuals who received preoperative anti-TNF therapy [36, 37]. Billioud et al. have reported an increase in the prevalence of infectious postoperative complications in CD patients with an OR of 1.45 (table 1), comparable to the risk related to the use of lower doses of systemic glucocorticosteroids [38]. Taking into account the large proportion of IBD patients who undergo surgery, these results are of great clinical importance. Therefore, anti-TNF therapy should be used with caution during the preoperative stage in these patients, and further studies are desperately needed.

Meta-analysis of studies involving UC has found that infliximab is associated with an increased risk of overall short-term postoperative complications [39]. This analysis was clearly underpowered due to the small number of studies assessed and the high degree of heterogeneity among them. Subsequent studies have failed to show a negative impact of anti-TNF therapy on postoperative outcome [40–46]. In their meta-analysis, Billioud et al. also failed to show an association between anti-TNF therapy in UC patients and adverse outcome. Thus, in UC patients on preoperative anti-TNF therapy, no postoperative complications related to this therapy are expected.

Conclusion and Future Directions

When CD patients on anti-TNF agents require surgery, a preoperative drug-free interval – if the clinical situation permits – is advisable and might

Table 1. Impact of preoperative anti-TNF antibody use on postoperative outcomes of Crohn's disease patients (selection of references according to Billioud et al. [36] and Ahmed Ali et al. [37])

Reference	Country	Period	N	Surgical resection	Design	Drug	Does drug increase complications?
Appau [25], 2008	USA	1998–2007	404	BR	R	IFX	Yes
Canedo [27], 2011	USA	2000–2008	225	BR	P	IFX	No
Colombel [28], 2004	USA	1998–2001	270	BR	R	IFX	No
Indar [29], 2009	USA	1999–2007	112	BR	R	IFX	No
Kasparek [30], 2012	Germany	2001–2008	168	BR	R	IFX	No
Marchal [34], 2004	Belgium	1998–2002	79	BR	R	IFX	No
Nasir [32], 2010	USA	2005–2009	370	BR	R	IFX	No
Tay [35], 2003	USA	1998–2002	100	BR, stric	R	IFX	No

BR = Bowel resection; IFX = infliximab; R = retrospective; stric = strictureplasty.
Although most studies revealed no increase in postoperative complications in IBD patients preoperatively treated with an anti-TNF agent, meta-analysis based on the above-mentioned studies revealed an increased prevalence of postoperative complications in IBD patients who received preoperative anti-TNF therapy (OR: 1.25; 95% CI: 1.02–1.53) [36].

reduce the risk of septic complications. There are no published data on the length of such an interval, but we suggest a lag of 2 weeks (adalimumab) to 8 weeks (infliximab). UC patients receiving preoperative anti-TNF treatment do not seem to be at an increased risk of experiencing postoperative complications. Surgeons should be informed about such complications, especially in CD patients, and specific operative strategies, including temporary ostomy, may be considered. Finally, CD patients undergoing surgery should be educated and counseled about the potential adverse outcomes of preoperative treatment with anti-TNF agents. Large prospective, randomized and placebo-controlled trials are needed to clarify the true risks and benefits of continuing anti-TNF therapy during the perioperative period.

Grant Support

The authors are supported by research grants from the Swiss National Science Foundation (33CSC0_134274 to the Swiss IBD Cohort Study Group, 320000-114009/3 and 32473B_135694/1 to SRV and 310030-120312 to GR, 314730-146204 and CRSII3_154488/1 to MS) and the Zurich Center for Integrative Human Physiology of the University of Zurich (to GR and SRV).

References

1 Delaney CP, Kiran RP, Senagore AJ, et al: Quality of life improves within 30 days of surgery for Crohn's disease. J Am Coll Surg 2003;196:714–721.
2 Gardiner KR, Dasari BV: Operative management of small bowel Crohn's disease. Surg Clin North Am 2007;87: 587–610.
3 Greenstein AJ, Lachman P, Sachar DB, et al: Perforating and non-perforating indications for repeated operations in Crohn's disease: evidence for two clinical forms. Gut 1988;29:588–592.
4 Bouguen G, Peyrin-Biroulet L: Surgery for adult Crohn's disease: what is the actual risk? Gut 2011;60:1178–1181.
5 Peyrin-Biroulet L, Oussalah A, Williet N, et al: Impact of azathioprine and tumour necrosis factor antagonists on the need for surgery in newly diagnosed Crohn's disease. Gut 2011;60:930–936.

6 Travis SP, Stange EF, Lemann M, et al: European evidence based consensus on the diagnosis and management of Crohn's disease: current management. Gut 2006;55(suppl 1):i16–i35.
7 Ng SC, Kamm MA: Management of postoperative Crohn's disease. Am J Gastroenterol 2008;103:1029–1035.
8 Regueiro M, Schraut W, Baidoo L, et al: Infliximab prevents Crohn's disease recurrence after ileal resection. Gastroenterology 2009;136:441–450.e1; quiz 716.
9 Unkart JT, Anderson L, Li E, et al: Risk factors for surgical recurrence after ileocolic resection of Crohn's disease. Dis Colon Rectum 2008;51:1211–1216.
10 Simillis C, Yamamoto T, Reese GE, et al: A meta-analysis comparing incidence of recurrence and indication for reoperation after surgery for perforating versus nonperforating Crohn's disease. Am J Gastroenterol 2008;103: 196–205.
11 Nos P, Domenech E: Postoperative Crohn's disease recurrence: a practical approach. World J Gastroenterol 2008; 14:5540–5548.
12 Caprilli R, Gassull MA, Escher JC, et al: European evidence based consensus on the diagnosis and management of Crohn's disease: special situations. Gut 2006;55(suppl 1):i36–i58.
13 Yamamoto T: Factors affecting recurrence after surgery for Crohn's disease. World J Gastroenterol 2005;11:3971–3979.
14 Froehlich F, Juillerat P, Pittet V, et al: Maintenance of surgically induced remission of Crohn's disease. Digestion 2007;76:130–135.
15 Filippi J, Allen PB, Hebuterne X, et al: Does anti-TNF therapy reduce the requirement for surgery in ulcerative colitis? A systematic review. Curr Drug Targets 2011;12:1440–1447.
16 Williet N, Pillot C, Oussalah A, et al: Incidence of and impact of medications on colectomy in newly diagnosed ulcerative colitis in the era of biologics. Inflamm Bowel Dis 2012;18:1641–1646.
17 Domenech E, Manosa M, Bernal I, et al: Impact of azathioprine on the prevention of postoperative Crohn's disease recurrence: results of a prospective, observational, long-term follow-up study. Inflamm Bowel Dis 2008;14:508–513.
18 Pascua M, Su C, Lewis JD, et al: Meta-analysis: factors predicting post-operative recurrence with placebo therapy in patients with Crohn's disease. Aliment Pharmacol Ther 2008;28:545–556.
19 Caprilli R, Corrao G, Taddei G, et al: Prognostic factors for postoperative recurrence of Crohn's disease. Gruppo Italiano per lo Studio del Colon e del Retto (GISC). Dis Colon Rectum 1996; 39:335–341.
20 Hesp FL, Hendriks T, Lubbers EJ, et al: Wound healing in the intestinal wall. Effects of infection on experimental ileal and colonic anastomoses. Dis Colon Rectum 1984;27:462–467.
21 Hesp FL, Hendriks T, Lubbers EJ, et al: Wound healing in the intestinal wall. A comparison between experimental ileal and colonic anastomoses. Dis Colon Rectum 1984;27:99–104.
22 Post S, Betzler M, von Ditfurth B, et al: Risks of intestinal anastomoses in Crohn's disease. Ann Surg 1991;213: 37–42.
23 Sands BE, Anderson FH, Bernstein CN, et al: Infliximab maintenance therapy for fistulizing Crohn's disease. N Engl J Med 2004;350:876–885.
24 Rutgeerts P, Van Assche G, Vermeire S: Optimizing anti-TNF treatment in inflammatory bowel disease. Gastroenterology 2004;126:1593–1610.
25 Appau KA, Fazio VW, Shen B, et al: Use of infliximab within 3 months of ileocolonic resection is associated with adverse postoperative outcomes in Crohn's patients. J Gastrointest Surg 2008;12: 1738–1744.
26 Kopylov U, Ben-Horin S, Zmora O, et al: Anti-tumor necrosis factor and postoperative complications in Crohn's disease: systematic review and meta-analysis. Inflamm Bowel Dis 2012;18: 2404–2413.
27 Canedo J, Lee SH, Pinto R, et al: Surgical resection in Crohn's disease: is immunosuppressive medication associated with higher postoperative infection rates? Colorectal Dis 2011;13:1294–1298.
28 Colombel JF, Loftus EV Jr, Tremaine WJ, et al: Early postoperative complications are not increased in patients with Crohn's disease treated perioperatively with infliximab or immunosuppressive therapy. Am J Gastroenterol 2004;99: 878–883.
29 Indar AA, Young-Fadok TM, Heppell J, et al: Effect of perioperative immunosuppressive medication on early outcome in Crohn's disease patients. World J Surg 2009;33:1049–1052.
30 Kasparek MS, Bruckmeier A, Beigel F, et al: Infliximab does not affect postoperative complication rates in Crohn's patients undergoing abdominal surgery. Inflamm Bowel Dis 2012;18:1207–1213.
31 Kunitake H, Hodin R, Shellito PC, et al: Perioperative treatment with infliximab in patients with Crohn's disease and ulcerative colitis is not associated with an increased rate of postoperative complications. J Gastrointest Surg 2008;12:1730–1736; discussion 1736–1737.
32 Nasir BS, Dozois EJ, Cima RR, et al: Perioperative anti-tumor necrosis factor therapy does not increase the rate of early postoperative complications in Crohn's disease. J Gastrointest Surg 2010;14:1859–1865; discussion 1865–1866.
33 Rizzo G, Armuzzi A, Pugliese D, et al: Anti-TNF-alpha therapies do not increase early postoperative complications in patients with inflammatory bowel disease. An Italian single-center experience. Int J Colorectal Dis 2011;26:1435–1444.
34 Marchal L, D'Haens G, Van Assche G, et al: The risk of post-operative complications associated with infliximab therapy for Crohn's disease: a controlled cohort study. Aliment Pharmacol Ther 2004;19: 749–754.
35 Tay GS, Binion DG, Eastwood D, et al: Multivariate analysis suggests improved perioperative outcome in Crohn's disease patients receiving immunomodulator therapy after segmental resection and/or strictureplasty. Surgery 2003; 134:565–572; discussion 572–573.
36 Billioud V, Ford AC, Tedesco ED, et al: Preoperative use of anti-TNF therapy and postoperative complications in inflammatory bowel diseases: a meta-analysis. J Crohns Colitis 2013;7:853–867.
37 Ahmed Ali U, Martin ST, Rao AD, et al: Impact of preoperative immunosuppressive agents on postoperative outcomes in Crohn's disease. Dis Colon Rectum 2014;57:663–674.

38 Subramanian V, Saxena S, Kang JY, et al: Preoperative steroid use and risk of postoperative complications in patients with inflammatory bowel disease undergoing abdominal surgery. Am J Gastroenterol 2008;103:2373–2381.
39 Yang Z, Wu Q, Wu K, et al: Meta-analysis: pre-operative infliximab treatment and short-term post-operative complications in patients with ulcerative colitis. Aliment Pharmacol Ther 2010;31: 486–492.
40 Bordeianou L, Kunitake H, Shellito P, et al: Preoperative infliximab treatment in patients with ulcerative and indeterminate colitis does not increase rate of conversion to emergent and multistep abdominal surgery. Int J Colorectal Dis 2010;25:401–404.
41 Bregnbak D, Mortensen C, Bendtsen F: Infliximab and complications after colectomy in patients with ulcerative colitis. J Crohns Colitis 2012;6:281–286.
42 Coquet-Reinier B, Berdah SV, Grimaud JC, et al: Preoperative infliximab treatment and postoperative complications after laparoscopic restorative proctocolectomy with ileal pouch-anal anastomosis: a case-matched study. Surg Endosc 2010;24:1866–1871.
43 Gainsbury ML, Chu DI, Howard LA, et al: Preoperative infliximab is not associated with an increased risk of short-term postoperative complications after restorative proctocolectomy and ileal pouch-anal anastomosis. J Gastrointest Surg 2011;15:397–403.
44 Kiran RP, Khoury W, Church JM, et al: Colorectal cancer complicating inflammatory bowel disease: similarities and differences between Crohn's and ulcerative colitis based on three decades of experience. Ann Surg 2010;252:330–335.
45 de Silva S, Ma C, Proulx MC, et al: Postoperative complications and mortality following colectomy for ulcerative colitis. Clin Gastroenterol Hepatol 2011;9: 972–980.
46 Norgard BM, Nielsen J, Qvist N, et al: Pre-operative use of anti-TNF-alpha agents and the risk of post-operative complications in patients with ulcerative colitis – a nationwide cohort study. Aliment Pharmacol Ther 2012;35:1301–1309.

Stephan R. Vavricka, MD
Department of Internal Medicine, Division of Gastroenterology
Triemlispital, Birmensdorferstrasse 497
CH–8063 Zurich (Switzerland)
E-Mail stephan.vavricka@usz.ch

Rogler G, Herfarth H, Hibi T, Nielsen OH (eds): Anti-Tumor Necrosis Factor Therapy in Inflammatory Bowel Disease.
Front Gastrointest Res. Basel, Karger, 2015, vol 34, pp 224–228 (DOI: 10.1159/000381610)

When and How to Stop Anti-TNF Treatment in Inflammatory Bowel Disease: Predictors of Relapse after Stopping Treatment

Edouard Louis

Department of Gastroenterology CHU Liège, and GIGA Research University of Liège, Liège, Belgium

Abstract

The global benefit-risk ratio of long-term anti-TNF treatment appears favorable. Nevertheless, reasons exist for contemplating treatment cessation, including patient preference, associated side effects, the development of infection in high-risk patients, pregnancy and cost. Several prospective studies have shown very consistent relapse rates of around 50% at 1 year. Globally, patients with a low risk of relapse are those with steroid-free, clinical, endoscopic and biological remission of Crohn's disease, while no clear predictor has been identified in ulcerative colitis. These studies as well as larger retrospective studies have also shown excellent responses and remission rates and very good tolerabilities of retreatment with the same anti-TNF agents, particularly when patients are concomitantly treated with an immunosuppressant.

Introduction

Inflammatory bowel diseases (IBDs) are chronic relapsing diseases associated with long-term consequences of chronic intestinal inflammation, including tissue damage, leading to impaired organ function [1] and the increased risk of cancer [2]. Furthermore, anti-TNF agents are used in the most severe IBD cases characterized by a high risk of disease progression, tissue damage and refractoriness to conventional therapies. It may thus seem risky or even irresponsible to contemplate anti-TNF withdrawal in this setting. Nevertheless, anti-TNF agents are able to induce full tissue healing and apparently full disease control in a substantial number of long-term treated patients, who represent the best responders to these drugs. Anti-TNF therapy may thus create a situation in which these patients, albeit still harboring their genetic predisposition, may be considered, at least transiently, to be disease-free. This situation may be considered similar to the post-surgical situation in some Crohn's disease (CD) patients because relapse-free survival may be observed in up to 1/3 of these patients at 8–10 years [3]. On the other hand, anti-TNF therapy is still associated with some risks, mainly infection, and may pose problems in specific situations, such as pregnancy. This therapy also currently represents a very significant proportion of the global budget for IBD management [4], justifying a careful consideration about the optimal use of resources. Therefore, because anti-TNF therapy has never been shown to cure IBD, available data suggest that a transient and sometimes prolonged treatment withdrawal may represent a reasonable option in selected patients.

Reasons for Anti-TNF Discontinuation in Inflammatory Bowel Disease

The risks of infection and cancer have been the main reasons for contemplating anti-TNF treatment withdrawal after achieving sustained remission. These risks are reviewed in other chapters of this book and may be somewhat lower than previously thought. The risk of infection has decreased since systematic measures to avoid the reactivation of latent tuberculosis have been widely recommended [5]. This risk can be even further minimized by promoting vaccination against preventable diseases and informing patients about the risks and preventative measures for these infections [5]. The most recent population-based data seem reassuring about the long-term risks of lymphoma and cancers associated with anti-TNF therapy [6]. Nevertheless, this therapy will always represent a threat justifying careful consideration, particularly in elderly people. Milder side effects may also be taken into account, the best example of which is probably skin lesions, which may affect up to 20% of treated patients [7, 8]. Although these eczematiform and psoriasiform lesions are usually mild to moderate in severity, they sometimes impact the quality of life of patients and may represent an argument for treatment cessation in a stable patient. Pregnancy is another situation in which anti-TNF withdrawal may be considered. This aspect is reviewed in another chapter of this book. Despite reassuring data about pregnancy outcome and newborn health, we should not forget that IgG1 anti-TNF agents (adalimumab, infliximab, and golimumab) are very effectively transported through the placenta as of week 20 and that more experience is required before we can consider it to be fully safe to treat a pregnant women with an anti-TNF agent throughout pregnancy.

Most cost studies of CD have essentially included direct medical costs. The first studies were based on models generated with data from the literature [9]. These studies indicated that hospitalizations and surgeries represented the majority of the direct medical costs (up to 80%) linked to CD. These results were further confirmed by several retrospective and prospective cohort analyses [10, 11], suggesting that a therapeutic strategy that would decrease the number of hospitalizations and/or surgeries in CD might have an important impact on direct medical costs. A recent study conducted in the Netherlands has indicated a major change in cost repartition, with anti-TNF treatment now representing up to 2/3 of the cost of CD management and 1/3 of that of ulcerative colitis management [4]. This finding was not associated with a global increase in the cost of IBD management because parallel decreases in surgery and hospitalization were confirmed. However, it indicates that anti-TNF therapy now represents a big part of the budget of IBD management. Therefore, it seems wise to think of the optimal use of these drugs, including carefully considered withdrawal.

Available Studies on Anti-TNF Treatment Cessation in Inflammatory Bowel Disease and Other Immune-Mediated Inflammatory Diseases

Anti-TNF agents are broadly used to treat patients with rheumatoid arthritis. A study of patients with risk factors for severe disease who started infliximab early in the disease course in combination with methotrexate showed that after 1 year, infliximab could be stopped in patients who reached remission and that the relapse rate over the following year was low at around 30% [12]. More recently, similar results were obtained with adalimumab [13]. After patients received combination therapy with adalimumab and methotrexate for 6 months and reached a low disease activity state, they were randomized into two groups, one continuing combination therapy and the other continuing methotrexate alone. The outcomes were similar in the two groups over 1 year of follow-up, suggesting the possibility of at least transient anti-TNF withdrawal in this clinical setting.

In CD, the first published study of anti-TNF treatment cessation was conducted in Spain [14]. In this small-sized, multicenter, retrospective study, the outcomes were very different in patients with luminal versus perianal disease. Patients had been treated for at least 1 year by combination therapy with infliximab and an immunosuppressant before infliximab withdrawal. In patients with perianal disease, infliximab withdrawal was associated with an almost systematic relapse within 1 year. These findings highlight the difficulties of full tissue healing and disease control in perianal CD. These difficulties have already been suggested in studies systematically comparing clinical remission and tissue healing on MRI [15] as well as in studies showing a relatively low rate of full fistulous track disappearance up to 10 years after the diagnosis of fistulizing perianal disease [16]. The situation in the patients with luminal disease was substantially different because approximately 50% did not experience relapse within 1 year after infliximab withdrawal. This finding has been more recently confirmed in a prospective cohort study of the GETAID [17]. A total of 115 patients with stable remission on combined immunosuppressant-infliximab therapy for more than 1 year stopped taking infliximab while pursuing immunosuppressive treatment. After 1 year, more than half of the patients were still in sustained remission. More recently, this proportion has been confirmed in three independent prospective cohorts, including both CD and ulcerative colitis patients. In a Hungarian cohort of 121 CD patients who stopped adalimumab or infliximab after 1 year of successful therapy, 45% had to restart anti-TNF therapy within 1 year due to relapse, and 9% had to undergo surgical resection. In another Hungarian cohort of 51 patients with ulcerative colitis, the relapse rate after 1 year after infliximab discontinuation was 35% [18]. Importantly, around 10% of the relapsers had to undergo colectomy [19]. In a mixed cohort from Finland, including 52 patients (17 with CD, 30 with ulcerative colitis and 5 with unclassified colitis) in a state of deep remission characterized by clinical remission, endoscopic healing and a fecal calprotectin level of <100 µg/g, a smaller proportion of relapsers was observed of around 30%. The same proportions of relapse were observed in CD and ulcerative colitis patients, and colectomy was necessary in 10% of ulcerative colitis patients who relapsed.

Predictive Factors for Relapse

Predictors of relapse after anti-TNF withdrawal were studied in the prospective cohort studies described above. For CD, in the initial prospective GETAID study, the parameters associated with the time to relapse in univariate analysis were the CD activity index (>20), CRP (>5 mg/l), fecal calprotectin (>300 µg/g), and hemoglobin levels (<14.5 g/dl) and smoking status (nonsmoker) [17]. Multivariate analysis enabled the construction of a predictive model, in which patients were stratified according to their risk of relapse. Four levels of risk were identified. The lowest risk group, representing around 20% of the patients with a risk of relapse of around 5% over 1 year, was characterized by no more than 3 out of 9 deleterious factors (the use of steroids between 6 and 12 months before stopping infliximab, male gender, no previous surgical resection, hemoglobin level of <14.5 g/dl, CRP level of >5 mg/l, fecal calprotectin level of >300 µg/g, CD endoscopic index of severity of >0, leukocyte count >6,000/mm^3, and infliximab trough level of >2 mg/l) [17]. Globally, these predictors led to the conclusion that this low-risk group of patients was characterized by deep remission, including not only clinical remission but also tissue healing and the normalization of biomarkers of inflammation. The Hungarian study also found that smoking status as well as the recent use of steroids and the past need for infliximab dose escalation were predictive of relapse [18]. In the Finnish study, no clear predictor of relapse was found, but these authors only selected and included patients who were in deep remission, with mucosal healing and a low fecal calprotectin level [19]. For ulcerative colitis, neither the Hungarian study nor the Finnish study found any predictors. Even mucosal healing, which was not an inclusion criteria to enter the Hungarian study, was not found to be associated with the risk of relapse [20].

Monitoring and Retreatment of Patients

Another important question to address when contemplating anti-TNF discontinuation is the possibility of restarting this treatment in the case of relapse. Available data seem very reassuring in this regard. In the STORI trial, almost all patients were in remission at 4 weeks and 4 months after resuming infliximab treatment [17]. No infusion reaction was observed, and no patient showed anti-infliximab antibodies at 4 months before the 3rd reinfusion. These remissions were sustained because the rate of the loss of response for the retreated patients was around 12% over 2 years. Other prospective studies have also shown excellent results for tolerance and the response to retreatment, with remission rate ranging from 60 to 90% for both CD and ulcerative colitis [18–20]. More recently, a large retrospective study of retreatment after infliximab withdrawal has been reported [21], which has described very high response rates in association with immunosuppressant co-treatment as a major predictive factor.

Further analyses of the STORI trials have also suggested that these relapses could be predicted by the longitudinal follow-up of patients using biomarkers. CRP and fecal calprotectin levels have been shown to increase significantly within 4 months before clinical relapse [22]. This ability to predict relapse could thus allow for patients to be retreated before the occurrence of the relapse, minimizing the impact of treatment withdrawal.

The Concept of Treatment Cycles

Anti-TNF therapy should not be withdrawn at the price of incomplete disease control or the risk of disease progression. Nevertheless, IBDs have historically been considered relapsing rather than chronic diseases. Population-based data indicate long periods of remission, sometimes without any treatment, and the follow-up of CD patients after 'curative' ileo-cecal resection has clearly indicated that up to 30–40% of these patients may present with relapse-free survival for up to 8–10 years after surgery [3]. This finding may lead to the proposal of treatment cycles instead of continuous treatment. The principle of treatment cycles is completely different from that of on-demand treatment. For the latter, the patient is only retreated in the case of relapse and only until achieving clinical remission. In the former, the patient is treated until reaching deep remission, including clinical remission and at least tissue healing. Following the withdrawal of anti-TNF treatment, patients should be actively followed-up using biomarkers and ideally retreated before clinical signs of relapse emerge, avoiding the consequences of disease relapse. The treatment should then be given for a new cycle, at least until sustained remission is achieved without steroids, in addition to tissue healing.

Conclusions

Globally, the decision to stop or carry on with anti-TNF treatment in IBD may be based on an estimation of an individual's benefit-risk ratio, including his or her preferences, and on the cost-effectiveness of long-term treatment. In perianal fistulizing CD and ulcerative colitis, the relapse rates and/or the potential consequences of disease reactivation, including proctocolectomy, render this option of withdrawal inappropriate in most cases. In luminal CD, long-term remission has been described after anti-TNF withdrawal in a subset of patients, characterized by a state of profound remission in association with clinical remission, mucosal healing and the normalization of biomarkers of inflammation. Furthermore, the retreatment of these patients in the case of relapse has been shown to be safe and effective in most cases. In this setting, the concept of cycles of anti-TNF treatment may be proposed and should be prospectively and thoroughly evaluated.

References

1 Pariente B, Cosnes J, Danese S, et al: Development of the Crohn's disease digestive damage score, the Lémann score. Inflamm Bowel Dis 2011;17:1415–1422.
2 Rutter MD, Saunders BP, Wilkinson KH, et al: Cancer surveillance in longstanding ulcerative colitis: endoscopic appearances help predict cancer risk. Gut 2004;53:1813–1816.
3 Rutgeerts P, Geboes K, Vantrappen G, et al: Predictability of the postoperative course of Crohn's disease. Gastroenterology 1990;99:956–963.
4 van der Valk ME, Mangen MJ, Leenders M, et al: Healthcare costs of inflammatory bowel disease have shifted from hospitalisation and surgery towards anti-TNFα therapy: results from the COIN study. Gut 2014;63:72–79.
5 Rahier JF, Ben-Horin S, Chowers Y, et al: European evidence-based consensus on the prevention, diagnosis and management of opportunistic infections in inflammatory bowel disease. J Crohn Colitis 2009;3:47–91.
6 Nyboe Andersen N, Pasternak B, Basit S, et al: Association between tumor necrosis factor-α antagonists and risk of cancer in patients with inflammatory bowel disease. JAMA 2014;311:2406–2413.
7 Rahier JF, Buche S, Peyrin-Biroulet L, et al: Severe skin lesions cause patients with inflammatory bowel disease to discontinue anti-tumor necrosis factor therapy. Clin Gastroenterol Hepatol 2010;8:1048–1055.
8 Fidder H, Schnitzler F, Ferrante M, et al: Long-term safety of infliximab for the treatment of inflammatory bowel disease: a single-centre cohort study. Gut 2009;58:501–508.
9 Hay JW, Hay AR: Inflammatory bowel disease: medical cost algorithms. J Clin Gastroenterol 1992;14:318–327.
10 Feagan BG, Vreelad MG, Larson LR, et al: Annual cost of care for Crohn's disease: a payer perspective. Am J Gastroenterol 2000;95:1955–1960.
11 Silverstein MD, Loftus EV, Sandborn WJ, et al: Clinical course and costs of care for Crohn's disease: Markov model analysis of a population-based cohort. Gastroenterology 1999;117:49–57.
12 Quinn MA, Conaghan PG, O'Connor PJ, et al: Very early treatment with infliximab in addition to methotrexate in early, poor-prognosis rheumatoid arthritis reduces magnetic resonance imaging evidence of synovitis and damage, with sustained benefit after infliximab withdrawal: results from a twelve-month randomized, double-blind, placebo-controlled trial. Arthritis Rheum 2005;52: 27–35.
13 Smolen JS, Emery P, Fleischmann R, et al: Adjustment of therapy in rheumatoid arthritis on the basis of achievement of stable low disease activity with adalimumab plus methotrexate or methotrexate alone: the randomised controlled OPTIMA trial. Lancet 2014;383:321–332.
14 Domènech E, Hinojosa J, Nos P, et al: Clinical evolution of luminal and perianal Crohn's disease after inducing remission with infliximab: how long should patients be treated? Aliment Pharmacol Ther 2005;22:1107–1113.
15 Van Assche G, Vanbeckevoort D, Bielen D, et al: Magnetic resonance imaging of the effects of infliximab on perianal fistulizing Crohn's disease. Am J Gastroenterol 2003;98:332–339.
16 Karmiris K, Bielen D, Vanbeckevoort D, et al: Long-term monitoring of infliximab therapy for perianal fistulizing Crohn's disease by using magnetic resonance imaging. Clin Gastroenterol Hepatol 2011;9:130–136.
17 Louis E, Mary JY, Vernier-Massouille G, et al: Maintenance of remission among patients with Crohn's disease on antimetabolite therapy after infliximab therapy is stopped. Gastroenterology 2012; 142:63–70.
18 Farkas K, Lakatos PL, Nagy F, et al: Predictors of relapse in patients with ulcerative colitis in remission after one year of infliximab therapy. Scand J Gastroenterol 2013;48:1394–1398.
19 Molander P, Färkkilä M, Salminen K, et al: Outcome after discontinuation of TNFα-blocking therapy in patients with inflammatory bowel disease in deep remission. Inflamm Bowel Dis 2014;20: 1021–1028.
20 Farkas K, Lakatos PL, Szűcs M, et al: Frequency and prognostic role of mucosal healing in patients with Crohn's disease and ulcerative colitis after one-year of biological therapy. World J Gastroenterol 2014;20:2995–3001.
21 Baert F, Drobne D, Gils A, et al: Early trough levels and antibodies to infliximab predict safety and success of reinitiation of infliximab therapy. Clin Gastroenterol Hepatol 2014;12:1474–1481.
22 De Suray N, Salleron J, Vernier-Massouille G, et al: P274 Close monitoring of CRP and fecal calprotectin levels to predict relapse in Crohn's disease patients. A sub-analysis of the STORI study. J Crohn Colitis 2012;6(s1):S118–S119.

Edouard Louis
Department of Gastroenterology, CHU Liège
Domaine du Sart Tilman
BE–4000 Liège (Belgium)
E-Mail Edouard.louis@ulg.ac.be

Rogler G, Herfarth H, Hibi T, Nielsen OH (eds): Anti-Tumor Necrosis Factor Therapy in Inflammatory Bowel Disease.
Front Gastrointest Res. Basel, Karger, 2015, vol 34, pp 229–233 (DOI: 10.1159/000381611)

Treatment Options after Anti-TNF Failure

Taku Kobayashi

Center for Advanced IBD Research and Treatment, Kitasato University Kitasato Institute Hospital, Minato-ku, Tokyo, Japan

Abstract

A certain proportion of inflammatory bowel disease patients do not respond to anti-TNF therapy. Switching to another option, such as a calcineurin inhibitor or an anti-integrin, should be generally considered for patients with primary failure. Avoiding the delay of surgery is also very important, especially in patients with severe ulcerative colitis. Secondary failure is a loss of response experienced during anti-TNF maintenance therapy, and it develops within 5 years in approximately half of patients with a primary response. In the case of a loss of response, the underlying mechanism should be investigated, and a corresponding strategy should be chosen according to the serum drug level and detection of anti-drug antibodies.

Introduction

A paradigm shift has occurred in the field of inflammatory bowel disease over the last decade, which has even been named the 'biologic era' because of the expanding use of biologics. Anti-TNF agents were the first biologics introduced to this field, and they are most widely used worldwide. Although these agents exert high efficacy and good tolerability, there is a certain proportion of patients remain who do not respond (primary failure) or who lose response after initially responding and maintaining a response for a duration of time (secondary failure or loss of response (LOR)). Approximately 10% of patients who have achieved remission once experience LOR to infliximab (IFX) each year, based on the previous studies of both ulcerative colitis (UC) and Crohn's disease (CD). In this chapter, the treatment options after primary and secondary failures for both UC and CD are discussed.

Treatment Options after Primary Failure in Crohn's Disease

Switching to another anti-TNF agent is generally not recommended in patients who do not demonstrate an initial response to an anti-TNF agent unless the failure of response is due to the development of anti-drug antibodies. Although the early development of anti-drug antibodies does not occur very often, its presence may suggest the possible usefulness of switching to another anti-TNF agent. Otherwise, another treatment option with a different mechanism of action should be considered after excluding other possible etiologies, such as a stricture, abscess, fistula or co-existing cancer, which may require surgical intervention. Anti-integrins, natalizumab and vedolizumab have been approved and are used in the US and Europe [1, 2]. Tofacitinib has failed to demonstrate significant efficacy in CD patients in contrast with UC patients, as recently reported [3].

Treatment Options after Primary Failure in Ulcerative Colitis

In general, moderate to severe steroid-refractory or steroid-dependent UC patients are indicated for anti-TNF therapy. In the initial clinical studies [4, 5], the response and remission rates were 69.4 and 38.8% with IFX and 50.4 and 16.5% with adalimumab, respectively. The efficacy of adalimumab might have been underestimated because this study included 40% of patients who had already failed to respond to an initial anti-TNF agent before being treated. Therefore, overall, these data suggest that the remaining 30–40% of patients may require rescue therapy after an initial failure to respond to anti-TNF therapy.

The most widely used 'second rescue therapy' agents after steroids and anti-TNF agents are calcineurin inhibitors (CIs), which inhibit the production of the pro-inflammatory cytokine interleukin-2. There are two options in this class, cyclosporine A (CSA) and tacrolimus (TAC or FK506). CSA has been used extensively to reduce graft rejection after organ transplantation [6]. In 1994, Lichtiger et al. first reported the efficacy of CSA for treating patients who failed intravenous steroid therapy [7]. Subsequently, many studies have demonstrated its efficacy in the management of steroid-resistant UC, with response rates of no less than 60% [8]. Despite a good initial response to CSA, many patients again relapse and eventually require colectomy because of the insufficient efficacy in maintaining remission. It has also been shown that the use of azathioprine after CSA-induced remission is correlated with a decreased colectomy rate [8, 9]. Recently, Laharie et al. conducted a head-to-head comparison of IFX and CSA as rescue therapies in steroid-refractory severe UC [10]. There were no significant differences in the short-term efficacy between the standard induction regimen of IFX (5 mg/kg at 0, 2, and 6 weeks) and intravenous CSA (2 mg/kg for 2 weeks, followed by oral CSA administration).

The other CI is TAC, which originated in Japan and has also been widely used to treat patients who have undergone transplant surgery. In the initial nationwide multicenter clinical trial of refractory UC in Japan, Ogata et al. demonstrated remission and response rates of 20.0 and 68.4%, respectively, with high blood trough levels of 10–15 ng/ml for 2 weeks during the initial induction phase [11, 12]. It is still unclear whether TAC also lacks efficacy in maintaining remission or whether it is more effective because its blood concentration can be maintained more stably than oral CSA. In Japan, there is some preliminary evidence (unpublished) indicating successful remission maintenance with oral TAC for up to a few years; however, long-term outcomes, including remission maintenance and safety, are unknown. Furthermore, there is no clear evidence of TAC efficacy in patients with prior anti-TNF therapy failure.

There are emerging treatment options that represent alternatives to these drugs. Vedolizumab is an anti-α4β7 integrin antibody that selectively blocks lymphocyte migration to the gut immune system. Its high efficacy and tolerability have recently been reported for both UC and CD [2, 13], and it is expected to be safer than the anti-α4 integrin monoclonal antibody natalizum-

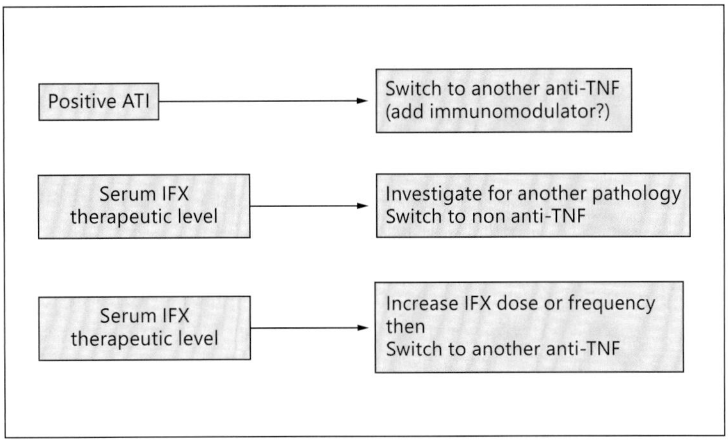

Fig. 1. 'Simplified' algorithm for Crohn's disease patients who experience secondary failure of infliximab. Modified from reference no. [17].

ab, the use of which is limited to refractory CD in the US due to the potential risk of progressive multifocal leukoencephalopathy. Tofacitinib is an oral Janus kinase inhibitor that has been reported to be effective for treating UC [14].

There is also a debate as to whether colectomy should be considered without sequential rescue medical therapy with CI (or other novel options) after anti-TNF treatment failure in moderate to severe UC. It is very important to keep in mind that failure of a second rescue therapy may simply result in an unnecessary delay of surgery. Furthermore, although several studies have demonstrated that a sequential medical intervention decreases the colectomy rate, a high incidence of adverse events (30%) has been shown [15, 16]. It is also unclear which CI and anti-TNF agents should be considered first in patients who fail to respond to steroids when sequential rescue therapy is required, although there is a trend of using IFX due to the possible favorable long-term outcome. There is also a concern that the long half-life of anti-TNF agents may cause profound immunosuppression when sequential rescue therapy with CI is conducted soon after anti-TNF therapy. In summary, up until now, the indication of sequential rescue therapy in moderate to severe UC needs to be discussed on a case-by-case basis.

Treatment Options after Secondary Failure

Secondary LOR occurs in approximately 10% of UC and CD patients who initially respond to anti-TNF therapy each year, resulting in the LOR of approximately half of these patients within 5 years. The main causes of LOR are decreases in serum drug levels or the development of a new etiology that is less related to TNF-α, such as an infection, stricture, abscess, fistula or cancer (fig. 1). Therefore, investigating the reason for an LOR is very important.

Therapeutic drug monitoring has been well studied for the use of IFX to treat CD. The best explanation for a low IFX level is the development of anti-drug antibodies, called human anti-chimeric antibodies or antibodies to IFX (ATIs). ATIs neutralize serum IFX and reduce the drug concentration, leading to an insufficient titer to control inflammation. Typically, patients suffering from an LOR feel that the effect wears off as they near the date of the next infusion of anti-TNF agent during the interval. Although there is no concensus on the optimal therapeutic level of IFX yet, if the trough level is below the therapeutic level, either (1) increasing the IFX dose to 10 mg/kg, (2) shortening the infusion interval, or (3) switching to another anti-TNF agent should be considered. In patients who are positive for ATIs, switching to another anti-TNF agent is more effective than optimizing the dose/interval [17–19]. If the serum level is above the therapeutic level, the possible causes of clinical worsening should be carefully investigated. When possible mechanisms unrelated to disease activity are excluded, switching to an agent from a different class, such as an anti-integrin, can be considered. More recently, it has been shown that higher trough levels are required to achieve mucosal healing, and it might still be beneficial to escalate the dose prior to switching to another biologic. In addition, a recent study has suggested the possible usefulness of adding an immunomodulator to eliminate anti-drug antibodies and restore sufficient blood drug levels [20]. Although most studies of the above-mentioned therapeutic drug monitoring strategy have involved IFX and CD, the underlying theory is believed to be similar for other anti-TNF agents and in UC [21, 22].

Conclusions

Because multiple novel drugs have emerged recently and also will be appearing in the future, we can and will be able to have much more medical options after anti-TNF treatment failure than ever before. However, we should keep in mind that the underlying pathology for refractoriness to this treatment should be carefully investigated before easily switching to the next option. Furthermore, it remains very important not to delay the decision for surgery by relying too much on medical therapy, especially for severe patients who require surgery.

References

1 Sandborn WJ, Colombel JF, Enns R, et al: Natalizumab induction and maintenance therapy for Crohn's disease. New Engl J Med 2005;353:1912–1925.
2 Sandborn WJ, Feagan BG, Rutgeerts P, et al: Vedolizumab as induction and maintenance therapy for Crohn's disease. New Engl J Med 2013;369:711–721.
3 Sandborn WJ, Ghosh S, Panes J, et al: A phase 2 study of tofacitinib, an oral Janus kinase inhibitor, in patients with Crohn's disease. Clin Gastroenterol Hepatol 2014;12:1485–1493.e2.
4 Rutgeerts P, Sandborn WJ, Feagan BG, et al: Infliximab for induction and maintenance therapy for ulcerative colitis. New Engl J Med 2005;353:2462–2476.
5 Sandborn WJ, van Assche G, Reinisch W, et al: Adalimumab induces and maintains clinical remission in patients with moderate-to-severe ulcerative colitis. Gastroenterology 2012;142:257–265.e1–e3.
6 O'Keefe SJ, Tamura J, Kincaid RL, et al: FK-506- and CsA-sensitive activation of the interleukin-2 promoter by calcineurin. Nature 1992;357:692–694.
7 Lichtiger S, Present DH, Kornbluth A, et al: Cyclosporine in severe ulcerative colitis refractory to steroid therapy. New Engl J Med 1994;330:1841–1845.
8 Kobayashi T, Naganuma M, Okamoto S, et al: Rapid endoscopic improvement is important for 1-year avoidance of colectomy but not for the long-term prognosis in cyclosporine A treatment for ulcerative colitis. J Gastroenterol 2010;45:1129–1137.
9 Cohen RD, Stein R, Hanauer SB: Intravenous cyclosporin in ulcerative colitis: a five-year experience. Am J Gastroenterol 1999;94:1587–1592.
10 Laharie D, Bourreille A, Branche J, et al: Ciclosporin versus infliximab in patients with severe ulcerative colitis refractory to intravenous steroids: a parallel, open-label randomised controlled trial. Lancet 2012;380:1909–1915.
11 Ogata H, Kato J, Hirai F, et al: Double-blind, placebo-controlled trial of oral tacrolimus (FK506) in the management of hospitalized patients with steroid-refractory ulcerative colitis. Inflamm Bowel Dis 2012;18:803–808.
12 Ogata H, Matsui T, Nakamura M, et al: A randomised dose finding study of oral tacrolimus (FK506) therapy in refractory ulcerative colitis. Gut 2006;55:1255–1262.
13 Feagan BG, Rutgeerts P, Sands BE, et al: Vedolizumab as induction and maintenance therapy for ulcerative colitis. New Engl J Med 2013;369:699–710.
14 Sandborn WJ, Ghosh S, Panes J, et al: Tofacitinib, an oral Janus kinase inhibitor, in active ulcerative colitis. New Engl J Med 2012;367:616–624.
15 Chaparro M, Burgueno P, Iglesias E, et al: Infliximab salvage therapy after failure of ciclosporin in corticosteroid-refractory ulcerative colitis: a multicentre study. Aliment Pharmacol Ther 2012;35:275–283.
16 Leblanc S, Allez M, Seksik P, et al: Successive treatment with cyclosporine and infliximab in steroid-refractory ulcerative colitis. Am J Gastroenterol 2011;106:771–777.

17 Afif W, Loftus EV Jr, Faubion WA, et al: Clinical utility of measuring infliximab and human anti-chimeric antibody concentrations in patients with inflammatory bowel disease. Am J Gastroenterol 2010;105:1133–1139.

18 Hibi T, Sakuraba A, Watanabe M, et al: Retrieval of serum infliximab level by shortening the maintenance infusion interval is correlated with clinical efficacy in Crohn's disease. Inflamm Bowel Dis 2012;18:1480–1487.

19 Hibi T, Sakuraba A, Watanabe M, et al: C-reactive protein is an indicator of serum infliximab level in predicting loss of response in patients with Crohn's disease. J Gastroenterol 2014;49:254–262.

20 Ben-Horin S, Waterman M, Kopylov U, et al: Addition of an immunomodulator to infliximab therapy eliminates antidrug antibodies in serum and restores clinical response of patients with inflammatory bowel disease. Clin Gastroenterol Hepatol 2013;11:444–447.

21 Frederiksen MT, Ainsworth MA, Brynskov J, et al: Antibodies against infliximab are associated with de novo development of antibodies to adalimumab and therapeutic failure in infliximab-to-adalimumab switchers with IBD. Inflamm Bowel Dis 2014;20:1714–1721.

22 Mazor Y, Almog R, Kopylov U, et al: Adalimumab drug and antibody levels as predictors of clinical and laboratory response in patients with Crohn's disease. Aliment Pharmacol Ther 2014;40:620–628.

Taku Kobayashi, MD, PhD, Vice Director and Associate Professor
Center for Advanced IBD Research and Treatment
Kitasato University Kitasato Institute Hospital, 5–9-1 Shirokane, Minato-ku
Tokyo 108–8642 (Japan)
E-Mail kobataku@insti.kitasato-u.ac.jp

Author Index

Subject Index